THE BLOOD CONSPIRACY
How to Avoid Getting AIDS and Hepatitis in a Transfusion

by

Joleen Swain Ottosen

Aspen Leaf Press
P.O. Box 220
Woodland Park, CO 80866-0220

Although the author and publisher have made every effort to ensure the accuracy and completeness of information contained in this book, we assume no responsibility for errors, inaccuracies, omissions, or any inconsistency herein. Any slights of people, places, or organizations are unintentional.

ISBN 0-9632963-3-7

LCCN 92-71818

ATTENTION CORPORATIONS, COLLEGES, AND PROFES-SIONAL ORGANIZATIONS: Quantity discounts are available on bulk purchases of this book for educational purposes or fund raising. Special books or book excerpts can also be created to fit specific needs. For information, please contact our Special Sales Department, Aspen Leaf Press, 743 Gold Hill Place, Suite #297, P.O. Box 220, Woodland Park, CO 80866-0220.

Dedication

To the memory of my parents

*For Jonathan and all those
who continue to suffer
from transfusion AIDS*

Acknowledgments

Many people have contributed their time and knowledge toward the publication of this book. I am indebted to Dr. Donald Francis, Dr. Leora Traynor, Dr. Julian Schorr, Dr. Theresa Crenshaw and Dr. Ronald Lapin. There are also several off-the-record physicians who know I'm grateful.

A number of organizations and companies have generously supplied information. Among them are: the National Hemophilia Foundation, the American Foundation for Safe Blood and Health Care, the Institute of Bloodless Surgery, the California State Department of Health, the American Association of Blood Banks, Haemonetics, Idant Laboratories, PSICOR and Electromedics, Inc. I offer special thanks to the following: Alan Brownstein, Allen Gelb, John de Graffenried, Mattie Massengale, Mary Muecke, John Rivera, John Schumann, Steve Oliver, Robert Garvie and Peter Milio.

I am deeply grateful for the support and assistance of my husband and children—especially my daughter Sheri who was certain she would be keying this manuscript into the computer for the rest of her life. I'm also appreciative of the patience of my editors, Teresa Boyer and Marilyn Ross.

I cannot overlook the heroism of the victims of transfusion AIDS and their family caregivers who shared with me their experiences, their pain and their courage. At the top of this list are my brothers Orvin and Von, my sister LaRee and those who love and care for Jonathan. And finally, I'm grateful for the undefeatable spirit of my father whose life helped me keep the promise he asked of me.

Foreword

The Blood Conspiracy is a well-documented account of a family and national tragedy. It is a story of strength, a story of weakness, and a story of betrayal.

It tells of the strength of the Swain family of rural Eastern Utah. The patriarch, Orville, like an old greasewood bush facing the harsh winter winds, bends with the onslaught of HIV after being infected through a blood transfusion. Within a year, his wife, Ora, is sexually infected and becomes ill. Two years before, in another state, his brother's grandson had been infected with AIDS by a blood transfusion given on the day of his birth. Despite the onslaught of this slow, painful and progressive disease, these people face their enemy with heroic fortitude. But, as if AIDS alone were not bad enough, the elder Swains are forced by their health-care providers to face it in blinded ignorance and Jonathan is kept from preschool by unfounded fears.

As the elder Swains' health dwindles, their medical and support needs become immense. The challenge is met by the heroic efforts of their children, whose names—Orvin, LaRee, Von and Joleen—are as typical of the area as the ever-present greasewoods. But this story is not just one which describes the challenges of providing complex nursing and medical care in isolation from urban support networks. It is a story of their united efforts to uncover their parents' true diagnosis and to find out how and why they contracted AIDS.

The Blood Conspiracy tells of the weakness of the people directing the American blood collection system. It reviews the history of transfusion-associated AIDS and notes that if the directors of the nation's blood banks had followed the advice of those investigating the AIDS epidemic, tens of thousands of people, including the Swains, would not have been infected with HIV. In early 1983, my colleagues and I at the Centers for Disease Control warned blood bankers that AIDS posed a real threat to recipients of blood and blood products. We outlined simple measures that should have been taken to prevent further spread. The leaders of the blood banking industry ignored those warnings and did not implement effective prevention measures. Instead, they told the American public that the "blood is safe."

Ultimately, and most disturbing, *Conspiracy* tells of betrayal. The Latter-Day-Saints (LDS) Blood Bank knew soon after Orville Swain's transfusion that the donor was infected with HIV. Yet, they refused to tell Mr. Swain, thus subjecting his wife to infection risk through sexual relations. Apparently in an attempt to prevent litigation, the doctors and the blood bank conspired to hide the blood donor's HIV status and Orville's AIDS diagnosis from the Swain family. Ora, who died first, died without the benefit of specific AIDS treatment. Only after persistent attempts by the family to find the proper treatment modalities for their father's "unknown disease" was Orville's true diagnosis uncovered—far too late for him to receive life-prolonging AIDS treatments.

At the heart of the story is the betrayal of the Swains by the very country of which they were proud citizens. Orville, a paradigm of the dedicated American pioneer spirit, was a devoted Republican. His elected leader, Ronald Reagan, could never find the will to confront AIDS. The President failed to understand his duty as chief executive to control epidemics. His neglect of the AIDS epidemic, throughout his two terms in office, set the stage for today's huge AIDS epidemic which is in the process of consuming more than a million Americans—including the old greasewood from Lapoint, Utah, his wife, and his brother's grandchild.

Joleen Swain Ottosen could have stopped after telling this chilling and deadly story of what government, blood banks, and doctors did to her family. But she did not. Instead, she empowers the reader with information that was not made available at the time of her family's transfusions. The consumer section of the book outlines a blood users guide which, in a very clear, step-by-step fashion, shows the reader how to minimize one's chance of getting transfusion-associated disease.

After finishing this book, readers have both reason to be concerned and the means by which to take control of their own blood transfusion safety.

Donald P. Francis, M.D., D.Sc.
Centers for Disease Control (retired 1992)

Table of Contents

Part I. The Swains—A Ravaged Family

Two family members were given AIDS-contaminated blood in separate transfusions. One was a baby transfused at birth. The second was an elderly man who sexually infected his wife after one of the blood banks knew he had received the blood of an AIDS-positive donor and concealed that information for years.

Part II. Exposé—The Truth about Blood Safety

Believing safe-blood propaganda is a high-risk behavior. During the past two decades the blood industry has given millions of hepatitis infections and tens of thousands of AIDS infections while public health officials and blood bankers lauded the safety of the blood supply. Blood safety claims are still exaggerated.

Part III. For Consumers—
Steps That Can Save Your Life

There are exciting advances in transfusion therapy that can usually eliminate the need for getting someone else's blood. However, few hospitals routinely provide ultrasafe transfusion for their patients. Assertive consumers must have medically accurate information and what-to-do lists which are provided in this section.

Introduction

I sat at my father's funeral listening to a quartet sing, "Not now but in the coming years . . . Sometime, sometime we'll understand." I knew it would take years of investigation to uncover the truth surrounding the events of his death. It would be a long time before our family "understood."

My thoughts riveted on that fateful day three and a half years before—January 4, 1985—the day Dad received 18 units of blood during coronary bypass surgery in Salt Lake City, Utah. Now at age 79 he was gone—not a victim of heart disease but of transfusion AIDS. Orville Swain died on the 4th of July, 1988. It seemed appropriate that as the nation he loved celebrated its independence, he had finally gained his freedom from those horrible years of suffering.

I tried not to think of my father's wasted body and to remember happier times. They seemed so long ago, crowded out by the dreadful happenings of the past several years. I fought back tears as I remembered my mother's AIDS infection and subsequent death just 11 months before—a death that mercifully had not been so long in coming, but one that was caused by the blood bank's callous irresponsibility.

Blood bank officials had learned five months after Dad's surgery that one of his donors carried the AIDS virus. But they chose to conceal this information. They knew that he was old and in poor health after major heart surgery and expected him to soon die. They were confident their secret would be buried with him.

As a result of the blood bank's deadly silence, Mother was later sexually infected with AIDS. Even after doctors diagnosed my father's AIDS-related illness 25 months after his surgery, the coverup continued. The family was still not told. Children and grandchildren were unknowingly exposed to HIV-infected blood and bodily fluids as they cared for the couple without taking precautions.

I listened to the eulogy. As the speaker mentioned my father's surviving brothers and sisters, my mind lingered on Darreld, his youngest brother who was the grandfather of another victim of transfusion AIDS. 'How painful this must be for him,' I thought. Six months after Dad's heart surgery, Darreld visited my parents, distraught over his two-year-old grandson's recent diagnosis of AIDS.

Little Jonathan Swain had contracted the virus from a tainted blood transfusion given after his birth in a Denver hospital. As my uncle talked about his grandson's tragedy, Dad lay on the couch exhausted from the unexplained illness that had dogged him since his surgery. It is incredible that none of us recognized the transfusion connection between Dad and Jonathan's ill health.

My parents' world had been isolated and simple. They lived their entire lives in a small farming town in eastern Utah, far from the battlefields of AIDS. Their lifestyle was seemingly risk-free. They had married as virgins and neither had ever had another sexual partner during their 54 years together. Nor had they used any type of recreational drugs, not even alcohol or tobacco. They were a conservative Mormon couple, devoted to their church, devoted to their children and grandchildren.

Yet here we were, closing the final unforeseen chapter of my father's life. Although I felt relieved that his torment had ended, I knew it wasn't over. Our family had too many wounds that would never heal. I also knew that our story must be told so others might be spared a similar tragedy.

★ ★ ★

During the years since my father's death, I have researched the medical literature, politics and economic interests that shaped the blood industry's slow response to the AIDS crisis. Through the Freedom of Information Act, I obtained copies of FDA inspections of the blood bank which supplied the blood for my father's transfusion.

The Utah facility had been lax in educating and screening donors who were at risk for AIDS. The donor who gave the blood which infected my father revealed that the blood bank did not give him any educational materials or question him about AIDS or its symptoms.

Nonprofit blood banking is unique. It is a big business receiving free labor from volunteers and free advertising from the news media. Altruistic blood donors provide its raw product in exchange for a glass of juice and a couple of crackers. Because nonprofit blood enterprises operate as local monopolies, they seldom have any competition. They pay no state or federal income tax and are essentially protected from lawsuits.

Most people don't realize that this large billion-dollar "nonprofit" industry is, in fact, highly profitable—with greater profit margins than America's largest corporations! Blood banks enjoy the image of charitable organizations. They are the revered institutions that supply the lifesaving gift of blood.

Unfortunately, a transfusion that saves a life may later take that life. In the United States millions of hepatitis infections and tens of thousands of AIDS infections have been transmitted by tainted transfusions. In the past, the majority of transfusion infections went undiagnosed while well-meaning doctors preached the safe-blood propaganda fed to them by the blood industry. Moreover, the government usually allowed that industry to act in its own self interest.

In addition, public health officials have slanted information on blood safety. For example, when health authorities argue against testing health care workers for AIDS, they emphasize the test's inability to detect all those who are infected. They maintain, "the test isn't reliable." However, when they discuss the blood supply, authorities describe the same test as "virtually eliminating every donation of HIV-infected blood." The ELISA test does not have the ability to distinguish between the blood of health care workers and the blood donated for transfusions. If blood does not contain antibodies to HIV, the test will be negative even though it might carry the AIDS virus. This is due to the "window period" between the time of exposure and the time the body produces antibodies to the virus.

Although the risk of getting AIDS in a transfusion was greatly reduced when blood banks began testing for HIV in 1985, an unknown number of infections still slip through. The inadequacy of the ELISA test is compounded by the continuing problem blood banks have with human and mechanical errors—errors that can cause either infected hepatitis or AIDS blood to be released.

According to Centers for Disease Control (CDC) reports there are 5,000 AIDS cases which were transmitted by blood transfusion. But the agency only recognizes 20 of them as being from blood that was tested for HIV. Those few cases give the misleading impression that since testing began in 1985, the risk of getting AIDS in a transfusion has virtually been eliminated. However, it is not known how effective the imperfect HIV test is for protecting the blood supply. Transfusion recipients who received blood that tested negative, but was actually contaminated with HIV, can be infected for up to a decade before symptoms appear. When they do become symptomatic, their cases are not reported to the CDC until they are *diagnosed* and reach the full-blown AIDS category. Doctors are often remiss in testing patients who received blood after 1985 for AIDS. The vast majority of all HIV infections given via transfusion *never* show up as AIDS cases in the CDC report.

Moreover, the 20 cases from tested blood lack creditability because, unlike the thousands of other reported transfusion AIDS cases, those given since the spring of 1985 have to be *confirmed by finding an HIV-positive donor*. Locating and testing up to 20 or more donors per case presents a roadblock to confirmation. Most disturbing of all, hospitals and blood banks are only required to keep records linking transfusion recipients to specific donors for five years. After a person is transfused with AIDS-tainted blood, the virus will incubate for an average of seven years. Consequently, before transfusion AIDS cases surface, donor records will likely be destroyed so that the cases cannot be confirmed. Even if records are still available, HIV-positive donors may have already died or left the area. And blood banks have a powerful incentive *not* to find positive donors because of fear of litigation.

Although not yet counted in the CDC 20-case number, a positive donor has been found for Bob Jones of Wilsall, Montana, who is suffering from AIDS-related illnesses. The 60-year-old Mr. Jones had a transfusion in late 1989—nearly five years after blood banks began testing for AIDS. Nevertheless, the blood supplied by the Red Cross' Pacific Northwest Regional Blood Center was tainted with HIV. "The Red Cross leads you to believe that its blood is now doggone safe," Mr. Jones said. "But I can tell you that it isn't. The public is being given a false sense of security about the safety of blood after it has been tested for hepatitis and AIDS."

Some experts privately agree with Mr. Jones. A doctor who has been in blood banking nearly 40 years recently told me that getting a transfusion with someone else's blood "is akin to playing Russian roulette." The doctor's concern was for the total infectious risk from all the diseases known to be transmitted by transfusion plus any new ones that may be going around.

In the summer of 1992 there is concern that a new virus may be creeping into the population—or perhaps an altered strain of AIDS virus other than the two strains blood banks test for. Something is causing a fatal AIDS-like illness that cannot be detected by various HIV tests. It could take years to determine the cause, identify a new retrovirus and develop a test to protect the blood supply.

The first step toward consumer protection is to strip away the conspiracy of silence and half-truth that has perpetuated the myth of safe blood during the past several decades. Education is a universal concern because eventually every family will have a member who requires a blood transfusion. Patients must understand that to not prepare for transfusion with their own blood may have life-threatening consequences. If safe options to regular banked blood were not available there would be no purpose served by writing this book. But they *are* available. Unfortunately, they are only used for a small fraction of the patients who could benefit from them. According to information provided by the American Association of Blood Banks (AABB), in 1992 just 5% of the blood being collected nationally was intended for the donor's own use.

There are now five options that can be used either alone or in combination to enable patients to give themselves a transfusion. Most frequently used are patient donation before surgery and collection of blood lost during and after surgery for return to the patient. It is tragic that these advances in transfusion medicine, which were available before the AIDS crisis, aren't routinely explained to patients. Uninformed health consumers aren't motivated to go to the inconvenience of making several donations of blood or ascertaining if a hospital has equipment and will *use it* to recycle their blood.

The Swain family had a high risk behavior for exposure to the AIDS virus. We trusted. We had no knowledge of the risks of blood transfusion. We accepted the exaggerated claims of blood safety and did not actively participate in our health care. Our family had a blind faith that the medical establishment would act in our best interest. It did not. Neither did the government. When the blood used for my father's transfusion was collected, FDA inspectors had not been in the blood bank for over two years.

Without grassroot involvement, medical change comes slowly. Dr. Philip Casper, head of a research group that compiles information on medical issues, told the press, "I have not seen the medical community take the bull by the horns and make changes. Sometimes it takes ruffling a few feathers to do that." This book is certain to ruffle more than a few feathers. It is shaped by personal experience and written from the victim/consumer viewpoint—a perspective that is never heard. A more balanced writing would do little to counter consumer complacency and the lopsided accumulation of safe-blood propaganda. Nonetheless, I have made every effort to present an accurate account.

Some readers will question how a lay person could presume to sound a call for advocacy in areas of such medical complexity. Although I cite endless medical studies and health authorities, it is my belief that the only real authorities on transfusion AIDS and its politics are those who have experienced it—those families who have plodded and staggered in the trenches where their loved ones died. The Swains received two AIDS-contaminated transfusions and had a third member infected because information was concealed. Perhaps by telling our story and offering sound solutions for reform, the carnage will not have been in vain.

A consumer section presents a large amount of health information which must be read carefully. There are suggestions on how to work with physicians and how to place responsibility on hospitals for providing safe transfusion therapy. There are detailed what-to-do lists for planning blood replacement for both high and low blood-loss surgeries. There are tips for handling emergencies and the transfusion needs of children.

Even in the worst case scenario, when it isn't possible to use the patient's own blood, the number of donors can be reduced by as much as 80%. Transfusion risks multiply with each additional donor. There are also instructions for making a *wise* selection of donors chosen from the patient's friends and relatives. An emphasis is placed on the importance of obtaining single donor plasma and platelets.

There is nothing more sad than knowledge acquired too late—the knowledge that three AIDS infections could have been easily avoided, three lives spared. This story never should have happened. Don't let yourself or your loved ones be similar victims.

Author's Note:

For full information on sources referred to throughout this book please see "Notes" in the back pages.

For the sake of simplicity, this book often refers to individuals who are HIV-positive as being infected with the AIDS virus. It may be easier for the reader to view those who are HIV-positive, those who have AIDS-Related Complex (ARC) and those with full-blown AIDS as *all* being in different stages of the same disease process. The term "ARC" is now rarely used and illnesses that result from immune dysfunction due to HIV are considered AIDS-related. The definition of full-blown AIDS is more relevant to CDC case reporting than to patient treatment.

Part I

*The Swains—
A Ravaged Family*

Chapter 1

Betrayal

I pick up the phone and dial 911.

"We need an ambulance sent to Lapoint. My father has to be taken to the hospital in Roosevelt."

"Can you give us directions?" the dispatcher asks. "We'll be coming from Vernal."

"Stay on the main road," I say. "Go two blocks past the post office. It's the house on the right with the rock work and bright flowers."

"You mean the Swain home?"

"Yes, that's right. Uh . . . there's something else you should know. Tell the paramedics the patient has AIDS."

"Well, they'll give him aid when they get there . . . if it's needed."

"No, you don't understand. He has AIDS, the infectious disease."

The dispatcher's confusion doesn't surprise me. My parents live in a remote farming area in eastern Utah. Known as the Uintah Basin, it's 150 miles from Salt Lake City. Residents here haven't had any prior experience with AIDS patients.

Our family knows that legally we could say nothing. We do not have to disclose our father's illness. We are well aware that going public with the diagnosis will bring misunderstanding and persecution. But we feel it is our responsibility to warn others of any risk. It is unconscionable to knowingly expose health care workers to this virus.

We have good reason for our strong feelings. Dad received AIDS-tainted blood in a transfusion during coronary bypass surgery two and a half years ago. But after the blood bank learned one of his donors was infected with the AIDS virus that information was concealed from us for two years. Blood bank officials never intended for our family to know the true cause of Dad's many illnesses. Our knowing was not in their best interest.

I look at Dad. He is in the living room lying in his hospital bed. The home I knew as a child is now a care center for my parents. The old-fashioned furniture has been pushed aside to make room for medical supplies and equipment—a strange contrast to the antique pictures hanging on the walls, five generations of our family's ancestors. Dad's appearance is that of the emaciated patients shown on TV, the ones who are dying of this plague. His eyes are glossy, temperature 104°, pulse 140. His breathing is labored. He is disoriented and unresponsive.

It is late July 1987, 10 weeks since we were told of the AIDS diagnosis—a reluctant disclosure we finally forced from Dad's local doctor. Three months before we learned of the AIDS, we were told Dad had hepatitis B and cytomegalovirus (CMV) infections. AIDS brought his total infections to three blood-borne illnesses, all passed by transfusion. Often the same blood donor will carry all three viruses.

Knowing Dad has AIDS explains a lot. It explains why during the years since his surgery our attempts to solve his perplexing health problems failed. It explains why doctors tried to convince us it was depression and anorexia that would kill him. It explains the inconsistent medical treatments. We now realize the coverup has prevented Dad from receiving proper treatment for AIDS when the progression of the disease could have been slowed.

I look out the window. The ambulance is taking longer than expected to travel the 18 miles from Vernal.

Three weeks ago Mother's test came back positive for the AIDS infection. We were stunned. My brother Orvin knew that for a long time after the heart surgery Dad was impotent. After Mother's positive test, Dad was questioned by his doctor. Dad said that about a year after his operation, he and Mother had intercourse only three times.

By the time the AIDS was revealed, eight children and grandchildren had been exposed to infectious blood as they provided care without taking precautions. Several others were exposed to bodily fluids. After learning of the AIDS, our entire family was traumatized. Recalling past exposures brought fear. Crippling fear.

When I arrived from my home in Colorado a few days ago, I was shocked over the rapid deterioration of my parents, especially Mom. Doctors rarely look for AIDS symptoms in women and their illness is often misdiagnosed. For over a year Mother's health problems were shrugged off as old age and senility. Dementia, a deterioration in mental function, is a well-known symptom of AIDS. So are hallucinations.

I remember the state Mother was in the night I came.

"Oh, it's awful," she said.

"What's wrong?" I asked.

"How can we take care of all those children? I can't do it, I'm too sick."

"Mother, there aren't any children here."

"Yes, there are. Over there by the closet. They're all sick."

"Mother, your mind is playing tricks on you again. Trust me. There are no children to care for."

"Oh, okay. Well, if you're sure. I just won't look over there."

I got in bed with her and held her. Mother had always been very nurturing with children. She couldn't stand to see a child suffer. One of her grandchildren had died of leukemia when he was six years old and Mother had provided much of his care. His illness and death had devastated her.

I turned Mother away from the closet so she couldn't see the suffering children. She had been in a state of nervous anxiety for many weeks, unable to sleep for more than a few minutes at a time. Tranquilizers and sleeping pills did her little good. Before she suffered motor dysfunction, she would pace the floor for hours at a time, day and night. Mother's diarrhea is now excessive. She complains of being unable to breathe and of constant headaches. Her life is hell and nothing we do brings relief.

We are in a crisis situation. We want to keep Mother and Dad at home but their care demands are horrendous. When I arrived from Colorado I thought I was prepared for what I'd find. I was wrong. For five years I have cared for my seriously ill, housebound daughter and I understand the stress of a caregiver. What I didn't understand was the emotional impact of AIDS and the unique problems that come with it. These must be experienced firsthand.

An AIDS death is the ugliest death known to medicine. The patient's mind can be reduced to dark pits of delusion and fear. Fever, nausea and pain are endless. Our parents have both lost control of their bladders and bowels. This incontinence, when combined with the infectious AIDS virus, causes us great stress. We wear rubber gloves when changing diapers and cleaning up vomit. But those who care for patients in hospitals do not also have to clean the bathroom, wash soiled laundry and rush back to the kitchen to finish cooking food. We must frequently change gloves and our hands are chapped and bleeding from continuously washing them in strong disinfectants. Everything takes twice as long to do. There is a nagging tension, a need to always be on guard against an invisible enemy.

For two and a half years Orvin has cared for our parents. The burden has consumed every hour of his life. Our sister, LaRee, and her family have also shared the responsibility. LaRee works at the hospital in Roosevelt as an inhalation therapist. She has a husband and three children, yet she spends many hours each week caring for Mother and Dad, taking time off work during emergencies. Recently the emergencies have been continuous. Last June, LaRee wrote in her diary:

"My brother and I care for Mother and Dad day after day with no relief. Sometimes I forget what day it is. I can't remember when I last slept in a bed."

The ambulance finally arrives with its crew in full protective dress: masks, gowns, bonnets, gloves and goggles. I think of all the times our family cared for this old couple without even using gloves. Long years before we knew.

Dad is loaded into the ambulance and our brother Von, who is here from his home in southern Utah, rides with him to the hospital. LaRee follows in her car. I stay with Mother and persuade Orvin to go to bed. He is exhausted and his own health is beginning to fail.

We have been trying to hire two nurses. We already have a nurse's aide who works 40 hours a week and another woman who cooks special food and delivers it to the house. Home Health Care has provided excellent assistance for well over a year. But there are 168 hours in a week and both parents are too much for one person to handle. Our efforts to hire nurses have failed. We aren't surprised no one wants the job.

Dad was released from the hospital just yesterday after a four-day stay. During that time, the doctor, with the consent of Dad and family members, had classified him as a "no code" which means code blue revival procedures would not be used at the time of his death. Dad has been on a downhill course for several weeks. When the doctor released him yesterday he said there was nothing more he could do for him.

When Von and Orvin brought him home and settled him into bed, he looked terrible. He saw Mother and became emotionally upset. Both parents are more distraught when they observe the other's debilitation. When apart, they worry incessantly over each other; but if together, they worry even more.

The short time Dad was at home was a nightmare. I prepared some food and attempted to feed him dinner. He took one bite, vomited and began to chill. It was difficult for me to look into his eyes. There was so much pain. Helpless pain. All his life he had been a rugged survivor. A fighter against high odds. Yet there he was, trapped by a strange virus, cornered by an unknown adversary. It robbed his dignity and mocked his independent spirit. To die from it would be the ultimate curse.

As the hours wore on, his breathing became more and more labored and his fever climbed higher. Orvin and I struggled throughout the night to bring the fever down and to relieve some of his distress. His condition worsened.

Night gave way to the first light of morning. Roosters crowed. The aide arrived and took Dad's vital signs.

"Why haven't you called the doctor?" she asked.

Her question was poorly timed. Orvin's anger exploded.

"Call the doctor? What good would it do? That's why he has AIDS. I called a doctor and they gave him a batch of poisoned blood. Then covered it up and Ma got it. Now they both have to die like a couple of lepers.

"The blood bank just gave it to us and washed their filthy hands of the problem. Well, I'll tell you what we did all night. We handled the problem they gave us. The problem no one else wants to handle."

I asked the aide to call the doctor. When she put down the phone she was angry.

"What did he say?" I asked.

"He yelled at me and said, 'we just sent him home yesterday. If you people can't take care of that old man, bring him back.'"

We decided to keep Dad at home. LaRee came and went in to comfort him. She was used to seeing death at her workplace but she was badly shaken by Dad's appearance. She found me in the kitchen where I was feeding Mother and pulled me aside.

"That's a dying man, Joleen. He can't last long."

Around noon the doctor called and asked to talk to me. Obviously he had heard I was in town. This local doctor was the bottom man on the coverup totem pole. Since the forced disclosure of AIDS, he had been in a very tight spot. He feared me more than he feared Orvin's sharp tongue. I had the nasty habit of calling national AIDS experts and pharmaceutical companies to check out his prescribed treatments.

"Well, where is he?" the doctor demanded.

"It was my understanding you didn't want him down there," I replied.

"Well, I'd like to run tests to find out why he is so much worse," he said. "We don't have to treat him."

"We'll decide what we want to do and call your office."

When I hung up the phone I was puzzled. Why did the doctor insist on running tests? For a week he had subtly pressured us to discontinue treatment. If the objective was to let Dad die, why put him through more tests? For months we had been confused by Dad's ambiguous health care.

From past experience we knew that the doctor's decisions were often orchestrated by the politics of Dad's case rather than his welfare. There was fear of a lawsuit.

Complicating these politics was the attitude that elderly people are expendable. Some doctors excuse coverups by saying "Why tell them they have AIDS? They're old and will soon die anyway." The message kept coming through. If someone had to get AIDS-tainted blood, it was good that he was old and that his sexual partner was his old wife.

As a family we couldn't allow our parents' care to be dictated by this attitude.

After the phone call, Von, LaRee and I looked at each other. We had to decide if Dad was going back to the hospital. There were many variables to consider but we all knew the deciding factor had to be the strong feelings of our brother, Orvin. After all the debate, he would call the decision.

Orvin has an uncompromising moral code and sees issues very simply: black and white. He insisted on telling everyone who rang the doorbell that the AIDS virus was in the house. I tried to tell him it was just the health care workers who needed this information but he was adamant. The right thing was to tell everyone. It then became difficult even to find a repairman who would come into the kitchen and fix the refrigerator.

Orvin's home was next door to our parents. He and Dad had worked together since he was a small boy. Their relationship was extremely close. Devoted.

Although Orvin agreed to Dad's no code status he did not approve of withholding antibiotics which are necessary to treat the various pneumonias and other infections that AIDS patients suffer. We knew Orvin wouldn't be able to stand by for long and watch Dad go untreated. As the primary caretaker he refused to bow down to this plague. He had fought it for two and a half years before he knew its identity. He wouldn't quit now. No, Orvin would continue to do the superhuman in an effort to heal what had not been healed before. To him, it would be the only moral thing to do.

There was no "right" decision but we couldn't delay any longer. I called the doctor's office. "We're going to bring my father back to the hospital," I said.

Since the ambulance left, Mother is very upset. The health care nurse tries to calm her by massaging her feet.

There is laundry that needs my attention. I go outside to get the blankets and sheets which we prefer to dry in sunlight. Mother has always said that sun kills germs and we are fighting the worst "germ" in the history of infectious disease.

On my way to the clothesline I walk past the shed used to store farm equipment. I notice an old saw hanging on the wall. It's covered with rust but it looks familiar. Then I remember. It's the same saw that, as a child, I watched Dad use to cut down greasewoods on his first 80 acres. Part of the land was undeveloped and had to be cleared before it could be farmed. It was covered with greasewood—straggly, thorny shrubs with heavy, twisted trunks, anchored by deep root systems. They grew higher than Dad's head—a formidable obstacle against cultivation.

The greasewoods were the tough survivors of dry, scorching summers and harsh, frigid winters, growing where nothing else could grow. The hardy shrub had claimed the land for centuries and refused to surrender to farmers without a fight. Each day for weeks Dad took that old handsaw and tore into their gnarly, cast-iron trunks. Stronger ones had to be chopped with his ax. Then Dad would dig deeply around each twisted root so he could pull it up with his team of horses. But a few of the more stubborn greasewood would start to grow back the next spring and Dad had to once again confront them with his saw.

As the years passed, Dad's annoyance with the tenacious greasewood slowly turned to admiration. He came to view their strength and indestructibility with respect.

I return to the house and sit Mother in the kitchen. As I fold clothes, we talk of her childhood. I am grateful that for a few hours her mind is sharp, without the dreaded hallucinations. Recently, she has spoken many times of her parents, as if she is being drawn back to them. Perhaps tonight will be easier.

Von calls and says he will be staying at the hospital with Dad so that Orvin can take a break. When either parent is hospitalized, LaRee and Orvin try to have a family member stay with them. It is especially difficult as there is always another ill parent at home to care for. I am concerned because Von and I have to return to our respective homes soon, and the care crisis is still going on as usual.

At 5:00 in the morning Mother is finally asleep. Two hours later she is awake and asking about Dad.

"Mother, we will go see Dad this morning."

"Then hurry. Get me ready."

"Not for awhile," I say. "It's too early."

I am not sure I should see Dad today. A badly upset stomach plagued me all night. I'm worried I might have a contagious flu. I decide that my upset is probably nerves, along with the burden of guilt I am carrying.

During the past year my daughter's condition has worsened and become very serious. The doctors aren't sure she will live. I have no choice but to return to Colorado and care for her. But how can I tell Mother and Dad goodbye?

I dress Mother and Orvin struggles to get her into the car. Although she can still stand and walk a few steps, she has no sense of how to bend or sit down. She holds her body rigid. Getting her up and down is a task, getting her into a car is close to impossible.

She enjoys the ride. It calms her.

"Mother," I say. "Last night we should have put you in the car, laid the seat back and driven you up and down the road all night. It would have been easier on us all."

When we get to the hospital, we are relieved to see that Dad's condition has improved. He is receiving nourishment and antibiotics through a tube in his nose. His nausea is better. The vomiting has stopped. He is lucid and able to speak a few short sentences.

Since I've been here, Dad has been too ill to talk. I sit by him. I feel he doesn't have much time left and there are so many things I want to tell him. I know he is concerned about a responsibility he will leave behind. I assure him that my husband and I will take care of it.

"Please don't worry, Dad. I promise you it will be handled in the way you want."

He nods.

"I'm going to promise you something else. I will find out how and why this happened to you and Mother. Why they didn't tell you."

Dad's answer is barely audible.

"Just see that no one else has to die like us. Do what you have to."

"I'll do all I can," I promise.

Dad seems convinced. He knows I inherited his genes. The determined, stubborn ones.

LaRee walks with us to the car.

"This can't go on forever, LaRee," I say.

"That's what I keep thinking," she replies. LaRee sighs and wearily returns to Dad's room.

We take Mother home and I spend the rest of the day with her. It is dusk. In a few minutes Orvin is going to drive me to the home of my husband's parents in Vernal. They are taking me back to Colorado tomorrow morning. Orvin and I get Mother back into the car and take her with us.

We pull into their driveway. Orvin carries my luggage into the house. I stay beside Mother.

"How I wish I didn't have to leave you," I say. "I love you."

"I love you, too." She holds onto me. "I'm so scared. Don't go. I'll feel more alone if you're gone."

I try to reassure her, to comfort her. She senses how upset I am and says, "It's all right. My parents are coming soon to get me in the wagon."

"Did you like riding in the wagon when you were a child?" I ask.

"Oh, no. The sun was hot and the road was long and bumpy."

★　　★　　★

It was the last time I saw Mother. She died two weeks later, but the pain I felt that night is still with me, whenever I think of her.

Chapter 2

A Harsh Life

When they were nearly 70 years old, both Mother and Dad recorded their life experiences. Mormons are encouraged to do this so that copies can be given to their children and grandchildren. My parents' lives would end the same way they began: with hardship.

My father, Orville Hatch Swain, was born in 1908 in Vernal, Utah, a small city located near the Colorado border. Even today, the area is isolated and sparsely populated for hundreds of miles.

Orville was one of 10 children. When he was a year old, his parents homesteaded 160 acres of brush-covered land in the midst of the Ute Indian Reservation. It was there, in Lapoint, a small town 18 miles west of Vernal, he would live the rest of his life.

The homestead was not fenced and, as a boy of four, it was Orville's job to herd the milk cows. At five he was old enough to help milk them by hand. His journal records, "My dad raised plenty of prickly cockleburs and the cows' tails were full of them. One night as I was milking this ornery cow, she swatted me in the face with her cocklebur tail. It made me mad. I grabbed her tail and wrapped it around my neck so she couldn't do it again. By the time she'd made two jumps, I knew I'd made a big mistake."

When Orville was 12, he was old enough to work in the small brick-making plant his father had set up to supplement the meager farm earnings. The plant produced about 5,000 bricks per day with a crew of seven. The work was heavy, the hours long. Orville would become so tired, he had to duck his head to hide the tears. No one was going to say he couldn't do a "man's job."

After completing eighth grade at the one-room schoolhouse, Orville had to quit. He was needed to work in the fields and the brick plant. Although his later accomplishments would show it to be inconsequential, he always felt ashamed of his limited formal education.

Growing up as a farm youth was harsh but not without pleasant times. Sometimes at the end of a long day, Orville watched his father and uncle grab their mandolin, jew's harp and banjo. They were talented musicians who played by ear and often provided boot-stompin' hoedowns for the neighbors.

My mother, Ora Mae Anderson, came from the same background as Dad. She too, was born in Vernal and moved with her family to Lapoint when she was four years old. She writes in her history: "We lived in a tent about three years before a one-room cabin with a dirt roof was built. Straw was put on the floor and a home-woven carpet was tacked down over it. When it rained the mud would run down the inside of the wall."

Being an only child, Ora had few playmates. Her mother made dolls for her out of corn husks, wooden spools and bell-shaped hollyhock flowers. Ora enjoyed playing with the farm animals. She told how she cried when her favorite baby pet pig was washed away in a flash flood.

Ora kept busy with family chores. As a young girl, she had to herd the sheep and cows. There were eggs to gather from the chicken coop and weeds to pull in the garden. She churned the butter and placed it in the ice house to keep it cool. Ora and her mother spent hours canning vegetables to add to the winter supply.

The only means of transportation for Ora's family was by horse or on foot. She badly froze her feet walking home from school one cold winter's day. She wrote, "When I was sixteen my father bought a Model T Ford and I will never forget how thrilled I was to go down the long driveway at night with the lights. We were used to riding in a buggy in the dark and this was a welcome change."

She rode in that same Model T to her wedding. Ora wrote, "I was married in the Salt Lake Temple to Orville Swain, June 14, 1933. My mother and grandparents made the long drive with us in my father's automobile. We were coming home after dark when the car lights went out so I stood on the running board to direct my new husband. A short distance from home, we came to a canal bridge. I told him to turn south but he kept going the other way. I finally grabbed the steering wheel and gave it a quick turn. We missed going off the bridge by a hair." It was not the last time during their long marriage that my mother did not let Dad ignore her advice.

After their wedding Mother and Dad lived with her parents. Dad helped his father-in-law build a five-room brick house that replaced the cabin.

I was born in 1934 during the depression, the oldest of four children. Dad considered himself lucky to get farm work for 25 cents an hour.

In the spring of 1935 he leased a house with 40 acres of farm land and moved his family. He borrowed $2,000 from the Farmers Home Administration to buy some equipment and 11 jersey cows. Dad spent three hours milking them before daylight, worked in the fields past dark, then milked them again by lantern light. The milk and cream were divided with a hand cranked separator. The milk was then fed to the calves and the cream was sold for $7.50 a week.

Dad was fiercely independent. The $2,000 loan really "stuck in his craw," as he would say. He hated being indebted to anyone. He had been ashamed to ask for the government assistance—something he had always abhorred. Dad wrote about his humiliation when the FHA loan representative visited them each month and took inventory of everything they owned. "They counted right down to each pair of socks and underwear and just stopped short of checking my waistline for any extra fat!" Within two years he had paid off the loan ahead of time and vowed he would never go in debt again. He never did. This experience shaped a lifetime of frugality and financial conservatism.

In 1938 my parents bought their first 80 acres and Dad built a nice stucco home with running water and our first bathroom. It was here that my brothers, Orvin and Von, and my sister, LaRee, were born.

Modern conveniences came very slowly. Eventually a diesel-powered tractor and six-foot disc plow replaced old Barney and Bess, our draft horses, and the 14-inch walking plow they had pulled day after day with Dad trudging along behind. I was nine years old before electricity reached our house. My parents didn't get a telephone until I left home to attend college.

Dad had always been progressive and community-minded. He served several years as president of Whiterocks Irrigation Company, and four years as County Deputy Assessor.

By early 1952, the roads to Lapoint were still unpaved. Each spring they became nearly impassable. I remember walking home in mud up to my knees when the school bus got stuck. Dad got so frustrated with this annual annoyance that he demanded an appointment with Governor J. Bracken Lee, whom he had never met. He invited two neighbor friends to accompany him to the meeting in Salt Lake City. He apprised the governor of their community's plight and made a convincing plea for assistance. The governor was persuaded. He picked up the phone and directed the State Road Commission to pave the 10-mile stretch of road from highway 40 north to Lapoint. Within three months it was complete.

That meeting was the beginning of a long association between Governor Lee and my father. A mutual respect grew between the big-city politician and the rough-hewn farmer.

Dad was influenced to try his hand at local politics. That fall he was elected to the Uintah County Commission as a Republican. He was re-elected three more times before retiring and served as Chairman of the Commission for the last three terms.

He accomplished many noteworthy things during his tenure. His leadership brought the county a new administration building and library. Bridges and roads were constructed or improved and the major water reclamation projects, Flaming Gorge Dam and Steinaker Reservoir, were completed. Television was brought into the county.

Dad conducted his political responsibilities much the same as he lived his life. He had a genuine concern for all of the people he represented and wanted each of them to be treated fairly. He was frugal yet progressive and a scrappy fighter for what he believed in. His critics saw him as headstrong and domineering, but he was always re-elected by substantial margins.

To describe my father as an "honest, hard-working man" is both trite and true. In the world he lived in, a man was judged more by these two characteristics than by any other. To be labeled by one's peers as lazy or untrustworthy was a stigma that could mark someone for life. Most of Dad's business dealings were done with a handshake, not a written contract. He saw contracts as something a slick lawyer could break. His word could not be broken.

My father had been a compulsively hard worker all of his life, doing heavy, exhausting work for long hours each day beneath the relentless summer sun or in the biting cold of winter. He continued to run the 260-acre farm during his years as County Commissioner. For many years he and Orvin did rock masonry work in the surrounding towns. While it started as a hobby, they soon had many requests for fireplaces, planters and fences. They found their rock in the rugged mountains and canyons nearby. Some of the masonry rocks weighed over 100 pounds and had to be carried long distances to the truck. The younger men left the heaviest rocks for Dad because he was the only one strong enough to carry them. He was strong even in his seventies and was accustomed to lifting heavy hay bales.

As Dad got older, we suggested he slow down and start to think about retirement. He refused to talk about it. Each time we brought up the dreaded "R" word, he grabbed his hat, jumped on his tractor and headed for the fields. His answer to "slowing down" was to get his real estate license so he could sell farm real estate and develop some of his own property into building lots. All of this in addition to running the farm and trying to keep up with the demand for rock work.

My parents never took vacations like most people. Farming was a full-time job. But somehow Dad found the time to do what he enjoyed most—fishing and hunting with the family in the beautiful Uintah Mountains nearby. One of Dad's favorite trips was riding 30 miles on horseback into the primitive high Uintahs with its many pristine lakes full of rainbow trout. He loved to raft down the Green River and take long hikes up the Whiterocks River to beaver ponds where he caught "brookies" on every cast. He often spoke of the time he hunted deer on Mosby Mountain—the day he shot the big four point buck.

It seemed like the fish got longer and bucks got bigger with each telling. Dad delighted in humorous tales and embellished his stories with great flair. His listeners laughed uproariously, encouraging the performer even more. Some stories raised eyebrows among church friends. My six-year-old son made the mistake of repeating one to his first grade class. The teacher asked her students to comment on different birds they knew. "My grandpa taught me about the Mile-er-more Bird," my son exclaimed. The teacher looked puzzled. "Oh. What kind of a bird is that?" He proudly recited, "It's a large purple bird with long legs and an even longer neck. When it buries its head in the sand and whistles out of its butt, you can hear it for a mile-er-more."

Some of Dad's most entertaining stories were about city people who moved to the Basin with no knowledge of farming. They bought a few acres and expected to be successful in agriculture. But it did not take long before reality set in. Over the years Dad befriended a number of these families. He loaned them equipment and taught them the basics of productive farming. If times got so rough for the newcomers that they couldn't feed their milk cow, Dad took them bales of hay.

Mother was skilled at making beautiful quilts. The women's organization was always working on one to be sold for a church fund-raiser. Our living room was used to set up the frames which held the quilts in place as they were stitched together. The older women who lived nearby came and quilted at our house every afternoon. The sewing took many days to complete. Dad and we kids weren't thrilled with this arrangement because we had to crawl on our hands and knees under the frames to cross the room.

My parents shared the abundance of their garden and orchard with their neighbors. During the long winters Dad took carrots and potatoes from the family root cellar to those in need. Neither of my folks ever forgot the severe poverty of their childhoods and often excused debts of those who couldn't afford to pay.

Mother and Dad donated much of their time to work in the Mormon Church. Each served in administrative and teaching positions. They possessed natural dramatic talent and during the '40s had leading roles in a number of plays which the church directed for the community. I remember hiding behind the shed and listening to Dad rehearse his accent as he milked the cows.

As we children married, three of us established our homes away from Lapoint. However, Orvin and his wife lived next door to my parents and in 1970 their son Rocky was born. He became the joy of his grandparents' lives. He rode with Dad on the tractor and followed him around as he milked the cows.

When he was two, Rocky's health began to fail. He was diagnosed with acute leukemia. For four and a half years his parents and grandparents helplessly watched him suffer the pain of this disease and its attendant treatments and tests—chemotherapy, spinal punctures and bone marrow aspirations. His medical care required incessant travel to Salt Lake City. When Rocky died in 1977, a bit of my parents died with him.

The strain had taken a toll on Orvin's marriage. He and his wife were divorced a few weeks after the death of their only child.

Chapter 3

An Ill-Fated Surgery

The tragic events that would eventually take my parents' lives made their entrance in January 1985.

On the evening of January 3, I called Dad's room at the LDS Hospital in Salt Lake City. Early the next morning he was scheduled for coronary bypass surgery. He was very frightened.

"I'm in bad shape," Dad said. "I don't have a choice. I gotta have the operation on three arteries—the whole works."

"Dad, wasn't it just three months ago you started getting the chest pain?"

"Yes, around then. But it wasn't bad. Just a mild pain once in awhile. It's only been the last few weeks that it got worse."

"Are you sure the pain couldn't be treated with drugs instead of surgery?"

"No. Dr. Jones said if I go home to think about getting the operation I might not make it back alive."

"I would feel better if we got a second opinion."

"Gosh, there isn't time. Besides there isn't anyone else as good as Jones. A young fellow just told me that Dr. Kent Jones is the best heart surgeon in Utah."

"Who was the fellow?"

"I dunno. He took some blood out of my arm. If I don't have the operation tomorrow I could die."

"Don't worry, Dad. The operation will go just fine. You'll be okay. Our prayers are with you."

I hung up the phone with an unsettled feeling.

The decision to operate seemed hasty but Orvin had told me earlier that the doctors hadn't discussed any options. Apparently this was emergency surgery.

Two days earlier Dad's local doctor had sent him to the LDS Hospital for evaluation after he failed a treadmill test. Studies were done to determine the condition of his heart and coronary arteries. After Dad and Orvin talked to Dr. Jones about the test results, they were certain surgery was necessary.

The doctors told Dad there was a five in 100 chance of death from the triple bypass procedure. They had also been honest about the risks of the tests, including fatal reactions to the dyes.

However, their candor did not extend to the subject of transfusion. It was never discussed. Neither the doctors nor any member of the hospital staff mentioned the large amounts of blood required for coronary bypass, with every unit increasing the risk of blood-borne diseases. Neither Dad nor family members were informed of the high risk of hepatitis or the risk of AIDS that transfused blood carried.

Other life-saving information was also withheld. We were not told that there were intraoperative autologous transfusion (IAT) procedures available to greatly reduce or eliminate the need for transfusing heart patients with someone else's blood. It was then possible to collect and filter the blood lost during surgery and transfuse it back into the patient. Large amounts of blood can be recycled in this manner without a risk of hepatitis and AIDS. Moreover, no effort was made to keep the number of Dad's donors to a minimum. Had we been informed we could have chosen one relative to act as a platelet monodonor to provide all the platelets Dad received from eight donors.

Without knowing the risks or the alternatives to unsafe transfusions, the next day Dad received the blood of 18 people. The blood was supplied by the LDS Blood Bank located at the large LDS Hospital complex. The 18 units had all been collected from local donors.

The hours seemed like days as the family waited for Dad's surgery to be over. LaRee and her husband were there with Mother, as were Von and his wife.

Orvin sat fidgeting on the sofa, running his hands through his hair in a compulsive motion. Why was it taking so long? He probably should have insisted on a second opinion. He stood up, unable to sit a minute longer, and paced around the waiting room. Orvin held a deep breath as he saw Dr. Jones approaching them.

"Everything went very well," Jones said.

Relieved, Orvin let go of the breath he was holding.

"He should have many good years left," the doctor continued. "He's in strong physical condition for a man his age."

The family was well aware of Dad's prime physical condition. During the 1980s Dad had continued to work like a miner in a cave-in. The previous year had been no different. In early spring Dad developed some of his land for sale as building lots. He sawed up old trees and hauled off rocks. He tore down old corrals and fences, burning the lumber he couldn't salvage.

During the summer Dad irrigated his 260 acres and baled hay. While helping him clean ditches along the fence lines, Orvin grumbled, as he had done for years, about Dad's concept of retirement. "You'll soon be 76 years old and you're working as hard as ever. You should think about my health—trying to keep up with you could kill me."

Dad just laughed. He had as much use for retirement as a duck had for a life preserver.

Orvin recalled that in the fall a teenager had lost control of his car and took out part of the fence in front of the house. He and Dad hauled rocks and gravel for the repair job. In late November, as they were doing the masonry work, Dad complained of the chest pain and shortness of breath that led to his surgery.

After his surgery, Dad spent three miserable days in intensive care. When he got back to his room he still vomited every day and took chills, asking for more blankets. Mother, Orvin and LaRee stayed in Salt Lake City to be near him. Either LaRee or Orvin was with Dad each night, sleeping on a cot in his private room.

Although Dad's heart functioned well while he was in the hospital, he had one scary episode of irregularity in the rhythm of his heartbeat which frightened him. The irregularity was brought under control with drugs and the doctors said he was doing fine. Dad didn't think the doctors were telling him the truth. "If my heart is okay why do I feel so sick all over?" he asked.

As the days wore on Dad's fatigue did not improve. "It takes everything I have just to sit up," he complained.

Mother tried to reassure him. "That's to be expected after a heart operation."

The family stay in Salt Lake City dragged on and on. When Dad had been hospitalized for 14 days my husband and son traveled from Colorado to visit him.

"I'm getting pretty discouraged," Dad told them. "The doctors say it could be the medicine that's making me throw up. That man down the hall had his heart operation days after I did and he's going home tomorrow."

My son could see his grandfather was depressed and tried to lighten the conversation. "Hang in there, Grandpa," he said. "It would take more than a heart operation to keep you down."

"I suppose so," said the old man.

"Grandpa, you're an expert on birds. What is the definition of a mugwump?"

"I dunno."

"A mugwump is a bird that sits on the fence with his mug on one side and his wump on another."

Dad smiled. "I met up with some of those birds when I was County Commissioner."

When Dad was released from the hospital, LaRee felt he should stay at her home in Roosevelt for a few weeks so he could be close to his local doctor. It took some persuasive effort but finally Dad agreed. LaRee also hoped her children would lift his spirits. Her little blond, blue-eyed girl of six was my parents' youngest grandchild. They adored her.

LaRee's husband shaved Dad each day and helped him shower. Though still very feeble, Dad's strength increased, enabling him to walk around the house without assistance. He no longer had spells of vomiting and there were no incidents with his heart. LaRee was relieved.

She stood at the stove stirring a pan of gravy. She was cooking all of Dad's favorite farm-style foods. He was a meat and potatoes man—hated those tuna fish casseroles. LaRee was concerned about his diet. When she asked the heart surgeon if Dad should be off high cholesterol foods he had said to let him eat the foods he had always enjoyed. That's what worried LaRee. Dad loved eggs, cream and butter—hated that loathsome margarine. As she stirred the gravy she consoled herself by remembering the pie they had served him while he was still in the hospital.

Orvin was concerned about Dad's emotional state—his nervousness and inability to cope. The doctors had explained this was not an unusual response after heart surgery but it was certainly unusual for Dad.

"Dad's a wreck," Orvin said. "Yesterday Ma and me took the bills down to him when we visited at LaRee's. He went all to pieces and she had to sit by his side and make out the checks for him to sign."

"Well, maybe he'll be more his old self when he gets back home," I said. "He's always like a caged tiger whenever he's away from Lapoint."

Dr. Gary White, Dad's local doctor, prescribed Ativan for him. It was the first time in his life that Dad had taken tranquilizers.

When Orvin and Mother took him home in early February, Dad was sure things would soon be back to normal. He expected to again take charge of his familiar surroundings and assume the old responsibilities. The work was still there. He could see everything that needed to be done but he could not will his body to do it. He was much too weak and fatigued. He panicked. It didn't matter that financially he didn't need to work. He wanted to work. It was his validation—all he had ever known.

Dad thought if he pushed himself harder he could build up his stamina by walking. The harsh winter left the country roads glazed with ice. Orvin took Dad to the elementary school and walked him through the halls and around the gym.

There were a few days when Dad had a bit more energy and could talk to the school custodians as he trudged along. He would be encouraged and optimistic about the future—only to be overpowered the next day by pervasive fatigue.

He longed for his former vitality and independence. The effort it now took to perform the simplest tasks, such as eating and dressing, left him feeling depressed and humiliated. All his life he had been iron-willed and hard as nails, able to accomplish just about anything he set his mind to, overcoming any obstacle that stood in his path. But despite all his efforts, he now feared he was losing the fight to regain his health.

Occasionally a spark of the old Dad would surface. Orvin sat him on the wooden kitchen stool to cut his hair. That stool had seen 50 years of family hair-cutting and some feisty exchanges between barber and patron.

Orvin finished the job and handed Dad the mirror. "Does that look better?" he asked.

"I look like an old buzzard with lopsided sideburns," Dad said. "Can't you cut hair better than that?"

"What do you expect?" Orvin asked with a teasing cackle. "You were my teacher."

Mother smiled. "It seems like old times," she said.

In late February, Orvin was alarmed when Dad had an attack of nausea and vomiting accompanied by a gnawing, persistent pain in his stomach. Dad shivered as though he were in a deadly chill. He had a rapid heartbeat. Orvin rushed him down to the emergency room in Roosevelt. The doctor diagnosed peptic syndrome and sent him home with two drugs for his stomach.

For the next three days Dad continued to feel miserable. He worried about a headache that wouldn't go away. He never suffered from headaches. "I can't stand to eat," he told me on the phone. "The sight of food makes me want to throw up. I feel like a limp rag."

Unknown to us or Dr. White, Dad was probably suffering the onset of hepatitis B which he got from blood transfusion during his heart surgery. Hepatitis B is caused by a virus that attacks the liver. The symptoms usually come on between six weeks and six months after infection. The severity of the illness varies. Some patients think they have a flu and their doctors can miss the diagnosis. Others are debilitated for nearly a year. Chronic liver disease develops in approximately 8% of hepatitis B patients and 1% die.

Dad called Dr. Jones in Salt Lake City and asked if the medications could be making him so sick. The doctor said that was a remote possibility and took him off one of his heart medications. "I think you can get along fine without it," Jones said.

Two days later Dad called out urgently, "Orvin, help me!"

"What is it?"

"My heart is about to stop. It's fluttering—jumping around in my chest."

Orvin and Mother frantically got Dad into the car and sped toward Roosevelt. Orvin's hands tightened around the steering wheel. He was convinced Dad was going to die.

"You're gonna be okay, Dad," he said, trying to steady the shakiness in his voice. "The doctors will give you some drugs that will control the rhythm. They did that after the surgery, remember?"

Silently, Orvin cursed the long distance they lived from medical facilities. And he knew better than to wait for paramedic assistance. Sixteen minutes later he pulled up to the hospital emergency entrance and was met by Dr. White. There was tension as the doctor and nurses worked to control the fibrillation. White called in his new associate, Dr. Ace Madsen, who had experience in handling heart patients.

In a short time, Madsen had Dad's heart under control. The crisis was over. In a few days, Dad was released from the hospital. Now Dad was Dr. Madsen's biggest fan. "I've found a doctor who is smart enough to figure out what's going on," he said. "He's sure a fine young fellow." Dad had a trusting faith in doctors—a great respect for their many years of education.

By mid-March it was evident to Orvin that Dad was not getting better. He was nauseated most of the time. His stomach was much worse than when he stayed at LaRee's home after the surgery. And he was sleeping nearly all day. Orvin recognized Dad's setback and thought there might be something else wrong with him. He cancelled an appointment Dad had with Dr. Jones for a checkup because he knew his father was unable to travel the long distance to Salt Lake City.

Orvin found it increasingly difficult to leave Mom and Dad while he picked up prescriptions, groceries and other supplies in Roosevelt or Vernal. He had been with them day and night since the surgery. Mother was now very upset about Dad and was afraid of handling an emergency by herself.

Dad's symptoms had him stumped. He had strange reactions to food and medications. Every time he tried to eat he went into sneezing fits and his eyes and nose ran—his stomach hurt and he became more nauseated.

Dad hated allergies and always prided himself on the fact that he didn't have any. His wife had them, his kids had them, and his grandchildren had them. But not him. He said they came from those "weak Anderson genes" on Mother's side of the family. Genes he put in the same category as "Anderson mush," the oatmeal he despised.

Dad gave my brothers allergy shots throughout their teen years and Mother cooked strange foods they weren't allergic to. Dad said the treatment was worse than the illness. He couldn't understand allergies. He suspected they were some form of weakness but now he feared he had them.

"The symptoms are the worst when I eat jello," he said. "Why would that be?"

Without knowing that Dad had been transfused with a potpourri of viral infections, I was grasping at straws in a futile attempt to help him. I thought for a moment. "Maybe the dyes injected into your veins for the heart studies left you sensitive to the dyes in foods," I said. "I'll ask Orvin to avoid buying foods that contain dyes."

Dad's country doctors were also having difficulty finding reasons for his vague and unrelated symptoms. He had a large lesion on his right lower lip which refused to heal and often bled profusely. His skin was dry and scaly. He said he itched all over.

In late March, Dad was admitted to the hospital because of severe abdominal pain. When he was released a few days later, the only treatment he had received was for constipation.

LaRee carried a large pot of homemade vegetable soup out to her car. She placed it in the center of a box so it wouldn't tip over and returned to the house for a shrimp and rice salad. Each weekend she prepared special foods for Dad's touchy stomach and took it to Lapoint. While she was there she would do some heavy housework and help Dad pay bills. He still depended on her to help with his finances—a task he handled efficiently before his surgery. If the weather was good she would go for a short walk with him.

LaRee drove back to her home wondering how long it would be before Dad regained his health. It upset her to see him so unlike the active, confident man he used to be. She worried about the strain it caused Mother. Her health was fragile. She was 73 years old and had suffered from migraine headaches and high blood pressure for years. The situation was a constant burden on Orvin. His life was on hold. LaRee thought of her own family. She worked during the week and the stress of Dad's condition was taking a toll on all of them—especially her children.

April was a better month. Dad's office visits to Dr. Madsen were confined to his unrelenting fatigue and an unexplained pain in his left leg and foot. Ativan had taken the edge off his nervousness but he viewed it with suspicion. "It makes me sick to my stomach and dizzy," he said. "I think it even makes me more tired."

It had been a long winter. Orvin felt he had to get Mother and Dad out of the house. He took them on short drives and stopped to let them visit with old friends. Some of the friends later voiced their concern about Dad. "That must have been one tough operation he had. You can sure tell he's still not feelin' good."

Dad felt as useless as a disabled baseball pitcher. It was time for spring farming to begin and he knew he couldn't do any of the work. He had high, demanding standards and worried that the farm would go to ruin. He fussed and stewed and stalled. Finally he signed a lease with the McKees, two brothers who ran large plots of land. They would take over all the planting, irrigating and harvesting.

As hard as it was for Dad to sit on the sidelines, he had confidence in the McKees. "They have all the big, fancy machinery," Dad said. "And they know how to farm. They're real wheeler-dealers."

Now that someone else was doing the farming, Dad was even more at loose ends—more humiliated by his slow recovery. "I guess I'm just a pantywaist. I'll have to do woman's work." He did laundry and some cooking. In his usual take-charge way he instructed Mother on how to prepare the food she had cooked for over 60 years. Tension built.

Mormon belief places husbands at the head of the family with authority over the wife. This was a belief Dad had always taken seriously and Mother ignored. During 52 years of marriage she had learned how to maneuver her way around the ruler of the roost. If Dad wanted to be the cook that was fine with her. She removed herself from the kitchen and worked on her genealogy. Tracing one's ancestors is another Mormon custom—one she enjoyed. She also enjoyed watching the soaps on TV.

"I don't know what's wrong with your mother," Dad said. "About all she does is watch TV. Could her mind be failing?"

"I don't think so," I said. "She's sharp enough to have you doing the cooking."

Instead of the usual large garden, Dad agreed to settle for just some green beans, corn and tomatoes. Mother kept an eye on the planting to make sure he stuck to his word. The last thing she needed was an enormous amount of vegetables to can. There were already more bottles of vegetables and fruits in the cellar than they could eat. Mother's nerves were frazzled. It drove her crazy watching her husband so sick and insisting on cooking. The only thing worse would be watching him can. She'd never get back in her kitchen.

One day as Dad was helping Orvin plant the hills of corn, he had mild chest pain. Any type of chest pain terrified Dad because he blamed all his health problems on his heart. Within the hour he was sitting in Dr. Madsen's office. The doctor was aware of Dad's anxiety and again encouraged him to be as active as he could. He reassured him that his heart was doing very well. But when Dad asked why he continued to feel so poorly, Madsen had no answers. Left without explanation for his problems, Dad found it impossible not to be concerned about his heart.

My brother Von, who lived some distance from Lapoint, kept track of our father's condition by telephone. Von was worried and puzzled. It was evident to him that at times Dad felt too ill to hold the phone and talk for longer than five minutes. And he often made strange grunting noises. When Von would ask where he hurt, Dad said he just felt sick all over. The last time he called home, Von told Dad he would be coming soon for a visit and they could go fishing together. He knew if fishing couldn't cheer the old man up nothing could.

At the time of Dad's transfusion, the AIDS virus crept into our lives as quietly as a poisonous spider spins its web. Although AIDS cannot be spread by casual contact, infected blood carries a risk to others. But during the 28 months before he was informed that he carried the infectious AIDS virus, we did not know we had reason to be cautious of Dad's blood.

For five decades our family members had cut each other's hair, sharing unsterilized barber tools. Manicure implements, fingernail files and clippers were also shared by the family. The same pincushion hung on my parents' wall for 40 years. If someone got a splinter in their hand they would take a needle from the cushion and dig it out. Then the needle would be returned to the pincushion without cleaning. After we learned of the AIDS, recalling these family practices brought an icy fear.

In summer, following his surgery, Dad resumed cutting Orvin's hair. Orvin would cut Dad's hair first, which was difficult because by then Dad's skin was scaly and scabby. Occasionally when cutting his sideburns the clippers would cause a scab to bleed. In a few minutes Dad would cut Orvin's hair with the same clippers.

Dad was feeble and shaky. There was one incident when he nicked Orvin's ear and his own finger with the scissors. Unaware of the danger they blotted their blood on the same tissue. For over two years the same barber tools were used to cut the hair of other family members, including grandchildren. But the LDS Blood Bank never notified Dad or his doctors that they had found one of his donors was infected with AIDS. They kept a deadly, voiceless silence, waiting for Dad to die.

★　　★　　★

The blood bank played a game of odds weighted in its favor. Most patients will die within a year of transfusion from their underlying condition. If recipients of AIDS-tainted transfusions live long enough to develop AIDS, there is a chance it will never be correctly diagnosed. Patients often die from AIDS-related illness with death certificates listing cancer or pneumonia, etc. as the cause of demise. And if transfusion AIDS *is* diagnosed, doctors may keep it concealed from the patient and family. If the unknowing victim's sexual partner has become infected with AIDS, that also can go undiagnosed. To this day, there is *no law* requiring doctors to tell patients they have AIDS or are HIV-positive. There is no national law requiring doctors to report full-blown AIDS cases, although they are supposed to report them to state health departments. However, the fine line between when a patient progresses from ARC to full-blown reportable AIDS allows doctors to avoid reporting many cases. Blood banks play with a stacked deck because the majority of those who contract AIDS infection from transfusions never find out about it.

★　　★　　★

Dad returned to Dr. Madsen's office in early June for one of his frequent visits. As he waited for the doctor he was very despondent. 'The chance of my getting better is as likely as a catfish climbing a tree,' he thought. He tried to think of how he could describe the strange feeling he had in his chest. He had to think about his breathing all the time now.

"My breathing has gone all haywire," he told the perplexed doctor. "I'm not breathing right."

The doctor listened to his chest for a long time. "Are you sleeping well?" he asked.

"I'm sleeping pretty good," said Dad, "but I take spells when I just start to cry and can't stop."

That day Dr. Madsen wrote in Dad's medical chart, "Mr. Swain is very difficult to figure out."

At the end of June, Dad's brother Darreld visited my parents. He was distraught because just a week before, his two-year-old grandson had been diagnosed with AIDS. He was shocked when he saw Dad, thinking Orville looked like he could fade as fast as their mother's lye soap on wash day. Darreld no longer believed that poppycock about the golden years. To him, life got tougher the longer it lasted.

Little Jonathan Swain was the child of Darreld's son, Dee, and his wife, Shiela. He was born prematurely in March 1983 with a strep infection. He was transfused with five units of blood supplied by the Belle Bonfils Memorial Blood Center in Denver, Colorado.

Though Jonathan developed normally, he was a sickly child and seemed to have a constant cold. He had recurring ear and skin infections and a bout of viral pneumonia.

When he was six months old, his mother read a magazine article about AIDS being spread through transfusions. She asked the pediatrician if her baby could have AIDS. Her question was brushed off as the irrational fear of an over-anxious mother.

Shortly before his second birthday, Jonathan was hospitalized and chest X-rays showed abnormalities. He had a chronic inflammation of the lungs called Lymphocytic Interstitial Pneumonitis (LIP) which is common in children who have AIDS.

It was the first day of summer when Shiela received the phone call that confirmed her worst fears. The doctor kept repeating "I'm so sorry," until the words became an empty echo. The sun's warm, genial rays faded. "His immune system is suppressed. If it worsens, he won't have long to live."

AIDS had come with the force of an earthquake, shattering everything the family knew before. At that moment Shiela realized nothing would ever be the same.

At the time of Darreld's visit, my parents knew little about AIDS. It was only something they had heard about on the TV news. Something that happened in large cities to those living lifestyles which they couldn't understand. But now the youngest of Dee and Shiela's three boys had AIDS. That hit close to home.

Hearing about Jonathan depressed Mother terribly. She knew all too well what it was like to watch a child die of a terminal illness. Nothing tore her heart like the tears of a child in pain.

Mother recalled that when Jonathan's older brother, Jeremy, was two, Dee and Shiela spent the summer in Lapoint living in Orvin's trailer. It was just one year after the death of Orvin's son, Rocky. Jeremy helped fill the void and eased my parents' pain. Mother smiled as she remembered how happy Dad was to once again take a little Swain toddler with him on the tractor.

The closeness with Dee's family had brightened that summer of 1978. It was the same year an unknown virus first entered America's blood supply—five years before Jonathan's birth and seven years before Dad's heart surgery.

The first week in July, Von and his thirteen-year-old son came from their home in Cedar City, Utah, to spend a few days with Mother and Dad. They encouraged Dad to go fishing. "It will do you good," Von said. "We'll go where we can drive to a lake so you won't have to walk."

Fishing with his children and their families was Dad's favorite pastime. He always enjoyed a high spirit of comradery with his grandchildren and loved to entertain them with his colorful stories.

Now Dad dreaded the thought of going fishing. He was so tired he could barely put one foot in front of the other. Doing anything took more effort than he could give. But he was afraid he'd turned into a helpless, complaining old man. How he hated it! He couldn't spend the rest of his life holed up in the house. He thought he would go and try to hide how badly he felt.

They drove into the mountains and got out of the pickup truck. A warm breeze wrinkled the lake. Dad cast his line far out into the water. The effort caused his legs to wobble with weakness and fatigue. Soon he put his fishing pole down and sought the shade of a tree. He lay under it, unable to fish or even recite his usual tales.

Von was alarmed. He knew his father was a gutsy man. Upon arrival he had been shocked at how his father's health had deteriorated since he last saw him. "I'm really worried about Dad," he told Orvin later that day. "Something is very wrong with him and it's more than psychological."

July 10 got off to a better start. Dad felt well enough to keep a long-delayed appointment for a checkup with Dr. Jones, his heart surgeon. Dad, Mother, and Orvin left early in the morning on the long drive to Salt Lake City. The visit with Dr. Jones went well. Dad was elated during the return trip—excited because Jones had been so pleased with the condition of his heart.

"You're doing very well," Jones had said. "I think you've turned the corner. Go home and enjoy life."

"I guess there's no reason I can't do the things I did before the operation," Dad said. "My heart's as good as new."

"That's wonderful news," said Mother.

Although Orvin did not voice his doubts, he did not share Dr. Jones's glowing prognosis. He had lived with Dad the past six months and knew his father was not a well man.

Later that night, after he got home, Dad's arms and legs began to jerk. He had no control over them. Loss of control was intolerable to him and he became very anxious. Orvin rubbed Dad's legs hoping he would relax. He debated taking him to the emergency room in Roosevelt. It seemed all he did was take Dad to doctors and there were no doctors in Lapoint.

He thought how much worse health problems like these were when you live out in the boonies.

Dr. Madsen examined Dad early the next morning. "Are you still on the Ativan?" he asked.

"No," said Dad. "I went off it about five days ago. It made me sick to my stomach and more tired. I've felt better without it."

"Your jerking is probably caused by benzodiazepine withdrawal because you abruptly stopped the Ativan." The doctor administered Tranxene, another tranquilizer in the benzodiazepine family, and in a short time Dad's jerking stopped.

But Dad eyed the Tranxene pills he was to take home like a wary fox would eye a trap. "Are these going to make me sick, too?" he asked.

"You'll just be on them a short time—then I'll taper you off gradually," the doctor answered. "You're going to be fine."

In the following weeks Dad tried hard to live up to Madsen and Jones's predictions of good health. He had bad days but there were other days when he definitely did feel better. He attempted to be more active—to do more. 'Perhaps part of my trouble is in my head,' he thought. Dad's mother, who was a midwife, had said that troubles were like babies—the longer you nursed them the bigger they got. It was time to wean the baby.

Dad hadn't driven a car since his surgery. He was totally reliant on Orvin to chauffeur him everywhere because his eyesight had deteriorated so rapidly. This was another blow to his independent spirit. Sometimes it was impossible for him to focus on anything either at a distance or up close. At times he couldn't read with or without his glasses.

Orvin took him to his optometrist in Vernal but tests indicated his glasses were still fine.

"Well, why can't I see?" Dad had demanded. "Why do my eyes hurt and feel funny?"

Even an ophthalmologist couldn't find a reason for his symptoms. "Perhaps they will go away," the doctor said.

★　　★　　★

A significant percentage of AIDS patients suffer from eye disorders and some become blind. Cytomegalic retinitis is common. It is caused by the cytomegalovirus virus (CMV) which preys upon AIDS patients because of their weakened immune systems.

★　　★　　★

"I don't wear my glasses much because they don't help anymore," Dad told me. "I guess Orvin will have to keep driving me everywhere."

In early September, Dad was helping Orvin pick corn in the garden and muttering about his eyesight. "My eyes are so bad I can't tell which ears are ready to pick. In fact, since my operation nothing on me has worked right."

Dad told Orvin he was impotent. Orvin was not surprised. "When someone your age has heart surgery that can be expected," he said.

"This has nothing to do with my age," Dad snapped. "It's just one more problem the operation caused."

By October it had been nine months since Dad had attended church. He recalled this was the only period in his life when he had not been part of the Mormon activities that were his roots. Getting back to church would probably get rid of this depression he kept feeling.

"I think I can sit through a meeting or two," he said on Sunday morning. He went to get dressed and became upset to find none of his suit pants fit. "I'm as skinny as an old crow. I didn't know I lost so much weight. I can't go."

Orvin rummaged through the back of his own closet and found some dress pants he hadn't worn for many years. "Try these on," he said brushing off the dust. "I wore these when I was real thin—before I gained 40 pounds." Dad put on the pants.

"See, under this sport coat they will do until I can take you to buy a new suit."

Orvin stood at the window watching Mother and Dad walk the block to the church. The chapel was fairly new. It had replaced an older one and was built on land Dad had provided—a piece cut out of the corner of his hayfield.

Although he was happy to see his parents attend Sunday services, Orvin had not gone to church since he was a teenager. He perceived a hypocrisy in organized religion, comparing it to some of the winter pears he picked in the orchard: good looking on the outside but disappointing at the core. This observation, which he enjoyed pointing out to the largely Mormon community, was not well received.

★　　★　　★

Mother was still upset over little Jonathan. He was being cared for at home by Shiela and a nursing service. The boy was tethered to an oxygen tank all the time. The doctors had him on antibiotics to fight infections, and gamma globulin to boost his immune system.

"I'll never understand why innocent children have to suffer so," Mother said.

I tried to comfort her. "Jonathan is holding his own," I said. "In spite of everything he looks healthy and is energetic."

Mother was concerned because Darreld had told them that AIDS was also destroying the lives of Jonathan's brothers and parents. The family's struggle to care for their ill child was hampered by fear of his disease. Medical expenses were mounting and it was difficult for Shiela to work part-time because a string of babysitters kept quitting. Even some professional health caregivers had treated the family like lepers.

Their children felt isolated. Many of the older boys' friends were no longer allowed to play with them. The situation had attracted the attention of the Colorado media, causing more problems.

"It's such a mess," said Mother. "I can't believe this happened. What are the chances of a baby getting AIDS from a transfusion?" LaRee shared Mother's concern for Jonathan. Like the rest of our family, however, she didn't see any connection between Jonathan's health problems and those Dad was displaying.

LaRee and Dad had always had a close and caring relationship. She understood him. She and her husband always invited Mother, Dad and Orvin to their home for holidays. But this year when LaRee mentioned Thanksgiving, Dad insisted that he prepare the turkey.

"You've done too much cooking for us," he said. "You bring food up here all the time." LaRee protested but he was adamant. "I won't come unless I cook the turkey and bring it."

Dad did even more. He baked pumpkin pies. However, the cooking drained him. When I called later that night he was exhausted.

"I used to get up before daylight and farm," he said. "Now I get up at dawn and stuff bread crumbs into a dead turkey. Even women's work wears me out."

"Maybe you've underestimated women's work all these years," I said. His response surprised me.

"It's awful. Fixing three meals and doing dishes can take all day. What's with this women's lib? Why would they want to do more?"

Earlier in November Dad was given his yearly flu shot. It appeared to bring on an episode of acute infection. Or as he put it, "That blasted flu shot gave me the flu."

Dad got a large knot under the left side of his chin. His neck hurt and his throat was extremely sore. He saw Dr. Madsen on November 14 and the doctor noted in his chart, "tonsils are very red and swollen." Madsen prescribed some medicine and in a few days Dad was feeling better.

In mid-December, Mother felt like she was getting a cold. She was very tired and her throat was sore. The glands in her neck hurt. I must have some kind of flu she thought. She wondered where she had picked it up. She hadn't left the house for over a week.

Six days before Christmas, Orvin took her to the doctor. Mother's lungs were clear but her ears and throat were red. She had symptoms of agitation, confusion and depression. Madsen treated her with an antibiotic for an upper respiratory infection.

★   ★   ★

In Denver, Jonathan was also treated in the emergency room and sent home with antibiotics for a respiratory infection.

Shiela was paralyzed with fear. "Oh, please. Not at Christmas."

But Jonathan responded well to the treatment. Santa Claus came to his house with a sack full of gifts. The small boy bounced around the living room playing with his toys and dragging his oxygen tank behind him.

Shiela was thankful the year would soon be over but she knew there were worse times ahead. She was convinced that this was Jonathan's last Christmas.

The family had been touched by an outpouring of concern and support from friends and strangers alike. Jonathan's Mother said, "AIDS has a strange way of bringing out both the worst and best in people."

★   ★   ★

Two days after Christmas Orvin was puzzled. "What's wrong with Ma?" he asked.

"I dunno," said Dad. "She sleeps almost all the time. She doesn't seem good. Maybe you'd better take her back to the doctor."

Dr. Madsen checked Mother and said her infection had improved since he last saw her. He suggested she could have a virus that was difficult to shake and noted in her medical chart that Mrs. Swain appeared fatigued. She was "sleeping too much."

Orvin and my parents spent New Year's Day with LaRee's family. My sister was glad to see 1985 come to a close and she was confident the next year would be better. For the past three months Dad had gained strength and Mother would soon be over her "flu."

Chapter 4

Unsuspecting Victims

Dad was sitting on the couch with Mother. "Do you want me to turn on the TV?" he asked. "You haven't watched your soaps for weeks now."

"I don't want it on," Mother said. "TV makes me nervous. I don't care about soaps anymore."

Dad was worried. She was obviously going downhill. She spent much of the day in bed and didn't seem interested in anything. She was forgetful. There were times when she would become very anxious and agitated.

"I still have this strange rash," Mother said. "I've had it for a week now."

Dad went over to the mirror and looked at his own face. It had a reddish hue and was peeling. The skin around his head, face and neck burned. It had been doing this off and on since early last spring.

He got a magnifying glass and peered at Mother's rash. There were red spots and little eruptions that looked like measles. 'Why in tarnation do we just have one thing after another,' he wondered.

On January 27 Orvin took both Dad and Mother to see Dr. Madsen. The doctor listed Mother's conditions as fatigue, agitation and a rash. He prescribed a tranquilizer for her and Kenalog for both her and Dad's skin problems. Dad was still on the same tranquilizer he had been given the previous July. His nerves were so on edge that he put up with its side effects.

★   ★   ★

We were later able to deduce that Mother probably contracted the AIDS infection from Dad around the first of December 1985. Although he had experienced impotency for eight months after his surgery, later in the fall he had a few months of improved health. Dad would eventually tell doctors he and his wife had sex about a year after his surgery.

The CDC states that within three weeks of exposure to the AIDS virus many people experience symptoms of acute infection. Dr. Madsen saw Mother the 19th of December and diagnosed an upper respiratory infection. She had a red throat and felt like she had the flu. She developed a heavy fatigue that would remain to her death. By late January she had a rash. Her memory worsened and she experienced periods of nervousness and anxiety which increased in severity over the next year and a half.

Information from the CDC also states that following the initial infection period most AIDS-infected persons are without symptoms for varying lengths of time. However, some patients have continued symptoms which can include rashes, recurring infections, swollen lymph glands, fatigue, fevers, nausea and diarrhea. AIDS can cause symptoms of the central nervous system including apathy, forgetfulness, motor dysfunction, full-blown dementia and hallucinations.

When the above symptoms occur in the aged, doctors often overlook AIDS as a cause. They tend to dump the complaints into the elderly waste basket with its categories of digestive problems, increased susceptibility to infections, senility and Alzheimer's disease. If the HIV-infected patient is a woman, proper diagnosis is even more unlikely because they have additional AIDS symptoms that men do not have. Doctors are not inclined to consider those symptoms as AIDS related.

★   ★   ★

During the third week of February Mother called me, mad as a hornet. Dr. Madsen had arranged for her to have a CAT scan in Salt Lake City.

"I don't need any scan of my head," she stormed. "They won't find anything wrong. Dad has been telling the doctor how bad my memory is and he believes him. They gang up on me."

"Even so, I think you should go ahead and have it—just to make sure."

"Then your dad should have one too. He's as forgetful as I am."

"Mother, I'm sure if you took Dad to a woman doctor and complained about his memory like he does about yours, she'd send him for one."

"Well, I guess so. That's what it would take all right."

Mother calmed down and had the CAT scan. When the results came back they were negative just as she had predicted. "I told you so," she said to Dad. "You think your Dr. Ace Madsen is so great but he really doesn't know his 'Ace' from a hole in the ground."

That line tickled Dad so much he repeated it to Madsen at his next office visit. However, young Dr. Madsen took himself seriously and was not amused.

Dad had gone to the doctor because there were several new skin lesions behind his ears and around his temples. Mother was there because her stomach was now always upset. She couldn't imagine what was wrong. Dr. Madsen gave her some medication for it.

Apparently he forgave Mother for her harsh judgment of his competency. He wrote in her chart, "Mrs. Swain is very pleasant—memory is okay."

For over two months Dr. Madsen ran tests in an attempt to find the cause of Mother's problems. Everything was negative: her chest X-rays, an echocardiogram, a liver scan, a CAT scan, thyroid tests, even numerous blood work. Yet my parents sat before their doctor with no answers for the cause of their ill health or the vague fear that gnawed at them. They both had an obsessive sense of "everything being wrong."

In March Mother and Dad were excited because Von's oldest daughter would soon be home from her mission. She had spent the last year and a half in Florida knocking on doors and explaining the beliefs of the Mormon Church to anyone who would listen. After a missionary is released from full-time duties, it is customary for him or her to give a report of their labors to the congregation of their home ward (church). Her talk would be given in Cedar City, Utah, and my parents wanted very much to attend. This granddaughter had always been especially close to them.

LaRee thought that Dad was strong enough to make the eight-hour trip by car but she worried that it would be too hard on Mother. She finally decided they would be more comfortable if she went and took her mini van. Early on Saturday morning she and Orvin left for Cedar City with our parents.

The trip went well and they stayed two nights with Von's family. Mother and Dad enjoyed listening to their granddaughter's missionary experiences. They were very proud of her.

Von, his wife and four children drove their guests to the neighboring city of St. George to see how the area had grown as a popular retirement community.

"You should move down here," Von told Mother and Dad. "Get away from those long cold winters."

Mother did not look forward to the lengthy drive back to Lapoint. She was not at all impressed with LaRee's mini van. 'Why would anyone buy one of these ugly things?' she wondered. It was so cheap it only had one door and she could not ever remember which side it was on.

Whenever they stopped at a restroom Mother went to the wrong side of the van, pounded on the window and yelled until LaRee came and led her out.

"I can't stand this newfangled thing," Mother said. "Why, the first Model T we had was nice enough to have doors on both sides."

An exasperated LaRee looked at Orvin. "My nerves are shot," she said. "I feel like blasting a hole right through the other side of the van."

★　　★　　★

Jonathan had been having ups and downs as he fought frequent upper respiratory infections. However, when he felt better he enjoyed the activities of healthy three-year-olds.

His brother Josh was five. As they played, Josh would help Jonathan pull his oxygen tank. The two boys were very close. Josh took the place of the friends his small brother didn't have.

Jonathan adjusted to the oxygen tank and found creative ways to coexist with it. He would sit on his tricycle and hook his arm through the cart's handle. Then he pedaled up and down the sidewalks of the condominium complex where they lived, the oxygen tank racing behind him. If the line became tangled he got off the trike and usually fixed it himself. He was a plucky, independent little boy.

Jonathan had a tube inserted into a large blood vessel in his chest. It required daily care but medicines could be easily injected into it without sticking the child with needles. Jonathan hated shots and wasn't fond of swallowing bad-tasting medicines either.

He was becoming very aware that his disease set him apart. He could take the reporters and cameramen in stride. But the behavior of parents who pulled their children away as he approached was difficult for him to handle. Kids would say, "I can't play with you because you have bad blood."

Jonathan's family struggled to make him understand that it was not because people didn't like him. They were just afraid of his disease. A difficult concept for a young child to comprehend.

Though the media attention was stressful, Shiela did not regret making their tragedy public. She was committed to publicizing the plight of AIDS victims and their families. She also hoped it would make the public more aware of the dangers of blood transfusions.

However, she always asked the media not to reveal their last name. The family feared possible retaliation and violence. Shiela thought it was incredible that people blamed victims for getting AIDS from blood transfusions instead of blaming the blood banks that gave it to them. She knew there were surrogate tests for AIDS which the blood banks had refused to use. Yet the homes of those who got AIDS from blood products and transfusions had been vandalized and even burned while the blood banks went untouched.

Shiela also knew they would soon have to prepare Jonathan for the fatal outcome of his illness. It tore at her heart. She lived every day with the knowledge that no amount of medical care or personal sacrifice would stop the progress of the virus of death.

She recalled how upset Jonathan was to find a dead fish in their aquarium. He had kept asking, "Why can't it swim with its friends? Fix it, Mommy."

★   ★   ★

By May it was evident to Orvin that his parents were on some crazy downward spiral. He had watched Mother's health deteriorate rapidly for the past five months. Orvin was especially upset over Dad because he had improved during the fall and winter only to take a nosedive in the spring. Misfortune seemed to be following them like a faithful dog.

Dad sat on the kitchen stool for his monthly haircut. "Be careful of those scabs," he said. "They're a lot worse."

Orvin tried to guide the clippers around the lesions behind Dad's ears. He had taken him to the doctor the week before and filled another prescription for ointment. Orvin couldn't understand why none of the medication did any good.

There was a similar problem with the ugly sore on Dad's lip. It, too, was worse; nothing helped. The sore had been on his lip for well over a year and bled when Dad ate.

The next day Dad wearily carried a plate of food to Mother who sat in the living room staring into space. She didn't seem to care about eating. "Did you take your blood pressure medicine this morning?" he asked.

"No, I don't think so." Mother got up and went into the kitchen. By the time she came back her food was cold.

"Did you take your medicine?"

"Of course I took it," she snapped.

Dad wondered if she actually had taken it. The strain of worrying about Mother was a burden he wasn't up to handling. He was getting more fatigued each day and his nausea was worse. He had a growing fear that he and Mother were going to need more care than Orvin could give.

This was a fear LaRee and I shared. She decided to talk to their doctor and request limited home nursing care. I felt guilty that my daughter's condition prevented me from being in Utah to assist with the increasing problems.

I wasn't sure, however, what was needed to bring about improvements in my parents' lives. I meticulously studied their medical histories and could not find any diagnosed illnesses that explained their baffling ailments. Yes, there was old age but that tag could not be stretched to cover all that was happening to them.

Could it be primarily psychological? Both Mother and Dad were obviously depressed and their environment was certainly unstimulating. They had become shut-ins in a small town without senior citizen support programs.

I felt if I could relocate them in Colorado Springs they would have opportunity for involvement in enjoyable activities and I could share in the burden of their care. I also wanted specialists in cardiology and geriatrics to take charge of their medical needs. I was concerned about the growing numbers of drugs they were taking and wondered if, under close supervision, the amount could be reduced.

However, I realized my parents would not move without Orvin. They couldn't stay alone and there was a mutual dependency and closeness between the three of them that should not be disturbed.

I made a search of retirement communities in Colorado Springs—facilities which were alternatives to nursing homes. They were impressive. One center had spacious two-bedroom suites with full kitchens. Housekeeping and linens were furnished and three well-balanced meals were served daily in a pleasant dining area. It had a beautiful lobby and recreation rooms. Many activities were available: crafts, group walks, bingo, fellowship, tours, movies, live entertainment and educational lectures. The management agreed to bend the rules so Orvin could live with Mother and Dad.

I was optimistic that this arrangement would eliminate cooking and cleaning responsibilities plus offer involvement and close medical care. But I knew I had a hard-sell job ahead. Even if Mother and Dad agreed to the move, I feared cultural shock.

I consulted a sociologist who worked with the elderly and explained my plan to her.

"Tell me about your parents," she said. "How many places have they lived? Have they had friends of varied backgrounds? How good are they at adjusting to change?"

I decided not to mention the mini van but as I talked she looked at me over her dark-rimmed glasses and her eyes got wider. Finally she shook her head. It was obvious she thought I could teach a couple of old centipedes to polka easier than to fit my country parents into a modern city retirement facility.

Nevertheless, I tried. I sent the brochures over to Utah and then talked with Dad.

"You can't leave a farm in the summer," he chided. "Even with a lessor I have to keep my eyes on things. And there are two large yards and an orchard to water and keep up. It has Orvin jumping."

"Then wait and come over in late fall. Just stay through the winter. Try it out."

I couldn't get any commitment out of Dad.

So I made my pitch to Mother. "It's only an hour's drive from our house. A drive through scenic mountains. Orvin can bring you to spend the day whenever you want and we can visit you easily."

"We'll have to wait and see," Mother said in that tone of voice that meant never.

★　　★　　★

Later that week Dad called me very upset. "Your mother is impossible," he said. "It's afternoon and I just took my morning medicines because she got up in the night and cleaned out the cupboard. She moved every one of my medicine bottles and didn't know where she put them. All morning I hunted high and low. I could have had a heart attack."

"Where were they?"

"In the bedroom. And you should see the mess she makes when she tries to cook. Yesterday she made hotcakes and forgot to put in the baking powder."

"Does she have trouble every time she cooks?"

"Just about."

As I loaded my dishwasher I wondered if Mother was as bad as Dad thought. She still sounded okay on the phone when she complained about him and his memory. They were getting on each other's nerves. 'Too much togetherness,' I thought. I knew Mother was sometimes confused but I also knew how she could push Dad's buttons just to irritate him.

During June and July Dad had several visits with Dr. Madsen because of his fatigue. He saw him another time complaining of a cough and the doctor diagnosed a viral syndrome. Throughout the summer Dad's legs and foot pained him. "I can barely drag around," he said.

Dr. Madsen requested that Home Health Care be provided three times a week for both Mother and Dad. Edith Page, the program's director, visited to determine their needs.

"My bypass surgery didn't help much," Dad told her. "I still have chest pain off and on and I'm so tired I can't take care of myself. My wife gets worse all the time and I can't care for her."

"Do you feel bad every day?"

"Some days are better than others but since my operation I've never felt a third as good as I did before I had it."

Mrs. Page asked Mother how she felt.

"I'm so tired all the time I could cry," said Mother.

"What do you do during the day?"

"I mostly lie on the bed or couch. I sleep a lot."

"Do you watch TV?"

"No, my nerves can't take it."

"LaRee says you're interested in making quilts."

"I can't work on them anymore. I don't see good enough. My eyes always hurt."

"Where else do you have pain?"

"In my head most of the time. I'm real dizzy."

The nurse went over all their medications and symptoms.

Both were on tranquilizers for their nerves.

Both took medicine for stomach problems.

Both were terribly fatigued.

Both said sometimes their legs were too weak to hold them up.

Both were depressed, had memory problems and trouble coping.

Both complained of not being able to see and having pain or a "funny feeling" in their eyes.

Both had suffered from viral syndromes the past seven months at different times.

Both had experienced skin problems but Mother's had gone away while Dad's became worse.

Both had headaches and dizziness. Dad's were infrequent while Mother's were almost constant.

Dad had angina chest pain.

Mother had high blood pressure.

The nurse noticed the similarity of most of their ailments and wondered, 'Is this couple just competing with each other to see who can be sicker?'

During the spring and summer, my parents had a number of visits from their out-of-town children, grandchildren and other relatives. They enjoyed seeing them all but were chagrined because they weren't well enough to fix the large family meals that were a tradition in their home.

Von's two daughters came and stayed several times. They were good cooks and prepared lovely meals but Dad fussed because they had to do it. Lapoint didn't have a single commercial eating place so it was either cook or perish.

When Dad's brother Darreld came, he and Dad went into the kitchen and manned the stove together. Darreld had been a chef and restaurant owner. Now he showed Dad some fast ways to prepare his meat and potatoes.

"Darreld fixes the best beefsteak I ever ate," said Dad.

But Dad's brother was sick at heart over his grandson, Jonathan, and the impact that AIDS was having on his son's family. Darreld lived near them and when Jonathan had acute infections he and his wife often took Josh and Jeremy into their home and cared for them.

The two older boys were emotionally upset over their small brother and feared he would die whenever he got sicker. They knew he was fragile and tried to tone down their usual rowdy play around him. It was difficult for them to have their friends over, even the few whose parents would allow them to come.

They felt like outcasts at school because many people feared AIDS could be caught from members of Jonathan's family.

"The fallout from this horrible disease is everywhere," Darreld said.

Jonathan recently had been sick with an ear infection and when Darreld went to see him, the child was jumping up and down on his bed.

"Hey, you can't jump around like that," his grandfather said.

"Yes, I can. I'm all better and Mommy's in the shower."

Darreld settled him down and straightened the oxygen tubing.

"Grandpa, will you take me to the park to feed the ducks? Go get some food."

"Jonathan is such a precious child," Darreld told Dad.

There were tears in Dad's eyes as he remembered another precious little boy who never had a chance to grow up.

★　　★　　★

My parents felt more secure after the Home Health Care workers started making their routine visits. Having their hearts, blood pressure and medications monitored relieved some of their anxiety. The aides assisted them with their showers and did light housework. Most importantly, they gave emotional support to an elderly couple whose growing desperation could not be understood by any of us.

Orvin stood at the kitchen sink and watched the dark come on. He dreaded the nights. That was when his parents were the most anxious and despondent. It seemed their physical symptoms also became worse as the day wore on. In the evening Mother often walked the floor until Dad would become so nervous he said he was ready to jump out of his skin.

When they asked Mother why she was walking she said, "It's worse at night."

"What's worse?"

"Everything."

At times Orvin debated about taking them to the emergency room but what could he say was wrong? Everything? He eventually learned that after midnight Mother and Dad were more likely to settle down and go to sleep.

* * *

In early fall, Dad's condition improved and his spirits lifted. "I haven't felt this good in a long time," he told the nurse.

But he wanted to discuss Mother's ailments. He was very worried about her. "She has a pain in her stomach and diarrhea," he said. "And she keeps cotton in her ears because they hurt even when the doctor says they look okay."

"I'll check her over carefully," the nurse said.

"I know she's not getting enough exercise," Dad said. "She won't ever walk with me."

"I'll encourage her. Try not to worry."

LaRee was beginning to understand Dad's concern. In August, the day of her own birthday, she realized how badly Mother was failing.

Dad and Mother had both forgotten the birthdays of their three children who were born in July. When they realized what they'd done they were mortified.

"We won't forget yours," Mother promised LaRee.

"None of us want you worrying about birthdays. We're too old to have them," my sister protested.

But a week later Mother called her. "I'm going to cook dinner for your family on your birthday," she insisted. "Come up after you get off work."

LaRee arrived with her family at the appointed time.

Mother came to the door. "For land sakes," she said. "What are you all doing here?"

"You invited us."

"I did. Whatever for?"

"For birthday dinner."

"Whose birthday is it?"

"Mine," said LaRee.

"Oh, dear. Is that today? Oh my, I'll really have to hurry."

LaRee followed Mother into the large kitchen. It was a disaster. Every cabinet was piled high with dirty dishes. LaRee got her children busy on clean up chores and went and looked in the freezer. She took out some chicken and put it in the microwave to defrost. Her husband peeled potatoes and prepared vegetables for cooking.

All the while, Mother was looking in the cupboard for a cake mix.

"We don't need cake," LaRee said. "Let's just have some of the ice cream that's in the freezer."

"No, you must have cake on birthdays. I want to do it."

Mother found a mix and emptied it into a bowl.

"Where are the eggs?" she asked.

"In the refrigerator," said LaRee.

Mother couldn't find them.

"Here they are." LaRee put the eggs in her hands.

Mother stood for awhile and watched LaRee fry chicken. Then she put the eggs down on the stove top and went over and turned on the mixer.

"You forgot to put the eggs in," LaRee said.

"No, I didn't."

"You left them here."

"I did? Oh, what's the matter with me? I can't do anything right. I'm a mess."

LaRee gently led Mother out of the kitchen. "Lie down for a few minutes. Let the kids finish the cake. They like to do it."

When LaRee sat down at the table, she was physically and emotionally exhausted. She hoped she never had another birthday dinner. The harsh truth of Mother's condition left her with a foreboding fear. Mother sat at the table barely picking at her food. There was a defeated hopelessness in her eyes. LaRee thought she looked as wilted as one of the pressed flowers she kept from her youthful days.

On October 15, Orvin took Dad to the dentist to have a tooth extracted. Afterwards they went to LaRee's home. Dad still had moderate bleeding and LaRee changed the cotton rolls in his mouth several times with her bare fingers. She and her husband wiped the bloody saliva off Dad's face with a washcloth.

The bleeding continued after Dad got back to Lapoint. Orvin applied ice to Dad's jaw and had him bite down on the pads. It was messy. No special precautions were taken with the blood.

One brisk morning in early November the caregiver found Dad out in the yard turning off water pipes before an expected cold front arrived. "I have to get out of the house," he said. "It's hard for me to be around my wife. Yesterday she didn't get out of bed all day. But I'm feeling better."

"Well, I'm glad one of you is having a good day," the aide said.

However, towards the end of November, Dad became more depressed and tired. He developed a terribly sore throat with severe pain in his neck.

Orvin took him to the doctor. Madsen felt the glands in Dad's neck and looked down his throat. He later told LaRee "Your dad has the ugliest looking throat I've ever seen."

Dr. Madsen put Dad on antibiotics and within several days, his throat and neck pain were considerably improved.

A few days later, Orvin drove Dad to his bank in Vernal to get into his safe deposit box. They tried to persuade Mother to ride with them because they didn't like to leave her alone.

"You don't need to get out of the car. We will hurry back," Dad said.

"I don't feel like sitting up," said Mother. "Just let me stay in bed."

They went without her but when they came back a short time later they found Mother wandering about the house in a very confused state.

"Orvin, come here," Dad called. "Mother is acting strange. Look at how she's walking."

Orvin watched Mother as she went into the kitchen. As she took each step she would swing her other foot up behind her.

"Ma, why are you walking like that?" he asked.

"I can't remember how," she replied.

Mother was running a low temperature and said she ached all over. Orvin thought she might be getting the throat infection Dad had a week earlier but by morning she was over the episode and walking normally.

Later that week, Orvin stood looking down at Dad as he lay under a pile of blankets with his teeth chattering.

"I'm freezing," Dad said. "I feel terrible and I've started coughing."

Orvin took Dad's temperature. "Ma, we're going to take Dad to the doctor. You'll have to go with us and stay at LaRee's."

He got our parents in the car and headed for Roosevelt. Chest X-rays indicated Dad had viral pneumonia. Dr. Madsen treated him with an antibiotic and sent him home. As Orvin drove Dad and Mother back to Lapoint, he wondered what they would get next. It was a long night. When the Home Health Care worker came the next morning, Dad was propped up on the couch.

"How are you doing? I hear you have pneumonia."

"I'm dizzy and I can't breathe very good," Dad said. "The new pills the doctor gave me kept me awake all night."

"Maybe you can sleep after your shower."

"My mouth is so dry I could spit cotton," Dad grumbled. He shoved his tray away. "This food has no taste."

Orvin cackled. "That's probably good," he said. "I fixed it."

"Gosh, he's an awful cook," Dad said to the caregiver.

By Christmas, Dad's pneumonia had responded to treatment. Although he was still weak and a bit wobbly he was feeling better again.

That holiday my parents refused to have a tree.

"We don't want the fuss or the mess of pine needles dropping on the floor," Mother said.

Dad agreed. "The only thing Santa is bringing here is a new car with seats we can lay back when we go to the doctor. Sometimes neither one of us feels like sitting up."

Two days later my father called several car dealers and compared prices and models. One dealer tried to persuade him to buy a Japanese car.

Dad was indignant. "A good American does not buy a Japanese car," he lectured. He and Orvin went to Vernal and traded in the older car for a new Dodge Lancer. Dad never sat behind the wheel but he enjoyed the reclining passenger seat.

★　　★　　★

In Denver another Swain family greeted the holidays with more enthusiasm. They were grateful that Jonathan was still with them. That year they celebrated as they had the previous year—like it would be his last Christmas.

Jonathan was taught to say his prayers. He had been told that when children become very sick they go to live with Jesus and have no more pain. The small child seemed to understand and freely talked of dying. His family wondered if it was his way of comforting them. Did he want them to know it was all right with him if he died?

During a previous painful illness, Jonathan was upset with Jesus. "I told him to come and get me so it wouldn't hurt anymore. He didn't come," he said. Now he looked at the Christ Child in a manger scene and said, "It's all right. You can come another time."

★　　★　　★

Early on New Year's Eve, Orvin sat on the couch between Mother and Dad. The TV was showing clips from news events during 1986. There was a segment from San Francisco on AIDS patients.

As Orvin watched the dying, emaciated men, he counted his blessings. 'No matter how hard it is for me to take care of Ma and Dad,' he thought, 'at least I don't have to deal with AIDS.'

Chapter 5

Unmasking the AIDS Coverup

The year of apocalypse began on January 1, 1987, with a heavy feeling in the back of Dad's head and neck. Soon he had pain that started under his ribs and went around to his back. By early morning it was intense.

"I can't stand this any longer," Dad gasped.

Orvin got Mother and Dad into the car and drove to the hospital. An emergency room doctor treated Dad for pleurisy and sent him back home.

Several days later, the pain subsided but Dad began running an intermittent fever with alternating chills and sweats. When the Home Health Care worker arrived, she found him depressed and crying.

"The pressure in my head won't go away," he said. "I either sweat or chill. I throw up when I try to eat."

Orvin took Dad to Dr. Madsen who thought he was seeing a flu. However, two days later when Dad wasn't any better, he admitted him to the local hospital for testing. The first night Dad was at the hospital Mother got up several times looking for him. She woke Orvin. "Dad's gone," she said. "He's not here anywhere."

"Remember, Ma, we took him to the hospital. LaRee's with him. He'll be home in a few days." Orvin put her back into bed and sat beside her until she fell into a shallow doze. By now Mother was very dependent on Dad because disorientation left her helpless and frightened.

Five days later Dad was released from the hospital. No cause had been found for his fever. Tests only revealed a small stomach ulcer. Madsen prescribed Xanax for Dad's nervousness and depression. The tranquilizer was in the same drug family as the Ativan which caused Dad's myoclonic jerking a year and a half before. The doctor observed that Dad's depression was the result of worry over his wife's condition.

Our family would eventually realize that our parents' depression and anxiety were the result of medical treatment which infected them with HIV. The AIDS virus can injure neurons in the brain causing emotional and mental disorders. Loss of memory may be one of the first signs of HIV infection.

Dad was home for the next eight days but his fever and cough continued despite antibiotic treatment. He took two falls because he was too dizzy to walk. The sight of food sickened him and his weight dropped.

One morning when the nurse arrived Dad's bed was wet with perspiration. He had vomited all night and Orvin was up with him. The nurse gave Dad a bed bath because he was too weak to get into the shower, then she started washing several loads of soiled bedding.

The next day Dad was hospitalized again for vomiting and fever. Dr. Madsen had exhausted all the tests that could be run at the small community hospital. On January 30, Dad was taken in an ambulance to Salt Lake City and admitted to the University of Utah Medical Center for evaluation of a fever of unknown origin.

LaRee stayed with Dad in Salt Lake City for a number of days before Mother and Orvin got there. Then all three of them stayed in a motel near the hospital and either Orvin or LaRee spent the nights in Dad's room. Von's oldest daughter was living in the city and would often visit her grandfather in the evenings and try to cheer him up.

The situation was very hard on Mother because change and worry made her worse. One night at the motel Orvin couldn't get her to lie down. She shuffled about the room until dawn.

"Ma, if you don't stay in bed I'm going to hold you down," an exhausted Orvin said.

Mother's dark eyes flashed. "If you do you'll be a mouse and I'll be the cat!"

Orvin laughed. "Well, why won't you stay in bed?"

"I can't breathe. I'm suffocating."

For several months the health care nurses and an occasional doctor had listened to Mother's chest and said it was clear. They thought her "breathing spells" could be from hyperventilation due to her frequent anxiety. LaRee finally took Mother back to Roosevelt and cared for her while Orvin stayed with Dad.

Von came to Salt Lake City during the second week of Dad's testing and stayed for six days. Von spent the first night at the hospital and called me the next morning. "Could Dad have AIDS?" he asked. "He looks exactly like those AIDS patients on TV. And he had transfusions two years ago."

"They would have discovered it by now," I said. "He's at an excellent teaching hospital. They would have tested for AIDS."

Von wasn't satisfied. "How do we find out?"

"Ask them. But ask more than one doctor."

My brother did. Von talked to one of the interns who was cooperative and answered all his questions.

"Oh yes," the intern said. "Now days the center always tests for AIDS if a patient has a fever of unknown cause. It's one of the first things we do."

But when Orvin asked Dr. Thomas H. Caine, the doctor in charge of Dad's case, the response was curt.

"Doctor, has my father been tested for AIDS?" Orvin had asked.

"Of course," Caine snapped and left the room.

Orvin shrugged it off as just a doctor with an attitude.

The next day the University doctors informed Dad he had chronic hepatitis B. My brother sought out the talkative intern. "All my father's problems started after his heart surgery," Orvin said. "Did he get the hepatitis from the transfusions?"

"Yes. You could safely bet that he did."

Orvin was furious. "Over two years of misery because of a bad transfusion," he said. "Jonathan got AIDS from one and Dad got hepatitis."

But when I talked to Dad on the phone he wasn't nearly as upset over the hepatitis as he was insulted because he had been evaluated by a psychiatrist. "These doctors think I'm a mental case," he grumbled. "They give me tranquilizers that make me confused. Then they open the barn door and sic a blasted psychiatrist on me."

It was evident that the doctors were looking for other plausible causes besides hepatitis to explain Dad's condition. An expert in infectious disease was brought in for a consultation. Dr. Zell A. McGee came to Dad's room and checked him. Dad anxiously searched the doctor's face for some clue to his fate. "What do you think I have, Doc?" he asked.

"Well . . . I think you might have caught a disease from your cattle," the doctor told the elderly rancher.

Dad accepted McGee's answer.

My brothers did not. "Dad sold all his cattle six years ago," they fumed.

During the 22 days Dad was at the University Medical Center, his fever and vomiting waxed and waned but the stressful discomfort of testing added to his misery. His body was subjected to nuclear scanning from stem to stern. His head was scanned in addition to his esophagus, chest, stomach, liver, spleen and leukocytes. He had painful biopsies, bone marrow aspirations and endoscopies. The blood tests were endless.

Dad's doctors were thorough. In addition to the AIDS they said they had tested him for, the doctors ordered cultures and studies for numerous bacteria, fungi, viruses, parasites and protozoa. They looked for a string of infectious diseases including toxoplasmosis, Q fever, tuberculosis, Chlamydia, Epstein-Barr, coccidioidomycosis, brucellosis, cysticercosis, mycoplasma pneumoniae, hepatitis and cytomegalic disease. A good number of these diseases can infect both man and animals. When a person becomes infected with them it is often because of a suppressed immune system. The doctors were looking for the opportunistic diseases that prey on patients who are infected with the AIDS virus.

However, Dad was told he had just two of the more common infections, cytomegalovirus and hepatitis B. AIDS, his major diagnosis, was never mentioned. Like a field of potatoes, it was buried underground.

The only medical record we had at the time of Dad's discharge was a sheet of instructions the doctors gave Orvin. After studying it and recalling prior conversations with specialists who examined Dad we were even more baffled. It was obvious the doctors were still reaching for a cause for Dad's fever. There was, they suggested, a chance it could be from a possible prostate infection. (The urology experts had not felt this was likely.) Or again maybe it was rheumatoid arthritis. (The specialist didn't think so.) Or . . . there was that insidious cattle disease. (But where were the cattle?)

The doctors appeared concerned with Dad's weight drop of 20 pounds. On the sheet they instructed our family to weigh him daily and take his temperature three times a day. A record was to be made of both temperature and weight and the University doctors kept informed.

I did not know that Dad had AIDS but I was, nevertheless, enraged. The medical center had taken a defenseless old man and for over three weeks tortured him with countless invasive tests, ran up a bill of $15,000 and discharged him in worse condition than when he was admitted. All without any solid explanation for his fever and no treatment to relieve his misery.

"We have an appointment in a week with Dr. Caine," Orvin said.

"The hell you do," I said. "That poor man is not going anywhere near those doctors or hospital again. Why should anyone so sick travel that distance for nothing?"

"You're right. It wouldn't do him any good. I'll cancel the appointment," Orvin said.

★　　★　　★

Looking back I am dismayed at how naive I was. I should have suspected we were involved in an AIDS coverup. In 1987 Jonathan had already been diagnosed with transfusion AIDS for nearly two years and Von had recognized the similarity of Dad's appearance to AIDS patients. But I was certain that, as the Medical Center doctors had told us, he had been tested for AIDS. It simply did not occur to me that if doctors found a patient had AIDS they would conceal it from him and his family.

I was then unaware that some blood banks around the country influence doctors to coverup the AIDS infections that are contracted from the contaminated blood they have supplied. The motive is fear of lawsuits and bad publicity. If the victims are told, it can mean trouble for the blood banks and have a negative impact on the local blood supply. And there has been a long-standing policy for doctors to report the AIDS infections of prior transfusion recipients to the blood banks that supplied the blood. An FDA investigation found that between 1985 and 1990, 235 such AIDS infections were reported to the Red Cross Washington, DC, Blood Center by the patients' doctors!

The LDS Blood Bank, which supplied the blood for Dad's surgery, is the main collecting and processing center for a large blood monopoly that supplies over 80% of all blood transfused in Utah. The state's health care delivery system is dependent on it, including the University facility.

Over the years blood from the LDS Blood Bank has been promoted as being exceptionally safe. Publicity about AIDS contamination could erode patient and donor confidence. Many people incorrectly think there is danger of getting AIDS from donating blood. If donations were to drop, Utah medical facilities would be forced to buy out-of-state blood at higher prices. Hospital costs would increase.

Although the University Medical Center has an in-house blood bank, it can only provide approximately 30% of the banked blood needed at the center. The other 70% comes from the LDS Blood Bank, according to a University spokesperson. There is an agreement between the two blood banks. The University Blood Bank is not allowed to recruit donors through the Mormon Church, which is the LDS Blood Bank's primary donor source. In exchange, the LDS Blood Bank does not recruit on the University campus.

For many years there has been a very close affiliation between the University Medical Center and Intermountain Health Care (IHC), the parent company of the LDS Blood Bank. While my father was at the University Medical Center, construction was underway on the new Primary Children's Medical Center, an IHC facility, located on the University campus. The agreements between the state-owned University Medical

Center and IHC's Primary Children's are, at the time of this writing, under investigation by the U.S. Department of Justice for possible violation of antitrust laws.

★　　★　　★

When Dad was released from the hospital in late February, Dr. Ace Madsen was contacted by the University doctors and asked to monitor the progression of his illness. Dad was to be sent back to the University Medical Center when his condition worsened. The center could depend on Dr. Madsen. He had graduated from the University Medical School just a few years before. (Six months later, Dr. Madsen would write in Dad's medical records that Dad had been a known carrier of HIV for six months, but we did not find out about the AIDS until May.)

★　　★　　★

Dad and Mother stayed at LaRee's home for the first two days after his release from the hospital. On the second day, an edgy Dr. Madsen came to the house and asked to see the instruction sheet the University doctors had sent home with Orvin.

"I'd like to know what they found out," the doctor said. He read the sheet and talked with Dad for awhile. LaRee thought the visit was most unusual. However, Dad was delighted to see his favorite doctor again. "It's so nice of you to visit me," he said.

The doctor looked around at all the stuffed animals and dolls in the bedroom where Dad was staying. It was the room of LaRee's youngest daughter who had been temporarily moved to another level of the house because Dad couldn't climb stairs.

As Madsen left he asked to talk to LaRee outside. They went and stood out on the front porch. The doctor was visibly upset. "What do you think you're doing?" he demanded. "You can't have him here with your family."

LaRee was startled. "What do you mean? He's my father."

"Well . . . it's too much stress. Your first responsibility is your children. Your father should be in the nursing home."

"We don't want him in a home."

"That's where he belongs—not here with your family."

There is one thing I will never be able to forgive the University doctors for. They sent Dad home with his family without one word of warning or instructions on how to avoid the spread of infectious disease!

The doctors had already told us Dad had hepatitis B which presented a perfect opportunity for emphasizing the dangers lurking in bodily fluids and blood. However, we had observed the hospital staff's cavalier attitude concerning precautions against the spread of Dad's hepatitis. With the exception of a student nurse, no one had worn gloves. When Orvin asked why they did not wear them, a male nurse told him it wasn't necessary. We now realize we were left with the wrong impression because the staff had been vaccinated against hepatitis B.

On the instruction sheet they sent home, the doctors could at the very least have told us to wear gloves when handling Dad's bodily fluids and blood. We would have just thought it was because of the hepatitis. But not one word was written on the sheet for the protection of our family. Neither was the family instructed to obtain hepatitis B shots.

There is an abundance of vomit, mucus and blood when caring for AIDS patients. Frequent diarrhea makes a dirty nursing job even dirtier. By 1987 many of the doctors at San Francisco General Hospital were wearing full protective dress as they cared for AIDS patients or performed surgery. That protective dress included waterproof gowns or suits, rubber boots, surgical masks, double surgical gloves and face shields. These doctors had witnessed the destructive wrath of the AIDS virus. They respected it.

While Dad was at LaRee's home he vomited and had a high fever with profuse sweating. She changed his bed twice the first night he was there. His nose ran a steady stream and he took sneezing fits. Soiled tissues were everywhere.

Mother had a miserable night and was unable to sleep, constantly worrying over Dad. Her diarrhea was worse. She soiled the couch and LaRee's two older children cleaned up the mess the best they could.

The next morning it took LaRee's husband over half an hour to shave Dad. Due to weight loss his face was as withered as an emptied balloon. It was impossible not to nick his sensitive, scabby skin. There was bleeding.

Dad was worried about being around LaRee's children. "I want to go home," he told Orvin. "I don't want to give these kids some awful germ."

"Just stay until tomorrow," Orvin said. "Give me some time to shop and get the house ready."

"No," said Dad. "That disease fellow, McGee, said I had something from cattle. Take me back to the farm."

Orvin went to the drugstore and refilled prescriptions and got supplies. At the grocery store he pushed a cart up and down the aisles looking for anything he thought his parents would or could eat. Dad's appetite was terrible and his weight was still dropping.

Orvin returned to LaRee's home and loaded Mother and Dad into the car. My sister watched them drive off with a sense that her family was whirling out of control. The only solid reality left in her shifting world at that moment was bone fatigue. LaRee had not been able to lie down once during the 48 hours her parents had been in her home. 'There's no way Orvin can manage them alone,' she thought. Each night is an eternity.

However, both Mother and Dad were more content at home. Although she usually made things worse, Mother tried to help care for Dad. She was able to fix his hot cereal because the task only took a minute. But her mind would drift away before it was time to remove his 3 1/2 minute eggs from the stove.

"These soft boiled eggs are like rubber," Dad said. "They bounce."

Dad's fever stayed under 100° for the first four days he was home. Though he was extremely weak and had "strange feelings" in his chest, he had a brief glimmer of hope. "I might lick this thing yet," he said.

But before the week was over, Dad was in another crisis situation. His fever went up, accompanied by severe vomiting. According to Orvin, Dad was "puking up his toenails." Dad's face was bright red and an angry rash spread across his body.

Dr. Madsen examined him, surprised to learn that he had not been taken back to see Dr. Caine as instructed. Orvin explained that the family no longer wanted the University Medical Center doctors to care for Dad. From the patient viewpoint their care had rated a zero. Madsen found this news as disturbing as a skunk at a picnic.

The doctor admitted Dad to the hospital in Roosevelt. He told us Dad's rash and vomiting were probably an allergic reaction to the drug, Bactrim, which the university doctors had prescribed. Dad was taken off Bactrim and by the next afternoon his condition started to improve. After three days, Madsen persuaded our family to transfer Dad to the nearby Cedar Crest Convalescent Home.

Orvin was very reluctant to leave Dad in the facility. He immediately asked the nursing supervisor if he could check over the orders for his medications. He was especially concerned about Dad's heart medicine because since the bypass surgery they had been given exactly on schedule to keep his heart regulated.

Orvin read the instruction sheet and went into a rage. Both of Dad's heart medicines had been left off the list. He asked the nurse to call Dr. Madsen.

"Why aren't his heart medicines on the nurse's orders?" he demanded.

"I'm taking him off as many drugs as possible to reduce toxic buildup," the doctor said.

"But why take him completely off both heart medicines at once?"

"I doubt that he needs them. That's why I want him close by so I can monitor him."

Orvin hung up the phone and thought back to the only time since Dad's surgery that his heart medications had been abruptly reduced. It was over two years before, after Dad had called Dr. Jones and told him the pills made him sick. Jones had taken him off just one drug and within two days it caused a medical alert because of severe fibrillation. Dr. Madsen had been brought in to assist with the emergency and afterward became Dad's regular physician. From that time on, Madsen had controlled Dad's intermittent episodes of irregular heartbeat with drugs. And he had always told Dad that he would have to take the drugs for the rest of his life.

Orvin returned to his father's room. Without his heart medicines he felt Dad should be in the hospital instead of the convalescent facility. He rang for the nurse and clocked how long it took before someone came to the room. Orvin was not reassured. And he knew that Dad was often too ill to even ring for help. "In an emergency Dad might as well be up on Mosby Mountain as here," Orvin muttered.

But Dad was upset for another reason. "Madsen told me I needed to get away from Orvin," he said to Mother. "The doctor thinks it's because of him that I'm depressed and sick. Orvin doesn't make me sick. He just takes care of me because I am sick," Dad fumed.

It was late before Mother and Orvin left the convalescent home. As Orvin drove to Lapoint a dark curtain in the back of his mind was rustling. "Something is not right, Ma. I'm getting bad vibes," he said. "There was too much maneuvering to get Dad into that home. Something weird is going on."

Mother was tired and impatient with Orvin. "Oh, for land sakes," she said. "What on earth could be going on?"

During the next week Orvin was relieved when Dad's heart remained stable. "I can't believe its doing all right without any medicine," he told me.

"Well, maybe his heart condition has not been as serious as we and the doctors thought," I commented.

"What do you mean?"

"Well Dad's had hepatitis B for a long time which explains the fatigue and weakness he always blamed on his heart. And not all his chest pain has been from angina—he's also had chest wall syndrome and pleurisy."

But Orvin was still concerned. "No, it's just a matter of time before Madsen has to put him back on the heart meds," he said.

The first week Dad was at Cedar Crest he had a severe pain in his head and his anxiety was worse. Dr. Madsen had taken him off Xanax and replaced it with the antidepressant Desyrel. Dad complained of being shaky inside and soon went into myoclonic jerking with his arms and legs jumping uncontrollably. He was terrified. He was having symptoms of benzodiazepine withdrawal just as he had done after stopping Ativan over a year and a half before.

Orvin was unable to get Madsen to go see Dad at the convalescent home. Finally he persuaded the head nurse to call the doctor and eventually Madsen came into Dad's room.

"What's wrong?" he asked my father.

"I'm shaking all over. I can't keep my legs or arms still."

"Has someone upset you?" the doctor asked Dad, glaring over at Orvin.

"I'm upset about this jerking," Dad answered firmly.

"I can tell you what's wrong," Orvin interrupted. "You took him off Xanax. He's going to keep on jerking until you give him more poison from the snake that bit him."

The doctor's face contorted with angry sarcasm. "Well, 'Dr. Swain' has made another diagnosis," he sneered and left the room.

In a few minutes a nurse came and gave Dad a high dose of Xanax. The jerking stopped and in a few days Madsen began tapering the dosage.

The day after the jerking incident, Dad felt well enough to watch the Brigham Young University (BYU) basketball game on TV. He was an enthusiastic supporter of BYU sports and was cheered by the team's exciting victory. LaRee and Orvin were happy to see him in such a good mood.

It would be two years before I reviewed Dad's Cedar Crest records. Dr. Madsen had informed the convalescent home that Dad was infected with cytomegalovirus and was a carrier of hepatitis B. The doctor had written incredibly strict instructions for infection control. Disposable eating utensils were to be used for serving Dad's meals. The staff was to wear gloves at all times when caring for him or changing his bed linens. The doctor warned against contact with Dad's blood or semen and noted the "potential for nocturnal emissions." All his bedding and clothing were to be bagged in plastic, labeled and washed separately.

On March 16, Madsen had a lab technician go to the Cedar Crest Home and draw some blood from Dad's arm. Unknown to us, it was mailed out to be tested for AIDS. On March 20, the positive results of this last test were reported back to Dr. Madsen. We, of course, were not told.

Madsen continued to have contact with the doctors in Salt Lake City regarding Dad's AIDS-related conditions. Later he would send blood for T-cell typing to the University Medical Center Lab. He wrote in Dad's medical records that the results indicated his T-cells were very low.

Dr. Madsen struggled to keep the lid on the growing coverup labeled "Swain AIDS." But ultimately the snake named Xanax would slowly inch away from him toward discovery.

Mother had been spending her days in a nervous blur. She complained incessantly of a hazy, funny feeling over her eyes. Anxiety and worry over Dad gnawed at her and she spent one wide-eyed night after another. Orvin had trouble keeping her in bed. Her tranquilizer was increased and she would drift in and out of a fitful, drug-softened sleep. Then she would get up and wander around the house in a confused daze. One night she went into Orvin's bedroom and woke him. "You're here in your bed," she said. "But I can't find where I am."

By the middle of March, Mother's voice became hoarse and soon she was ill with another viral syndrome. The nurse noted her cheeks were red and she had a cold and cough. As Orvin divided his attention between his two failing parents, a gray cloud of premonition hung over him.

★   ★   ★

Jonathan lived to celebrate his fourth birthday with a cake and new toys. However, his isolation left him a lonely, little boy. Each morning he sadly watched his brothers go off to school leaving him without anyone to play with. His mother wanted to put him in a preschool but was afraid none would take him.

"But Shiela, wouldn't he catch more infections from the other kids?" I asked.

"Yes, but he needs to be with children. We want his life to have quality. He doesn't have much time left."

"How is he doing?"

"It depends on the week or even the day," she answered. "His infections come and then get better with treatment."

"Could he keep up with the kids in school?"

"Sometimes he's very sharp when he plays games and works puzzles. Other days he's what I call AIDS dull. The virus causes his comprehension and coordination to vary."

Since Jonathan's diagnosis, Shiela had spent a good amount of time in the medical school library researching AIDS. One night she saw one of her son's doctors there and asked him a medical question.

The doctor sighed and shook his head. "Shiela, by now you know as much about childhood AIDS as I do."

★   ★   ★

For 10 days, Dr. Madsen decreased Dad's dose of Xanax. As the amount reached a very low level, my father's arms and legs again started to jerk wildly. This time the doctor tried a moderate Xanax increase and the results were erratic and unpredictable. The jerking would subside for awhile and then make another attack causing Dad to exist in a state of fear. He never knew when it would strike.

After four days of this misery Orvin decided to take Dad out of the convalescent home and care for him himself. "I can give the Xanax on schedule and observe him real close," said Orvin. "And I know I can get more food down him." He was concerned with Dad's continued weight loss.

After being in Cedar Crest for three weeks Dad was delighted to be back at home. He knew it was easier for Mother if he was there so Orvin didn't have to take her out to visit him. He hoped his condition wouldn't get worse and they could stay together.

However, Dad's jerking continued off and on after he was at home. I wanted to contact the pharmaceutical company which manufactured Xanax but I knew Madsen would not appreciate my intervention and Dad enjoyed a good relationship with his doctor. "Ask Dad what he wants me to do," I told Orvin.

That evening Dad talked to me on the phone. He spoke in the low, weak voice of desperation. "Do whatever you can," he said. "I can't stand this. I'm sick all over but this jumping is the worst."

"I'll call early tomorrow morning," I promised.

It was 9:38 a.m. on March 30 when I reached the Drug Experience Department of Upjohn Pharmaceuticals in Kalamazoo, Michigan. I was referred to Sheri M. St. Clair and I explained to her the predicament my father was in from use of the company's widely prescribed drug.

"Xanax makes his nausea much worse," I said. "His doctor has repeatedly tried to taper him off it but he always goes into myoclonic jerking when the dose gets real low."

"How long has he been on Xanax?" she asked.

"Just since January. A little over two months. But I think it would be in the best interests of all concerned if you could tell the doctor how this withdrawal can be done. My father is far too ill to go through this."

St. Clair said she would call Dr. Madsen immediately. During the previous night Dad had suffered from excruciating pain in the back of his head. Orvin arrived with him at Madsen's office right after the doctor received his call from Upjohn. Their timing was poor.

The doctor's face was blotchy red, his eyes flashing with anger. "The drug company said I was handling the Xanax right," he stormed. "They said I could try taking him down more slowly." He put Dad back on the higher dose and the detox crisis was over—at least for awhile.

April was not as chaotic as the three previous months and Orvin cared for both Mother and Dad at home. The major emergency occurred when Dad's heart rhythm went out of control and Orvin had to make a mad dash with him to the emergency room in Roosevelt. As my brother had predicted, Madsen put Dad back on his two previous heart meds. The next day Orvin told the health caregiver, "Well, he's back on the heart medicine just like I said he'd be. I guess 'Dr. Swain' was right again, huh?"

Orvin faithfully gave Dad all his medications and shoved soft food down him at least six times a day in addition to giving him Ensure, a nutritionally balanced supplement of around 300 calories a can. Dad complained to the Home Health Care nurse. "If I can go to sleep Orvin wakes me up and gives me medicine and that Ensure stuff. He woke me up at 2:00 a.m. this morning."

Dad had no appetite and everything he swallowed made his nausea worse. One afternoon I waited a long time before he could talk on the phone. "You must be worse," I said.

"Oh, I just stay in the bathroom as long as I can so Orvin won't feed me," he confided.

It seemed to Orvin that he and his parents were players in a silent movie being run in slow motion. The movie went on for 24 hours a day, then the reel would rewind and play over again.

Orvin was obsessively devoted to his parents. Now he made their care a crusade that sometimes irritated the Home Health Care workers. Never one to keep his opinions to himself, Orvin expressed to them his growing mistrust and criticism of the medical profession which did not set well.

The friction originated in the propaganda that was being spread to convince our family that Dad's health problems were caused by depression. One family member was played against another. Orvin and I were convinced that it was medical treatment that had brought about Dad's tragic decline. But Dr. Madsen cornered LaRee at the hospital where she worked and explained in detail how life-threatening depression can be—how it can lead to serious weight loss.

"It's the depression that will kill your father," he warned. And there was always the inference that somehow Orvin was responsible for the depression. Caught in the middle, LaRee was inclined to believe Madsen, the professional she worked with.

The depression line was also fed to the Home Health Caregivers along with an attempt to discredit Orvin. They were led to believe that, in addition to being depressed over his wife's deteriorating health, Dad's overprotective son was also having a negative effect on him.

Orvin was shouldering the responsibility of his parents' demanding care under the most difficult circumstances. There were so many obstacles that he felt like he was pushing jello up a mountain while fighting the whole world to do it. He was not in any mood to tolerate disapproving glances behind his back. He minced no words when telling LaRee what he thought of the health care system she worked in. "You can't trust doctors," he fumed. "They talk out of both sides of their mouths to cover their asses. Are you so stupid you can't see through it?"

LaRee was furious. "I'm looking at stupid," she shouted. "You don't know a thing about the medical profession or what goes on in it."

"Well, I'm smart enough to know it isn't depression that's killing Dad. It's doctors!"

But we were as oblivious to the cause of our problems as a bat is to darkness. While the depression campaign was going on, we remained ignorant of the AIDS connection.

★   ★   ★

Orvin preferred using an electric razor to shave Dad but it would become clogged from the scabs on his face. One morning he took a long darning needle from the pincushion and used it to push dried blood and whiskers out of the shaver. The needle slipped and Orvin got a deep stick in his finger.

Later that week at 5:00 a.m. Orvin called LaRee for help.

During the preceding two months, Mother had had a few incidents with loss of bladder and bowel control. The incontinence had been infrequent and dismissed as that which can accompany old age.

But this night Mother had gotten out of bed and tracked feces throughout the house. Bedding and carpeting were so badly soiled that it took LaRee and Orvin four hours to hose down rugs, shampoo carpets and wash bedding. We later learned that loss of bowel and bladder control occurs in the vast majority of AIDS patients toward the end of the disease.

A week later Von, his wife, and four children arrived for a visit with Mother and Dad. Von found his parents beaten down from illness. The threat of death hung over the house. He took Orvin into the kitchen. "I didn't know it was this bad," Von said.

"Oh, it isn't," said Orvin. "It's worse."

Von and his family pitched in and worked for four days doing yard work and heavy house cleaning. They cooked food and cared for Mother and Dad.

Dad's mind was sharp at times and confused at others. He tried to put his foggy perceptions into words. "Sometimes I can't tell the difference between my dreams and what goes on in my house," he said.

It was day 38 of the long Xanax taper when Dad's arms and legs again began to jerk uncontrollably. Orvin took him to the emergency room in Roosevelt and he was given a Valium IV. The jerking stopped and after a few hours he was sent back home. But as the night wore on, the wild jumping started up again. Early the next morning Orvin took Dad back to the emergency room and Dr. Madsen admitted him to the hospital.

On the fateful morning of May 8, 1987, I once again called Upjohn and spoke to Sheri St. Clair. "It's obvious that my father cannot be tapered off Xanax," I said. "Every time the dose reaches a very low level he goes into myoclonic jerking. Can you give me the name of a detox center that has experience with Xanax addiction?"

There was a stunned silence followed by nervous hedging. "Well, er no . . . I don't know of any center that does Xanax detoxes. Your doctor is doing it correctly."

"Then you're saying this poor man can't be taken off Xanax. Right?"

"No, I don't mean that. I'll call your doctor again."

After Madsen talked with St. Clair he weighed his options. None of them were good. He had put Dad on Xanax despite Upjohn's warning in the Xanax Product Information Sheet that it was not to be used in patients who had known problems with benzodiazepines. Nearly two years before, Madsen had cared for Dad when he had experienced allergy and jerking caused by Ativan, another benzodiazepine.

The doctor knew Dad's family was getting more frustrated and angry with each passing day. His take-no-bull son was blaming all his father's problems on Xanax and Madsen's management of the drug, threatening a lawsuit. And now Upjohn was on his back.

Telling Dad and his family that AIDS was the primary cause of his illness would take pressure off the Xanax problem but would shake up powerful vested medical interests in Salt Lake City—interests that preferred to have our family remain unaware of Dad's HIV infection and his death certificate to list causes other than transfusion AIDS. The ambitious doctor no doubt wished he had gone into something safe like South American politics. Nevertheless, he slowly walked down the hall and into Dad's hospital room.

Sleep had finally nudged its way into Dad's weary mind. Madsen woke the old man, and in a voice reserved for dreaded things, told his trusting patient that he had ARC, which is one category below full-blown AIDS.

Chapter 6

Total Disillusionment

After talking with Upjohn, I was sure we needed expert help to get Dad off Xanax. In between making calls to drug treatment centers, my telephone rang. It was Orvin.

"I don't know what's coming down now," he said. "I had just brought Ma home when Dad called all upset. Dr. Madsen went into his room and told him something terrible. But Dad isn't allowed to tell us what it is until Madsen talks to the family tonight at 6:00."

"Didn't you get any clues as to what this is about?"

"No, but our old fear of him having AIDS is eating at me again. I have this strong feeling that is what Dad's been told he has."

"It must be major or Madsen wouldn't demand that he keep it secret."

"I'll wait until the caregiver comes to be with Ma and then I'll go back to the hospital and talk to Dad face to face. He won't be able to keep it from me."

"Call me the minute you find out," I said.

The horror my parents had been living was obviously going to get worse. I spent several hours studying AIDS symptoms and CDC classifications. When Orvin called at 5:00 I was braced for the news.

"I was right," Orvin said. "Madsen told Dad he has ARC. I guess that's not as bad as AIDS, is it?"

His words blew out my last flicker of hope. "There's very little difference when someone has as many AIDS symptoms as Dad has. If he doesn't have full-blown AIDS now, he soon will."

But there was something I had to do. "Orvin, I'm going to call Dr. Caine and then call Dad's room and talk to you before Madsen gets there. I think this explains the weird care Dad had at the University Medical Center."

It was 5:45 when Dr. Thomas Caine answered his page at the University Hospital in Salt Lake City. I got right to the point, carefully phrasing my question so he couldn't dodge it. "Doctor, when you evaluated my father's fever in February did you find that he was infected with AIDS?"

There was a pause but, to his credit, he didn't lie to me. "Well, we knew there might be a problem. We asked Dr. Madsen to monitor him closely." This doctor was a master at leaving much unsaid.

"Thank you," I responded. "That's all I need to know."

Orvin answered the phone in Dad's hospital room. LaRee and her husband had just arrived, still unaware of why the meeting had been arranged.

"The University doctors have known since February," I told Orvin.

"Madsen just came into the room," he said.

"Put him on the phone," I said.

"Now?"

"Right now."

Again I phrased the question so it could not be avoided. "Dr. Madsen, how long after you sent Dad to the University Medical Center was it before you knew he was infected with AIDS?"

"Oh, they didn't discover it there," he said. "I diagnosed it. I tested him for AIDS."

I thanked him and hung up the phone. Madsen had no way of knowing what Caine had just told me and was going the whole nine yards to protect the University doctors. 'He deserves all the heat he'll get from Orvin,' I thought.

LaRee stood listening to Madsen explain that Dad had ARC. She felt everything inside her go silent. Fear knotted her stomach as she thought of the many exposures to Dad's blood. She thought of her children.

Madsen paused and studied the family with a look that was troubled and still. "You must realize that at the time of Orville's transfusion there was no blood test available for AIDS," he said.

It was then Orvin started yelling. Because of our ties to Jonathan's AIDS case he knew there had been surrogate tests available that would have weeded out much of the AIDS contaminated blood. "There were other tests that could have been used," Orvin shouted. "High risk groups should have been deferred. It was 1985, for God's sake. What about the hepatitis B he got? There were tests for it."

Madsen stepped out of the room—a wise thing to do when Orvin gets riled.

Orvin turned his anger on LaRee. "I've tried to tell you for months that the doctors were lying to us. And you said I was paranoid. Are you still going to defend those bastards?"

Something in LaRee snapped. With all her strength, she hauled off and kicked Orvin square in the butt. Then she ran from the room.

Dr. Madsen scurried down the hospital corridor after LaRee and her husband. "Now you do understand why you can't sue," he huffed. "The blood bank would drag your father's sex life through the mud."

His statement carried the threat of a shark's tooth. This was a manipulative ploy that some blood banks used to fend off lawsuits. They threatened their victims with exposure of past sexual indiscretion. It was often very effective.

In Dad's case, however, it wouldn't fly. This conservative old man had been married for 54 years and had never had sex with anyone but his wife. His children would not fall for the blood bank's sick tactics. We did not fear exposure of Dad's sex life. He had lived the high moral code taught by the Mormon Church and the Mormon-named blood bank could never make us believe otherwise.

Nevertheless, the LDS Blood Bank continued its efforts to discredit my father. Three days after the AIDS disclosure I called the lab that had run the HIV test on Dad's blood that Madsen had drawn. The lab was at the Utah Valley Hospital, a large IHC facility in Provo, Utah. I asked to talk to Dr. J. J. Anderson whose name appeared on the test results.

"About two months ago you tested my father's blood for AIDS and it was positive," I said. "He got it from transfused blood supplied by the LDS Blood Bank. I'm wondering if you can answer a couple of questions for me."

"Oh, I can't discuss any AIDS tests at all. There are laws against it."

I noticed that he had a speech impediment—a slight stutter. "Not even questions about the test's accuracy?"

"I don't think so. The confidentiality laws are very strict. But leave your number and I'll check it out."

I gave him my phone number, sure that I would never hear from him. Already I was learning that the confidentiality laws passed to protect the privacy of AIDS patients or carriers provided excellent shields for blood banks to hide behind. They made it impossible for recipients of AIDS-tainted blood transfusions to obtain information.

However, to my surprise, Dr. Anderson called me back a few hours later. But now his stutter had dramatically worsened, which was unfortunate because he was most anxious to discuss my father's AIDS.

Apparently the confidentiality laws had been repealed for a few minutes. Dr. Anderson had a message for me from the blood bank and he struggled, like a good soldier, to get it out.

"I c-c-called the blood b-b-bank," he said. "The d-d-doctors said to t-t-t-tell you your father d-d-d-didn't get AIDS from his t-t-transfusion. He c-c-couldn't have s-s-symptoms this early. It t-t-takes f-f-five years for them t-t-to come."

His disjointed words reflected off my ear drum with the punch of a machine gun.

I protested, "The incubation period can last for many years or can be very short."

"No. The d-d-doctor said your father g-g-got AIDS from his l-l-l-lifestyle. He g-g-got it in some other w-w-w-way."

I was stunned and wondered how many other hapless doctors the blood bank would use to do its dirty work. Did the LDS Blood Bank and IHC control every medical professional and institution in Utah?

They had us coming and going. I didn't know where to turn for medical care or honest information. I called some AIDS hotlines around the country but they were not staffed by doctors. I thought of San Francisco General Hospital. I knew they were very involved in AIDS research and patient care.

On a hunch, I asked information for the number of the San Francisco hospital. I dialed, asking to talk with the department that cared for AIDS patients. I explained the political nightmare our family was experiencing in the state of Utah and asked if I could please talk to one of the doctors.

A doctor was paged and he kindly answered my questions. "Your father's HIV test has been confirmed by the Western Blot," he explained. "You can consider it 99% accurate."

"How long does it take for AIDS symptoms to appear after someone is transfused with contaminated blood?" I asked.

"It can be within a few weeks, although most people will go for years. The time it takes for symptoms to show varies widely between patients; we don't understand why. But the blood bank was trying to intimidate you for obvious reasons."

The doctor paused. "I think most of the AIDS patients in Utah are cared for by a woman doctor. I believe she's associated with the Catholic hospital in Salt Lake City." That last piece of information would prove to be very significant for our family.

★   ★   ★

The LDS Blood Bank trampled over us with all the soul of a microchip. If the Xanax incident had not forced disclosure, we never would have known Dad had AIDS. The silence the blood bank had maintained for years denied Dad proper diagnosis and treatment in the early stages of his disease. It caused the members of his family to be repeatedly exposed to his infected blood. Mother's sexual infection with AIDS was a direct result of the LDS Blood Bank's cold, calculated power play.

For years the blood bank had told the Utah press that it supplied exceptionally "clean blood donated by clean people." It was well known in the largely Mormon communities in the Uintah Basin where my parents lived that the majority of the blood bank's donors were recruited in Mormon Church meetings. It was difficult for people to believe that Dad got AIDS from blood supplied by the LDS Blood Bank. A few called the blood bank and were told by a spokesperson that there hadn't ever been problems with either hepatitis or AIDS contamination.

Many people believed that Dad got AIDS in "some other way." His reputation was ruined. Garbage was thrown on the lawns during the night. Orvin would try to clean it up before his parents noticed.

Copies of FDA inspections of the LDS Blood Bank, which I eventually obtained under the Freedom of Information Act, proved the blood bank's rosy PR picture of blood safety to be a sham. The blood bank had considered its regular donors above the behaviors that spread AIDS and had been extremely lax in educating and screening donors.

But a conservative local population cannot compensate for unsafe practices in a blood bank. Within just a few months after HIV testing of blood began in March 1985, the LDS Blood Bank identified six donors from their donor pool who were positive for AIDS. The six donors' positive status was confirmed with triplicate testing by two methods. Dad's donor was one of them. Over the years, the FDA had cited the blood bank for numerous deviations from FDA Safety Regulations. These deviations are discussed later in detail.

★   ★   ★

Dad retained his sense of humor even after being told about the AIDS. The next morning he was laughing over the swift kick LaRee had given Orvin. "You should have been here to see it," he told me.

"Who knows, Dad," I said. "Maybe you will be the CDC's first case of psychosomatic AIDS—all brought on by nerves and depression."

"Yeah," Dad said. "That was some smoke screen they built."

I was surprised his mind was so sharp and he was taking it so well. However, as the days went by, the reality of his illness sank in and darkness pressed down, smothering him in gloom. His was a heart without hope, fearful of the disease process that he faced.

Dad's knowledge of his diagnosis made him feel better in one respect. Now he understood why, after his surgery, he had not regained his health and had been unable to again do heavy farm work. There had been a valid reason—AIDS. Dad took some comfort in knowing that he wasn't a pantywaist after all.

After he came home from the hospital, Mother was upset by the new infectious measures that were implemented.

Having no idea she was already infected with HIV, Orvin tried to get her to wear gloves when she helped Dad walk to the bathroom or cleaned up his dishes, which often had blood on them from the lesion on his lip. There was a special, liquid soap for washing hands and Mother could not remember to use it. All Orvin's nagging did was make her more anxious and upset.

"I don't know what to do about Ma," he said.

"Maybe it's better not to worry her over it," I said. "She does very little clean up and the virus has already been in the house for nearly two and a half years."

The day after Dad got back home, a Home Health Care nurse came and Orvin showed her where the box of gloves was kept. Later he noticed she wasn't wearing them. "You do know he has AIDS don't you?" Orvin asked.

"Oh, he does not have AIDS." The nurse was annoyed. "Wherever did you get such a crazy idea?"

"Ask Dr. Madsen."

The nurse must have reported the conversation to her supervisor. When it was realized that Home Health Care had provided care for several months after Madsen knew about the HIV infection, the nurses were outraged. They confronted Dr. Madsen. "Why did you send us into that home without telling us to glove? Why weren't we informed that he had ARC?" they demanded.

The doctor's flippant reply was, "It wasn't necessary. I didn't think you'd have sex with the old man."

Our family didn't try to conceal that Dad was infected with AIDS. In fact, Orvin strongly felt that anyone who came to the house should be told. "I won't knowingly risk any person's life," he said. His anger over the coverup grew with each passing day.

After Dad's diagnosis became public knowledge, Orvin went to the drugstore in Roosevelt.

The pharmacist handed him Dad's medicine and said, "Some things work out for the best. Your father has been ill and depressed for so long over his family problems. With AIDS he won't have to live much longer."

Not only did this licensed health professional fail to connect Dad's prior poor health and depression to the AIDS virus, but he thought AIDS brought on an easy, storybook death. His comment was one the family would often remember during the remaining 14 months before Dad died.

★　　★　　★

How to handle Dad's Xanax addiction presented a dilemma. One of the drug treatment centers I talked with was the Height Detox Center in San Francisco, California. I had explained to Greg Hayner that my father always went into myoclonic jerking as his Xanax dose was reduced.

"Your father's case is a tough one," the pharmacist said. "Some people can be tapered off Xanax without difficulty, but others have to be hospitalized and taken off cold turkey. We put them on phenobarbital and then taper them off it. How old is your father?"

"Seventy-eight."

"The detox would be rough on him. The other alternative is to just leave him on the drug."

After I knew Dad had ARC, I talked with an AIDS specialist and was told that Xanax or similar drugs were often necessary to calm AIDS patients. I was afraid if another tranquilizer were substituted it might not be any easier on Dad than Xanax.

I called Dr. Madsen. "Our family prefers that Dad be left on Xanax at the level that will prevent further jerking," I said. "We don't want any more attempts made to get him off the drug by a taper." I left Greg Hayner's phone number with Madsen who was not at all appreciative of my assistance.

My parents' care was overwhelming. Some of the Home Health Care workers were frightened and refused to come back into the house. The burden fell on the program's director and two other faithful workers. LaRee helped Orvin on the weekends and drove to Lapoint with supplies after she got off work. I arranged for a woman to cook food and take it to the house. However, all the efforts did not sufficiently reduce the incredible load Orvin was carrying.

A hospital bed was moved into the living room for Dad. He would sit propped in it and make grunting moans, unaware he was making them. When asked where he hurt he'd say he was "sick all over." Most days he suffered from nausea and vomiting. His fever went up and down. "I'm going to die soon from this AIDS disease," he told the nurse.

Mother made a gallant effort to help Dad. "I would never ask for another thing," she said, "if he could just get well." Although she was in and out of her own mental fog, she compassionately fussed over her husband, taking him food and comforting him.

There was one week during May when Mother's diarrhea became so bad the caregivers had to keep disposable diapers on her. She was humiliated. "Why do I have to wear these? We never had to live like this before," she said. One contaminated transfusion had turned her world into a bewildering abyss of despair.

★   ★   ★

I often talked with Jonathan's mom, Shiela, after we knew that Dad had AIDS.

"We are going to be in *Money* magazine soon," she said. "They are writing an article on the high cost of AIDS."

During the two years since Jonathan had been diagnosed with AIDS, his medical costs had totaled $229,912. When the article came out in the November 1987 issue of *Money*, the magazine broke Jonathan's AIDS costs down as follows:

Items	Expense
Home care	$143,690
Hospitalization	50,692
Prescriptions	18,276
Gamma globulin service	10,840
Physicians	6,414
Total	$229,912 for two year's care

This total did not include costs for the first 27 months of Jonathan's life which were fraught with illness. Five years after the *Money* magazine figures were computed, Jonathan's lifetime medical costs have skyrocketed to nearly a million dollars. For a considerable length of time he and his mother made weekly flights between Denver and Bethesda, Maryland, so he could be treated with the experimental drug DDI at the National Institutes of Health.

Jonathan's million dollar cost for health care does not include the lost wages of family caregivers.

Shiela reflected on the emotional and financial roller coaster that had been her family's life since Jonathan was transfused with AIDS blood when he was 18 hours old. "The only way our lives could become normal again would be if we no longer had to cope with this disease," she said. "But we can't bear to think of that either. We can't imagine life without Jonathan."

Shiela tried to educate me in the politics of transfusion AIDS but I was a slow learner. I could not understand why health officials had so little concern for the plight of these victims. During the summer of 1987 I was told repeatedly by state and local health departments that we, "did not have AIDS" in our family and even if we did, "it couldn't be discussed." Actually Dad's ARC condition left him as ill and infectious as someone with "reportable AIDS."

On May 21, 1987, I called the Utah Department of Health in Salt Lake City and was told the two doctors in charge of AIDS were away attending a convention. A spokesperson suggested I have Dr. Madsen request the LDS Blood Bank to trace Dad's donors. This person said the department was aware of our situation but explained that my father was not an official AIDS case. "People can die from ARC but not be counted as an AIDS case if they haven't met strict CDC criteria. And even if they do meet the criteria they won't be reported unless their treating physician turns in the paperwork."

I got more information from this unguarded assistant than I would have received if I had spoken to the doctors. I talked with Shiela. "How do we know Dad doesn't now meet the CDC guidelines for reporting?" I asked.

"You don't," she said. "Not with the physicians he's had. They took extreme measures to keep his AIDS infection from him. They certainly don't want him reported as a transfusion case. They can just keep him in the ARC category until he dies."

The next day I called Dr. Madsen. "The family would like you to ask the LDS Blood Bank to trace Dad's donors," I said. "The State Health Department says the request must come from you."

The doctor was upset. "What for? So you can call up the donor and yell at him?"

"We aren't asking for the infected donor's name. We just want information on how this happened. We have a right to know."

Madsen grudgingly said he would contact the blood bank. Later he told us it would take an inordinate amount of time for them to do the tracing and give us any information. He was right. Blood banks have great expertise in stonewalling. Of course, at that time we did not know Dad's AIDS-positive donor had already been found by the LDS Blood Bank two years before.

I was in a quandary over how to get Dad under the care of a competent doctor who would not be influenced by the blood bank. I felt he should be cared for by an AIDS specialist in Salt Lake City but it would be a major family upheaval to move my parents there. The other doctors in Roosevelt practiced in the same office as Madsen. None of the doctors in the Basin had cared for AIDS patients and we knew they would not accept Dad without a specialist in Salt Lake to consult with.

For us, getting an acceptable specialist was a difficult task. IHC, the parent organization of the LDS Blood Bank, provided 60% of all health care in Utah, and the University Medical Center was another major provider. We did not want a doctor affiliated with either organization. Madsen tried to get Orvin to take Dad to an infectious disease expert within the power structure and had been refused. "From now on," my brother said, "our family will choose Dad's doctors ourselves."

But there weren't many choices. I had been talking with AIDS patients in Utah and learned that most of them were cared for by two doctors who were associated with the two other Salt Lake hospitals. I called one and asked if he would take Dad but made the mistake of saying too much about our situation. The next day his office called and told me the doctor wasn't taking any more AIDS patients.

The specialist who cared for most of Utah's AIDS patients was Dr. Kristen Ries, affiliated with the Holy Cross Hospital in Salt Lake City—a facility without apparent IHC ties. Dr. Ries' patients praised her integrity and warm sensitivity. "She is a very supportive and compassionate doctor," I was told. By this time we were in desperate need of some compassion. We had learned firsthand that there were no support groups in Utah for old Mormons with AIDS.

Initially I hesitated to call Dr. Ries because of her heavy patient load but when I did talk with her she graciously consented to take Dad as a patient on one condition—his present doctor would have to make the request.

This presented a dilemma. Madsen was anxious to refer Dad to a specialist chosen by IHC's inner circle but he was not receptive of the specialist we chose—even though she was Utah's top AIDS doctor. He stalled and said that he could probably care for Dad in Roosevelt. We left Dr. Ries' phone number with Madsen and asked if he would use her as a consultant on Dad's case. We knew that he still consulted with the University doctors regarding Dad's condition which made us uneasy.

"If we wanted the University doctors involved we would have taken Dad back to them," Orvin said.

★   ★   ★

Dad's health worsened throughout May. It was well into June before his long time friend, Dick Hackford, got up the courage to visit him. The elderly man was a devout Jehovah Witness who lived in Lapoint. In their younger days he and Dad had argued over religion, each trying to convert the other. Finally they had given up and just become good friends. They hadn't discussed religion in years.

Mr. Hackford went over to the hospital bed and gazed down at Dad as he lay emaciated and pale in wordless misery. All Dad could manage for a greeting were a few moans.

Badly shaken, his old friend went to the other side of the room and sat down, too emotional to talk. Finally he got up from his chair, walked over and shook his finger under Dad's nose. "Orville, it's your own fault," he said. "You wouldn't listen. If you had joined the Witnesses this never would have happened. Our God doesn't allow blood transfusions!"

Dad's condition continued to worsen during June. He was still losing weight and when his nausea and vomiting were bad, all he could tolerate was 7-Up. It was difficult for him to walk or even stand. He had trouble breathing and the yeast infection in his mouth and throat was worse. He spent much of the day fighting through the cobwebs of a nightmare-filled sleep. His existence had become a bitter, painful struggle brought on by complex events he could not comprehend.

On June 18, Dr. Madsen admitted Dad to the hospital in Roosevelt. On the same day, blood was drawn from Mother's arm to be tested for AIDS.

During June, the Home Health Care workers had noted how Mother's health was declining. She complained of stomachaches and a constant pain in her eyes. Both eyes were very red and watery.

Early on the morning of June 22, Orvin took Mother to the hospital emergency room. She was running an unexplained temperature of 100.4°. The ER doctor noted that an episode of incontinency was brought on by diarrhea. Mother was confused and the doctor thought perhaps she had suffered a small stroke.

Orvin took Mother to LaRee's home and then went back and stayed at the hospital with Dad. It was 3:30 a.m.

For the next few days, LaRee cared for Mother with a sense of troubled apprehension. One evening she prepared special food she hoped Mother would eat. Mother had been sitting in the same chair for two hours, awake but with her eyes closed.

"Open your eyes and see how good this baked fish looks," said LaRee as she started to feed her.

"My eyes hurt too bad to open," she replied.

For several weeks her memory had been drawn to the past. "My mother and father would sure be upset if they knew how sick I am," she said.

LaRee put down the plate. "I want to put you into bed so you can rest." But my sister knew that even Mother's brief periods of sleep were cruel.

"I don't want to go to bed," Mother protested. "If I sleep I dream that Dad dies and is carried off in a pine box."

The day after he left Mother with LaRee, Orvin took Dad home from the hospital. However, Dad was not any better. His voice was barely audible. "I feel terrible all over," he said. "But I can't describe it." A sensation of intense sickness and desolation was always with him.

Two days later LaRee took mother back to Lapoint. She had been worrying about Dad, wanting to see that he was still alive. Mother was glad to be home but shortly before midnight Orvin called LaRee.

"You'd better come get Ma and take her to ER," he said. "I can't wake her up and she hasn't been able to eat anything all day."

LaRee arranged for Dr. Madsen to meet them at the hospital. The doctor carefully examined Mother. Perplexed, he told LaRee, "I've never seen anything quite like this before."

Madsen admitted Mother to the hospital and called a technician to come from home in the middle of the night to do a CAT scan. The scan did not provide any definite answers. It indicated that Mother could possibly have had three small strokes but it was not conclusive. (AIDS patients, including children, often suffer strokes.)

During the four days Mother was kept in the hospital, she ran a low-grade fever of unknown origin. Blood and urine cultures were normal and chest X-rays were clear. She was given physical therapy because since December she had experienced intermittent difficulty with walking.

The nurses noted that Mother complained of being nauseated. She was often alert, lucid and talkative, but she had periods of hallucination. One night Mother insisted there was a rabbit under her hospital bed and a mouse on the ceiling.

On the first day of July, Mother was released from the hospital and taken to LaRee's home. During the night Mother couldn't sleep. She nervously paced between the bed and couch and all around the house. By morning LaRee was ready to buy padded wallpaper, but the worst was yet to come.

That afternoon my sister, her husband, and three children had appointments to get hepatitis B shots. When they arrived at the doctor's office Madsen asked to talk to LaRee and her husband privately.

Two weeks earlier the entire Swain family had gotten HIV tests and they had all come back negative except for Mother's. Her results were still pending and I had called the lab about the delay although I was not too concerned. I didn't realize that positive AIDS tests were then sent to

California for confirmation and I assumed my parents hadn't been sexually active. No one in our family was prepared for the next bombshell.

It was my brother Von who called me. "Joleen, Mother's AIDS test came back positive. Madsen told LaRee this afternoon."

A wave of numbness swept over my mind as I fought to reject his words. "That's not possible," I said.

"Well, the test is positive and Dad doesn't deny they had sex a few times—about a year after the surgery."

"It's unthinkable. They're close to 80 years old. Are they both to die from a sexual disease?"

"Well, Dad is too upset to be questioned now," Von said. "He and LaRee are crying something awful."

"Does Mother know?"

"Yes, but I'm not sure how much she understands. At least she's not sobbing like the others."

My hand shook as I hung up the phone. An icy fear engulfed me. Was it never going to end? How could Mother and Dad be cared for? How long would they have to suffer their agonizing deaths?

I thought of the arrogant, callous blood bank and my tears were dried by a burning anger. Someday, I silently promised my parents, this carnage will stop.

LaRee wrote in her diary: "Dad was brought to our home the day he was told about Mother. He refused to come in the house because of his fear of being infectious. He sat outside on a lawn chair and sobbed and sobbed for his wife. We brought Mother out and sat her next to Dad.

"It was such a beautiful day. The sun was shining. But the world had come to an end for my parents. I felt like we had been put into a dark hole and were spinning around without light.

"I told Mother that her HIV test was positive. She responded for a few minutes then slipped into her own little world. Sometimes I wondered if she went into that world to escape the horror that was unfolding around her."

Now our family fully understood the health care problems ahead of us. Extra help would have to be hired to work in my parents' home but caregivers weren't anxious to be around the AIDS virus.

Dr. Madsen suggested that Mother stay in the convalescent home in Roosevelt until other arrangements could be made. Unlike when he admitted Dad to the home, the doctor told the management that Mother was AIDS-positive. Unaware they could refuse to take AIDS patients, the management agreed to accept Mother. This was an unfortunate mistake because the facility was totally inexperienced in handling AIDS.

The summer heat was at its worst. Mother's small room did not have air conditioning. Her door was to remain open so the cooled air from the hallway could keep her room temperature comfortable. This worked well if the family stayed and cared for her. After they left, it was a disaster.

The workers had never cared for an AIDS patient and the majority were terrified of Mother. They shut her door and wouldn't let her out of the room. Von arrived at the home and found Mother leaning over her bed, trembling violently. "I can't get into bed," she gasped. "I've been standing here for hours."

LaRee started checking on Mother several times a day. One afternoon she found her drenched in perspiration in the closed, overheated room. Her luncheon tray, which had been delivered three and a half hours before, was by the door with the cover still on. Mother had to be fed her meals, but the aide had set the tray down and run from the room.

"Why is everyone so mean to me?" Mother sobbed. "They won't talk to me. It's so hot. They yell at me to stay in here and shut the door. Why do they treat me like this?"

LaRee fought back tears.

"Mother, I'm going to take you home. Now."

This was a lesson in the reality of AIDS. In that rural area, we couldn't depend on adequate care for our parents without constant family monitoring. Many workers gave excellent service but others were scared to death. The quality of care varied dramatically from shift to shift.

When Mother returned to Lapoint, Susan, an experienced medical aide, was employed to work the night shift in my parents' home. It was a challenging job. However, she quickly adjusted to my parents' demanding care and the AIDS precautions.

Mother liked her. "Susan reads to me from the *Bible*," she said. "She is always good to me."

But it was difficult for one person to care for both Mother and Dad. Orvin had to be up many of the nights assisting with Dad during endless emergencies. The strain on my brother was horrific. When we talked on the phone his voice was flat with weariness. I knew even if we could get more caregivers the responsibility would still be on his shoulders. He was there 24 hours a day and the problems were continuous.

I called nursing homes in the state of Utah and in the area of Colorado where I lived. I only found one home that accepted AIDS patients. It was in Salt Lake City which was inconvenient because none of us lived there.

During 1987 five of my parents' grandchildren were teenagers. They had been taught by their parents and the Mormon Church that living a clean life prevented becoming infected with sexually transmitted diseases. It was heartbreaking and confusing for those teenagers to watch their grandparents die of AIDS. Obviously chastity and refusing drugs were not adequate preventive measures.

The grandchildren's belief system toppled. They were upset over the behavior of the blood bank in its efforts to conceal their grandfather's AIDS infection. At school and church meetings rumors were passed around about their grandparents' lifestyle. Some classmates made cutting wisecracks. Others were afraid to come near them, thinking they would get AIDS.

It was a year of disillusionment. The LDS Blood Bank and IHC decision-makers were respected doctors and executives. They were not street criminals. They, like most of the nation's blood bankers, merely desired to preserve their safe-blood image and revenues.

Perhaps, for the tens of thousands of transfusion and blood product recipients who were nationally infected with AIDS, this is the most disheartening aspect of their tragedy. Their past and future deaths are by the hands of such good people.

Dad's eyes reflected the betrayal he felt. He knew that most of the blood bank and IHC executives were active Mormons. "What's all this religion good for?" he asked me.

On July 13 I called Dr. Craig Nichols at the Utah Department of Health and asked him if he knew how the donor trace we had requested was progressing.

"I'm not able to discuss that with you," he said.

"Are you aware that my mother has tested HIV-positive and my father's condition worsens with each passing week?"

"I cannot discuss the situation," he said.

"You're saying that the LDS Blood Bank can give my father AIDS and a collection of other viruses and the health department can't discuss it?"

"I'm not allowed to," he said.

"Can you tell me how many AIDS transfusion cases Utah has, or is that classified information?"

"We have only three transfusion AIDS cases. There have been no new cases in 1987."

A few days later I called the Uintah County Public Health Service and talked with Joseph Shaffer. We had a problem with clogged bathroom drains in my parents' home and plumbers were afraid to work on the lines or clean out the septic tank.

"Could you talk to this plumber about any AIDS risk that he would have in cleaning the drain lines?" I asked.

"That's the stupidest thing I've ever heard," Shaffer snorted. "You cannot get AIDS that way. There isn't a single AIDS case in Uintah County, just fear because of your family."

This attitude of the health departments was as sure to move me to anger as an onion does to tears. I knew that Dad and Mother were not considered full-blown AIDS cases but they were certainly HIV-positive and seriously ill with AIDS-related conditions and the lack of CDC reporting could not alter that fact. It was obvious that public health officials did not want to become involved with our problems and would have preferred that we had kept our situation secret so they didn't have to deal with public concern or "panic."

"The health officials' main interest is in making their jobs easier," Orvin stormed. "I'd like to see them care for our parents for one week."

Chapter 7

Blood, Thunder and Confrontation

When I arrived in Lapoint in late July, Dad was in the hospital. The night before he had vomited in his bed and the aide got him up and stood him by her. As she reached for a clean nightshirt, Dad pitched head first into the rock fireplace, suffering facial abrasions and a broken nose. Orvin and the aide worked 45 minutes to stop the bleeding. The next morning Dad was admitted to the hospital.

The bathroom of the farmhouse where I'd lived as a child reeked with the smell of laundry bleach. Used as a disinfectant, it was our family's main line of defense against the AIDS virus.

I thought how ironic it was that my parents' lifestyle had remained frozen in another time until AIDS came and dragged them into the late 20th century. HIV had been called the fast-lane virus but our parents were dying a slow-lane death. And all we had to fight with was a laundry product—one step up from the lye soap Mother used to make.

"Orvin, aren't you mixing the bleach solution too strong?" I asked.

"I'm using twice the amount they say to use," he confessed.

Although my brother insisted he did not worry about catching AIDS, his actions spoke otherwise. He's as scared as the rest of us, I thought.

The protective rubber gloves the family was using could get small holes in them which allowed skin contact with bodily fluids and blood. Orvin's hands were chapped and had deep cracks through which, I feared, the AIDS virus could enter his body. But I knew that to care for his parents Orvin would willingly risk his own life and deny his fears.

Unspoken fear was part of the AIDS legacy. Every time a family member got a fever or an unexplained symptom, the anxiety was always there in the back of our minds. The grandchildren's health was discreetly monitored by their parents but the younger generation was sharp enough to pick up on our tension. One grandchild got the flu and asked, "Do I have AIDS too? My chest hurts just like Grandpa's." When we learned that Mother had been infected with HIV we were badly shaken. AIDS was not supposed to be spread that easily.

"It's terrible to be afraid of your own parents," LaRee said. "You feel so guilty."

★   ★   ★

From the advantage of hindsight and medical studies, our fear of caregivers catching HIV was an overreaction. Although the risk was not zero, it was certainly very slight. However, the chances of a family getting two AIDS-contaminated transfusions and an elderly woman contracting HIV sexually were also slight. It is understandable why we did not wish to take another "chance" with this virus.

★   ★   ★

Mother was upset. "This place is a mess," she said. "My whole house needs cleaning."

"But Mother we cleaned this morning."

"I know, but then someone dumped raisins all over. Look at them, piled over there by the couch."

"There's nothing on the floor by the couch," I insisted.

"Oh yes there is. A whole bushel basket of black raisins got scattered on the rug."

Earlier that morning Mother was distraught because all the legs on the kitchen table were crooked and needed fixing. She often saw "glasses and little lights all over everything." Hallucinations were common in advanced AIDS but I wondered if some of her faulty perceptions could be due to CMV infection of the eyes.

Later that day a violent thunderstorm raged for the third consecutive afternoon. The lightning crackled the sky apart.

"Mother, I don't remember the electrical storms here being this bad. Are they worse this year?"

Her quick response carried an air of authority. "Yes, they're worse. This year there are more devils to be thundered down under." I marveled how in her confused mental state Mother still made perfect sense.

Dr. Madsen considered putting Dad on azidothymidine (AZT), a drug which inhibits replication of the HIV but does not cure AIDS. By 1987, side effects from AZT's high toxicity were well known. The first time AZT had been given to an AIDS patient was two years before on July 2, 1985.

I feared that Dad's condition had deteriorated so badly during the time his infection was concealed that AZT would be of little help. And Dad was now so ill I doubted he would be able to tolerate the drug's side effects.

However, I called a number of AIDS patients around the nation. Most of the ones who could tolerate AZT reported improvement in many of their symptoms and in the quality of their lives.

"I think we should try anything that has a chance of relieving Dad's suffering," Orvin said.

While our father was in the hospital after his fireplace fall, Madsen put him on AZT. Within a day the lesion that had been on Dad's lower lip for years began to heal.

Dad was taken home the following Sunday but Madsen felt it would be impossible for the family to care for him because of the "magnitude" of Dad's problems. The doctor wrote that most of them were "due to the insidious nature of the AIDS virus in causing a slowly progressive dementia."

It was just three weeks since we learned of Mother's AIDS infection but we were certain her mental condition was also due to the virus. We were aware of her rapid decline after the onset of an acute illness late in 1985.

We wanted Mother under the care of an AIDS specialist and appropriate tests run. However, it was apparent to us there would undoubtedly be interference from blood bank interests. They would not be anxious to have the extent of Mother's AIDS-related conditions investigated and confirmed. Dr. Madsen was showing an obvious indifference to her health problems.

On Monday, after Dad had been home less than a day, he developed severe pneumonia and was returned to the hospital by ambulance.

Mother sat in her wheelchair and watched the paramedics lift Dad onto the gurney and carry him out of the house. She was confused and frightened. She thought Dad died and kept asking me when we were going to have the funeral. Poor Mother. Just looking at her broke my heart.

When the health care nurse arrived, Mother was still anxious about Dad.

"They took Orville away," she said.

The nurse tried to calm her. "I know. He's in the hospital being cared for."

"Is everyone in my family going to die from AIDS?" Mother asked.

"No, Ora, that won't happen. Try not to worry."

"Well, why can't they do something?"

"The doctors are learning more all the time. They'll soon have a cure for this."

When the nurse left the room, Mother was angry. She was always able to see through pretense and get to the truth. "Don't you believe her," she said to me. "I know we're going to die."

I took her outside into the yard. Rain had cooled the afternoon air. I pushed her in her wheelchair the short distance to the Mormon church, wheeling her around and around in the empty parking lot. The motion soothed her. She stopped fussing about Dad.

As we returned to the house, the phone rang. LaRee was calling from the hospital.

"How is Dad?" I asked.

"They took new chest X-rays," she replied. "A radiologist examined them. He suspects Dad has pneumocystis pneumonia."

Mother was more relaxed after her wheelchair ride. She was alert, talkative and irritable. I made another attempt at getting her to eat. She quickly voiced her displeasure.

"I wouldn't mind eating if you didn't give me the same awful food every meal."

"That's not true, Mother. This chicken soup was just delivered to the house. It's homemade—delicious."

"Well, it tastes just like the stuff I had for breakfast and lunch and all the days before."

Two days later Dad's chest X-rays indicated he had pneumocystis carinii, the AIDS pneumonia which was often fatal. In 1987 pneumocystis carinii pneumonia (PCP) caused 60% of all deaths from AIDS.

A week of ambivalent medical care followed as tension mounted between Madsen and family members. Madsen put Dad on Septra and kept him on the AZT. Septra was a drug used to treat PCP but it caused severe skin rashes and anemia in 50% of the patients who took it. Dad had previously suffered an allergy to Bactrim which is another brand of the same drug as Septra. Madsen was aware of Dad's history of Bactrim-Septra allergy but our family missed the connection of the two drugs. At that time, all we knew was that Dad was on Septra, a drug used to treat PCP. We did not realize he had a known allergy to it or that there was an alternative drug called Pentamidine.

Dad's nausea and vomiting rapidly became unmanageable. I picked up my "hot phone" and began calling more AIDS doctors. I was distressed to learn that Septra and AZT have the same type of toxicity—they both cause anemia. The message I got from the doctors was that only one drug that eats bone marrow and causes anemia should be given at a time. Two drugs with the same toxicity could kill the patient.

Von and LaRee were taking turns staying at the hospital with Dad. The family again requested Dr. Madsen to consult with Dr. Ries—this time on the problems of mixing AZT with other drugs. A couple of days later LaRee had a head-on argument with Madsen over his reluctance to do so.

Von expressed his concern over Dad's care. "Joleen, we've got to get Dad with a better doctor," he said. "This one doesn't know what he's doing. But Dad's too sick to take to Salt Lake now."

Madsen had become increasingly concerned about the size of my phone bills. "Tell your sister," he said to Orvin, "that calling all those doctors is unnecessary. Her long distance phone charges must be awful."

During Dad's hospitalization for PCP, Madsen had repeatedly told our family that Dad was too ill to send to Salt Lake City. He said that although the local hospital was not able to do a bronchoscopy it would be of little value and too hard on Dad to take him to Salt Lake to get one. Later Madsen told Orvin he could not obtain Pentamidine, the other major drug used against the protozoa that caused PCP, without confirmation by bronchoscopy.

★   ★   ★

We would eventually learn that Pentamidine was easily available to any doctor and was used to treat those allergic to Bactrim-Septra. Nearly three years before, in October 1984, the FDA had approved Pentamidine for the treatment of PCP. According to Fujisawa Pharmaceutical Company, the drug's manufacturer, a doctor could get Pentamidine for a patient without any documentation whatsoever.

In fact, the use of aerosol Pentamidine had proved to be very effective in preventing PCP as well as in treating it. By 1986 Dr. Joseph Sonnabend, Dr. Donald Armstrong and other New York City and California doctors were advocating aggressive treatment with Pentamidine and other drugs during the early stages of AIDS infection. It was during this time period that Dad could have most benefited from treatment which the coverup had denied him. To say that by August 1987 it appeared that Dad's treatment was still being delayed is to say the least.

★   ★   ★

Unlike Von, neither Orvin nor I doubted Madsen's competency as a doctor. But we worried about the political pressure he was under. We were made more nervous by Madsen's response to our efforts to place Dad under the care of Dr. Ries. It was obvious he did not want us to take Dad to a Salt Lake City doctor of our own choosing. Our question was why?

Orvin and Madsen enjoyed a mutual loathing but I had a bit of empathy for the doctor. When he had agreed to monitor Dad's AIDS and keep it concealed, he never realized he would be left alone standing in deep muck. He could not have anticipated our refusal to return Dad to the care of the University doctors. Doctors are authority figures and most people go along with whatever they say. The University doctors said, "Bring him back in a week." We didn't.

There was an urgent need to complete arrangements for a change in Mother and Dad's health care. It was imperative that they were both cared for in the same area. One could not be in Salt Lake and the other in the Uintah Basin.

For several weeks I had been having discussions with the directors of the one nursing home in Utah which accepted AIDS patients. I felt if we could get both Mother and Dad under Dr. Ries' care they could be shuffled between that nursing home, which was located in a suburb of Salt Lake, and the Holy Cross Hospital. Orvin would stay in Salt Lake City to be near them.

On August 3, Mother was admitted to the South Valley Health Care Center and two days later Dad was taken to the Holy Cross Hospital. However, it took an explosive showdown with Madsen before Orvin got Dad extracted from his care.

Von and I had returned to our respective homes and early the morning of August 5 he called. He had just talked with Dr. Madsen who strongly recommended taking Dad off antibiotics. Madsen had told Von Dad's condition was so poor that he could not possibly live more than a week if left on the antibiotics and would die within three days if they were discontinued.

"If you can get Orvin to agree to take him off the antibiotics, I'll go and stay with Dad until he dies," Von said.

I could not reach Orvin because he had already left for the hospital with the determination of a grizzly headed to protect her cub.

Orvin's fury had been building for over a week. Now he raged around the hospital like Satan with a toothache. He found Madsen and told him he was taking Dad to the Holy Cross Hospital.

Seeing how resolute Orvin was, Madsen did one of his about-faces, this time on the availability of Pentamidine. "It isn't necessary to take him to Salt Lake," he said. "I can get the drug for PCP and treat him right here."

"Then why did you tell us you couldn't get it and let him get within an inch of death?" Orvin yelled. "I've had enough of this bullshit. I'm taking him out of here."

Madsen tried another approach. The previous day Dad's right leg had become swollen and painful. Tests had indicated he had two blood clots in the veins of his leg.

"You can't move him," the doctor said. "It's too dangerous. The ambulance ride could cause a clot to loosen and go to his lungs. It would kill him."

"Well, isn't that your objective? You want to stop treatment and let him die," Orvin shot back. "A blood clot would be a much easier death than discontinuing antibiotics and waiting for the end."

When my phone rang, Orvin was the angriest man in the state of Utah. "It's been like this for the past six months. Dad's as safe as a cow in the slaughter house. They want to bury this transfusion mistake as soon as possible."

Orvin's outraged voice reverberated throughout the room. I held the phone a few inches away from my ear.

"In March Madsen couldn't wait to get Dad into the nursing home, away from me, so he could take him off his heart medications. But Dad fooled them and lived. And the last few weeks we've been fed nothing but crap."

My head throbbed. It was a medical situation no one should have to face. The blood bank and doctors' long, sorry track record left them without credibility. They could not be trusted and I personally felt much of what Orvin said was true. Ulterior motives had been a factor in Dad's care.

However, there were two other factors complicating the situation. Madsen was fearful of a lawsuit against him, which could explain some of his erratic behavior. Also weighing on Dad's treatment was the fact that he was both terminally ill and elderly. Society has never defined how much care should be given to seriously ill AIDS patients or to people over seventy years of age. This subject causes sharp divisions of opinion among doctors, hospital staffs, organizations and families.

Dad's four children were not of one mind on this issue. Von and LaRee leaned toward less aggressive treatment while Orvin was a strong believer in the right to life at any age. He knew the vast majority of AIDS patients survived their first bout of PCP and that Dad had not received full treatment for the illness.

I was more neutral—very uncomfortable with playing God. I empathized with the feelings of all three of my siblings but I wanted Dad to have fair treatment regardless of how he had been given AIDS and regardless of his age. I was deeply disturbed by a medical system and a society that valued a man less for each year he had lived and would go to such lengths to protect the safe-blood image.

Orvin paused in his tirade, waiting for my response. I found myself saying what Dad had told me two weeks earlier. "Do what you have to do."

Orvin had his last confrontation with Madsen. "You have not done all you could for my father," he said. "Are you going to discharge him to Dr. Ries' care or do I just take him? You could be sued for inconsistent and inadequate treatment."

Madsen made the arrangements. LaRee was on duty that afternoon and watched as the doctor took Dad's medical records to an area behind the nurses' station and began dictating his lengthy discharge summary with the urgency of a rabbit running ahead of a prairie fire.

At 4:00 the next morning, Dad was loaded inside an ambulance. A nurse from intensive care took her place beside him.

"You're going to Salt Lake," Orvin told Dad. "The ride will take about three hours. I'll be following in the car, right behind you."

Dad was far too sick to respond.

A blurred and blood-red sun rose above the horizon as the ambulance streaked across desolate Strawberry Valley. It traveled on through Heber, down Parley's Canyon and finally entered beautiful Salt Lake City.

The ambulance turned right onto Wasatch Boulevard, weaving its way through the early morning traffic. In the distance, at the mouth of Emigration Canyon, stood a monument marking the spot where, in 1847, Brigham Young proclaimed, "This is the place."

Ten minutes later the ambulance pulled up to the emergency entrance of the Holy Cross Hospital. Dr. Kristen Ries, a small woman with a short utility hairstyle was waiting. Instead of the doctors' white coat, she wore a sweater, trousers and sturdy walking shoes. A Utah Physician of the Year recipient, she was considered in medical circles to be one of the city's busiest doctors.

Dr. Ries' practice of medicine was influenced by her Quaker upbringing. She was very sensitive to the needs of minorities, often providing care to groups unpopular with some doctors. The elderly had always been one of her major concerns and during the past five years she had cared for many gays who were stricken with AIDS. Her patient load was said to be slanted toward "gays and grays."

Now Dr. Ries examined "an unfortunate elderly gentleman" who was near death from an AIDS-related illness. He was not gay but he had what was mistakenly considered to be the "gay disease."

When Dad was wheeled into the emergency room he was unresponsive and cool all over. Dr. Ries warmed him and administered oxygen. She discontinued the Septra and treated him with Pentamidine. (Orvin made a mental note that the drug did not require documentation.) Because of Dad's persistent vomiting and the family's concern, Dr. Madsen had discontinued AZT the preceding day. Dr. Ries did not resume its use.

Dad was admitted to the AIDS ward and within a short time showed remarkable improvement. By the next afternoon he was able to talk with Orvin and mentally follow what was on television.

Dr. Ries sat on the edge of Dad's bed and hugged him. Hugs were one of her therapies. She had a demeanor that quickly bridged the treatment-trust gap that had so traumatized our family. We never questioned the motives of Dad's new doctors. They never gave us any reason to.

Dr. Ries ordered a bronchoscopy so that a small bit of Dad's lung tissue could be studied for diagnosis.

"I'm certain your father has had pneumocystis carinii," she said. "But it's probably too late to get a positive test result because of the antibiotics he's been on the past week." Dr. Ries was right—the bronchoscopy results were negative.

During the summer of 1987 the CDC had not yet expanded the guidelines for documenting AIDS cases. There was a narrow range of qualifying conditions which included PCP. But what we had not known was that it required documentation by bronchoscopy.

"Unlike Madsen told us, bronchoscopy was not needed to get 'the other' drug to treat pneumocystis," Orvin fumed. "It was needed to get counted as a transfusion AIDS case. There was a stall to keep him in Roosevelt where he couldn't be tested and documented. A stall to keep him on a drug he was allergic to."

I found myself agreeing with what my brother was saying. I thought back to the previous March when Madsen had treated Dad for a severe allergic reaction to Bactrim, the same drug as Septra. Why had he ever put Dad on Septra instead of Pentamidine?

I hung up the phone wondering how Utah's three transfusion AIDS cases had ever lived long enough to be documented.

Chapter 8

Homecoming

At night Orvin stayed in Dad's hospital room and during the day he spent time with Mother at the nursing home. I spoke with Dr. Ries and explained how anxious we were for her to see Mother. The doctor said she was scheduled to visit AIDS patients at the home the first weekend Mother was there and she would examine her at that time. However, by Thursday night Mother had a temperature of 101°. Dr. Monty McClellan, the nursing center's doctor, put her on an antibiotic and ordered a chest X-ray.

Dr. McClellan told me Mother had a slight case of pneumonia. He was a bit annoyed that the medical records Madsen sent at the time of Mom's admission were so scanty. "I have very little medical history for your mother," he said. "Her chart has Alzheimer's written on it but I don't think she has Alzheimer's disease."

"That makes two of us," I said. I knew that she had to be tested for AIDS-related conditions and properly treated.

Two days later when LaRee arrived in Salt Lake City she found Mother's pneumonia responding well to treatment but her mental condition seemed to have deteriorated. The next morning Mother didn't know LaRee and was unaware of her surroundings. She refused to eat. However, by afternoon she was painfully aware of reality and asked, "Oh, whatever happened to us that our lives could end this way?"

My sister left the home in tears.

An emergency prevented Dr. Ries from getting to the nursing center that weekend but she assured us she would see Mother very soon.

On Thursday, August 13, Dr. McClellan told me that Mother's pneumonia had improved and her temperature was normal. That evening Mother knew Orvin and responded to his conversation as he pushed her around the halls and lobby in a wheelchair.

When I called the next morning to inquire about her condition, I asked Dr. McClellan if he would have some blood drawn for a second HIV test, for verification. He agreed. A vial of blood was drawn and sent to the lab.

That afternoon the doctor was surprised when the nursing home called and told him Mother had gone into a coma. McClellan examined her and the family was notified that he doubted Mother would live through the night.

LaRee was at work when her husband called. Stunned by the news, her mind fought through a maze of medical cobwebs. Two days before, when she was at the nursing home, the doctor had said Mother's chest was better and she was without fever. But Mother had experienced low grade fever since June—unexplained fever that would leave and then come back.

LaRee and her husband left immediately for Salt Lake City. "The nursing center said they didn't know if she would be alive when we get there," he said.

Grief replaced the numbness in LaRee's brain. Mother was dying and the only family member near her was her husband of 54 years who lay in a hospital bed across the city. It was Friday and earlier in the day Orvin had left for Lapoint. LaRee had planned to spend the weekend in Salt Lake with her parents.

"I don't dare drive any faster," LaRee's husband said as a heavy rain pelted down. "Visibility is too poor." 'The heavens are weeping,' LaRee thought. There was nothing as sad to her as raindrops on a new grave.

Mother died 30 minutes before my sister reached her bedside. Each of us was now stricken with guilt and self-incrimination. For the past two hectic weeks our attention had been focused on Dad. AIDS puts families in a no-win situation. There is nothing you can do right. If you insist on aggressive treatment you feel guilty because suffering is prolonged, but if you don't fight with all available ammunition there is guilt because enough wasn't done.

It's difficult to know how you feel on this issue. Positions can shift. A family member who was upset because Dad was taken to Holy Cross for aggressive treatment was now the one most upset because Mother didn't have it. "You should have seen that she had better care in a hospital," I was told.

I talked with Dr. McClellan. "Your mother had sudden failure of vital bodily systems," he said. "It was her time to die."

I knew he was right. She died a peaceful death and, if she had lived, a far uglier death would have awaited her. But I was racked with guilt because she spent her last 11 days in a nursing home and died alone. I should have brought her to Colorado, I thought. I could have cared for both her and my daughter for that short time.

The telephone rang, bringing an unwelcome consideration. "Joleen, do you want an autopsy done?" my brother, Von, asked.

My mind scrambled to put all the pieces together. I knew that because Mother died before Dr. Ries could examine and test her, an autopsy would be necessary to prove her death was due to AIDS. However, at that lonely moment I was sure we could not get an honest autopsy in the state of Utah. The power of the LDS Blood Bank and IHC was too pervasive. We were one family against the giant medical monopoly responsible for Mother's preventable AIDS infection. That monopoly would not hesitate to use its influence to prevent a death by AIDS documentation. To get a report we could trust, her body would have to be flown into San Francisco.

Standing there across the Continental Divide, isolated from my family, I made the decision. There would not be an autopsy. But even in that emotional moment I knew the reason for my decision was irrational. I couldn't bear the thought of flying her body out of Utah. Mother had always been afraid to fly.

When LaRee told Dad of Mother's death he was devastated. Her AIDS infection haunted him. He blamed himself for infecting her. Seeing Mother suffer had been terrible for him but now that she was gone he thought he was to blame for her death as well.

Dad was disconsolate. He felt he had to attend the funeral. "There are some things a man has to do," he said. "And going to his wife's funeral is one of them."

The service would be held in Lapoint and it was impossible for Dad to travel that distance and go through a stressful public appearance. But Orvin didn't have the heart to tell him. He let Dad slowly come to that conclusion on his own.

My husband drove to Salt Lake City to stay with Dad so Orvin could return home. Unfortunately it was the same day Dad was being discharged from the hospital and admitted to the nursing home—more emotional trauma.

Dad had grown very fond of Dr. Ries, the nurses and the Catholic Sisters who provided supportive care and encouragement for the patients in the ward. The staff was well trained, having volunteered to work on the AIDS floor. It was difficult for Dad to leave the hospital where he was shown so much compassion. It was even more upsetting for him to think of going to the nursing home where Mother had died three days before.

Dad was taken to the large convalescent center in a mini-ambulance and efforts were made to comfort him. My husband stayed the night and was surprised that, in new surroundings and with a new family caregiver, Dad was oriented and frequently called out to him by name.

My husband and father's relationship had been close for 34 years. As the new day began to dawn they fondly reminisced about the past which had so abruptly come to a halt. Dad's son-in-law attempted to divert the old man's grief by recalling their prior hunting and fishing experiences. Dad finally relaxed as sleep softly enfolded his anguished mind.

★　　★　　★

Mother had moved to Lapoint when she was four years old and had lived in that small town the remaining 71 years of her life. Yet fear of AIDS prevented many people from attending her funeral or viewing. Those who did come sat in the back of the Mormon Church while the family sat at the front. The middle pews were vacant—as empty as our hearts.

After the service, Orvin left for Salt Lake City to be with Dad. He got permission to stay at the nursing home with his father and slept on the other bed in Dad's room.

★　　★　　★

Two weeks after Mother's death, Dr. McClellan called. "Your mother's test for AIDS infection came back positive. The results were the same as the results of her previous test of two months before."

"Then it couldn't be discounted as a laboratory error," I said. "Doctor, I have a question. Do you think any of Mother's health problems could have been due to Alzheimer's disease?"

"Oh, no," he answered. "Alzheimer's is a specific disease which requires confirmation over a long period of time. That was never done. Alzheimer's is used as a dumping box for mental symptoms in the elderly. Your mother didn't have it."

I spoke with the Centers for Disease Control. "My mother's death certificate lists pneumonia as the cause of death," I said.

"What kind of pneumonia?"

"It was never determined," I said.

"Then her death certificate should have also indicated that she was HIV-positive," the CDC spokesman said. "If listed as 'Pneumonia—HIV-positive,' a death is assumed to be the result of an AIDS-related condition even though it was not documented for CDC reporting purposes."

★　　　★　　　★

The summer had not brought as much heartache to the other Swain family with AIDS. In Denver, Jonathan had his good days and bad days but he enjoyed having his brothers home to play with him. He was excited because his mother had applied for him to attend a preschool for the physically handicapped which was operated by their local school district.

"I'm going to school," Jonathan said. "Just like the other kids."

Shiela winced. The school district had been stalling and had not yet accepted Jonathan. She feared he would be crushed if school started and he was left at home. "His main wish in life is to do the same things other kids do. That's asking a lot for an AIDS patient. But the little time he has left shouldn't be wasted."

Shiela paused, shaking her head. "Everything about this disease is so political. How do you explain that to a child?"

★　　　★　　　★

The South Valley Health Care Center was in a suburb of Salt Lake City. A large, new and beautifully maintained facility, it was well equipped to handle patients with infectious diseases. At that time the center was caring for nine people who had AIDS in addition to its many disabled and elderly patients.

The standard of care at the facility was generally good on the day and evening shifts but could be inconsistent at night. There was the usual problem of high staff turnover which made it difficult to keep new personnel trained in the care of AIDS patients.

Dad did not mind staying at the home if Orvin was with him but he became depressed and his condition worsened if Orvin left for Lapoint to take care of the yards. However, Dad did not want the yard full of flowers to go unattended and took pride in the buckets full of beautiful blossoms Orvin always brought back to the care center. Dad insisted that Orvin drive across the city and take some of the flowers to Dr. Ries and to the AIDS ward at Holy Cross Hospital. Both the staff and patients marveled at the enormous size of the many varieties of vibrant flowers.

My brother worried continually when he was away from Dad for a few days. He knew it was not possible for any facility to provide the type of care he gave his father. He rubbed Dad's back, applying hot or cold packs. He kept special foods on hand to feed him and used humor to lighten his grim days. He wheeled him up and down the halls to relieve his nervousness.

It was that extra-mile care that reduced Dad's pain and anxiety. Orvin could not leave his father in a nursing home to suffer the agony of an AIDS death alone. He decided that he would stay with him day and night.

Dad benefited from the whirlpool baths and physical therapy he received at the nursing center. He was able to walk with assistance and pedal an exercise bike for a surprising length of time. He enjoyed watching television with Orvin and his sense of humor returned.

However, after a few weeks, his fever shot up to 104° and he became confused and unresponsive. He was admitted to the Holy Cross Hospital where Dr. Ries treated him for an early pneumonia. Within 24 hours Dad made an amazing recovery and was able to get out of bed. After several days he was discharged to the nursing home.

I encouraged Orvin to rent a furnished apartment in Salt Lake City which the family would pay for.

"I wouldn't ever use it," he protested. "For the last ten months I've spent most of my time in hospitals and rest homes."

"You could get away for a few hours a day. Leave between 6:00 a.m. and noon when Dad usually feels better." I was afraid that Orvin was approaching burnout from the constant stress of the past two and a half years. But he never did rent the apartment.

★   ★   ★

During September 1987, the CDC expanded the guidelines under which patients with AIDS-related illnesses could be counted as AIDS cases. Dad's condition now qualified for CDC reporting and Dr. Ries prepared the paperwork and sent it to the Utah Department of Health.

Dr. Ries listed blood transfusion as the transmission category—the way Dad caught the disease. But because of our past experience, I wanted proof that his case reached the CDC in the proper category. The media has access to a state's AIDS statistics and it occurred to me that the blood bank could use its influence to have the category switched to another transmission route. The more transfusion cases a state has, the more the safety of the local blood supply is questioned.

I knew that for all practical purposes it made no difference to us how Dad's case was listed—he would still die of AIDS. But it was now a matter of principle with me. I consulted with Shiela. "How can I find out if the paperwork was accurate when it reached the CDC?" I asked.

"The cases are sent in with identifying numbers instead of names," she said. "The only way you could know is if the health department would give you the case number. I have contacts at the CDC who could then check it out."

"Will the health departments give out case numbers?"

"I don't know, but we have Jonathan's."

Something in Shiela's voice told me I was a novice at playing the system. "The Utah Health Department has never given me the time of day," I said.

Nevertheless, on September 27 I called and talked with George Usher. I asked if my father's AIDS case had been documented and sent to the CDC.

"That's confidential information. I can't discuss it with you."

"Can you just give me his case number?"

"Oh, no, I can't do that. Everything is confidential."

I couldn't understand how a case number betrayed a confidence when the health department knew Dad's AIDS was public knowledge. I understood the need for confidentiality laws but I had seen how those laws could be ignored if the blood bank wanted to send us the "lifestyle" message. A lab could then discuss Dad's case at length but the same laws were strictly enforced to prevent me from obtaining information.

There had been no forthcoming information during the three months since I had requested the blood bank to do a trace on Dad's donors. Years later I still don't have a response to that request which the health department advised me to make. To ask the LDS Blood Bank for donor information was like poking a marshmallow—nothing happened. And the health department never lifted a finger to help me.

I wrote to the CDC asking if they could confirm that my father's AIDS case was reported in the transfusion category. I was informed they could not.

There are numerous reasons why the number of reported transfusion AIDS cases is so small compared to the number of AIDS infections given through blood transfusion. These reasons are discussed in a later chapter.

★　　★　　★

The Denver news media was reporting the disagreement between parents, the school board and Jonathan's family over his acceptance into preschool. As Shiela had feared, the small boy watched the other kids go off to school without him. Parents had filed a petition objecting to the school admission of HIV-positive children.

I sat in my home watching Jonathan and his mother on the evening news. He was not yet five years old but there he was at the center of controversy, voicing his impatience at the injustice of the delay.

I wondered how we got to be the chosen family. Would anything be changed by our assertiveness? The majority of people with transfused AIDS go home and quietly die in secret.

★　　★　　★

On October 12, Dad's birthday, he was back in the Holy Cross Hospital sitting propped up in bed.

Orvin helped him open a brightly wrapped gift. "Hey, look at this fancy sweat suit."

Dad squinted at it with puzzled disinterest. "I'm too old to wear that."

"No, you aren't. You're only 79. You are in better shape than the AIDS patient across the hall who is 29. And Dr. Ries says your heart is strong."

Orvin always kept up a steady flow of optimistic dialogue around Dad. He believed hope could stem the course of the virus and continued to search for a rainbow in the dark night of AIDS. There was something in Orvin that would not give up.

Dad was being treated at the hospital for another bacterial infection. Once again he had shown dramatic improvement after one day on the appropriate antibiotic. During this hospitalization he was more physically active and Dr. Ries put him back on the AZT that had been discontinued two months before. It was obvious that the drug helped his nervousness and general mental condition. By the weekend he was watching BYU football and following the plays.

Orvin began to question the wisdom of keeping Dad at the nursing center. He was certain he would be more content at home in Lapoint. "I'm caring for him all the time anyway. In some ways it would be easier to have him home."

"But in other ways it would be harder," I said. "At the center you don't have to worry about food preparation, housekeeping chores or shopping."

"Well, it would be easier than when we were taking care of Ma, too."

"What about leaving his physical therapist and Dr. Ries?"

"Yeah, it's the doctor problem that bothers me," Orvin conceded. "It's only taken Dr. Ries a day or two to pull him out of each one of the last three crises."

After weighing the pros and cons, the family decided to return Dad to his own home. LaRee offered to take a leave of absence from her job at the hospital in Roosevelt and help Orvin care for him. Home Health Care agreed to resume their service.

I tackled the dilemma of finding a local doctor. There were few family doctors in Roosevelt and after our conflict with Madsen I hated to return Dad anywhere near the old battlefield. For most of their lives my parents had gone to doctors in Vernal, the one other community in the Basin that offered medical care. Dr. Larry Wilcken in Vernal had cared for Dad a number of years before and we decided to ask him to take his former patient back.

But would Dr. Wilcken accept Dad now that he had AIDS? More importantly, why should he? Our story was well known in Vernal. Why should county health care providers be saddled with a burden given by the state's large blood monopoly?

I waited for Dr. Wilcken to come to the phone. I took a deep breath like someone about to plunge into icy water. If he said no, we were left without options. Dad would have to remain in Salt Lake City.

When the doctor came on the line, I explained the family's desire to care for Dad at home and how difficult it was for him to be away from the area where he had always lived. "If we bring him home, would you consider being his local doctor if his Salt Lake specialist is available for consultation?" I asked.

"Well, I can't understand why you wouldn't want Dr. Madsen to resume his care."

I tried to keep my voice casual as if I were discussing an ingrown toenail. "I was sure you would ask that," I said. "The politics of Dad's case caused some friction between Madsen and family members. But all those politics are over now. We're in still waters and want to keep it that way without old feelings impacting on Dad's care."

Wilcken didn't hesitate. "I'll be happy to do what I can," he said, "but I don't know much about AIDS."

"We understand that. Dad has an excellent doctor in Salt Lake who is willing to consult with you. She is very easy to work with."

Dr. Wilcken was a native of the Uintah Basin and my mother-in-law had taught him in the second grade. He still farmed and had a large fruit orchard. He was a man of the soil with a medical degree and proved to be the type of doctor we needed—compassionate without an attitude.

LaRee prepared the house for Dad's arrival, purchasing medical supplies and foods he could eat. She was certain that this arrangement would not be of long duration. LaRee had expected Dad to die at any time during the past five months.

Orvin wanted to take Dad home in the car and avoid another ambulance trip.

"You'd better wait until tomorrow when someone can go with you," I protested.

"No, we'll just take off while he's feeling better."

However, checking out and loading the car took longer than Orvin anticipated and it was dusk as he left Salt Lake City with Dad. It was also Halloween and a good number of patrolmen were on duty. Unfortunately, in the confusion of the past months, Orvin's drivers license had expired and had not been renewed.

A couple of hours into the trip, Dad worsened and became very nauseated. Orvin lay him down, gave him a pan to vomit in and sped through Strawberry Valley like a bat out of hell.

A siren pierced the air. "Damn," Orvin said. "I'm going to get an awful fine. Dad, just moan and look sick."

"How could I look anything else?" Dad gasped.

Orvin nonchalantly handed the patrolman his drivers license. "My father is very ill," he explained. "He's got AIDS. I've had him in Salt Lake for treatment. Have you ever seen an AIDS patient? He's about to vomit all over everything."

The patrolman leaned forward and stared at the pale, gaunt, old man. Without a word he tossed the license in Orvin's lap, ran to his car and took off in the opposite direction.

"Good work," Orvin said wiping the vomit off Dad's chin. "He didn't even glance at my license. You're the spookiest Halloween ghost he's ever seen."

My brother kept his eye on the rear view mirror and a heavy foot on the accelerator. It was a desolate, dreary time of year and the passing scenery revealed only the gray bones of trees. Orvin had an eerie sense of unreality.

The road stretched on. Finally the car stopped in front of the house Dad thought he would never see again. He was home.

As they settled him into the hospital bed in the front room, Dad perked up—delighted to be back. He looked around at the familiar objects and studied the rock in the fireplace he and Orvin had built.

But something was not the same. "Where's your mother?" he asked LaRee.

"She isn't here right now."

Then Dad remembered. "Is she buried in the back yard?"

"No, she's buried in your cemetery plot in Roosevelt."

Dad's mind ebbed in and out around Mother's death. Sometimes he realized she was gone and other times he worried she wasn't being cared for. "Stop fussing over me and attend to your mother," he would say. "Go give her some of this custard."

Chapter 9

Death in the Slow Lane

A cold Uintah Basin wind brought the promise of snow. LaRee parked her car in front of the old brick farmhouse and carried in two bags of groceries.

The aide was already feeding Dad breakfast—soft boiled eggs and hot cream of wheat cereal. Dad had kept his life-long food preferences. He wasn't about to be fed any of that "oatmeal Anderson mush."

LaRee put away the groceries. "What time did Orvin get to bed?" she asked.

"It was after 6:30 this morning," the aide said.

"Did Dad have a bad night?"

"Not particularly. But he isn't constipated anymore. He kept soiling the bed and Orvin had to change it three times. This morning your Dad's in better shape than your brother."

LaRee shook her head. She could imagine the stories Orvin would have telling about the experience. A few nights before, Dad had slid to the floor when Orvin was transferring him from the wheelchair to his bed. Dad had laughed so hard at Orvin's futile attempts to get him back into bed that it took an hour to accomplish the task.

'We wouldn't survive this ordeal without the Swain sense of humor,' LaRee thought. 'It's good we can laugh at awful things.'

November had gone fairly well. Dad gained weight. He was stronger. He had enjoyed being at home and having some visitors—the few who had overcome their fear of AIDS. Martin Huber, the Mormon bishop in

Lapoint, often came with his wife who brought a casserole or homemade soup.

Dad was able to sit up in his wheelchair for a couple of hours a day and walk to the bathroom with assistance. He used oxygen when lying down. His appetite improved and he was often in good spirits despite some discomfort and pain.

The health caregivers found Dad pleasant to care for and concerned over their welfare. "Make sure you wear gloves," he told them. "So you won't get this AIDS thing."

LaRee took the day shift but Orvin was alone with Dad during the night when his symptoms were the worst. He had more hallucinations in the evening which made his care emotionally draining. Orvin spent the nights giving reassurance, massages and medications.

In mid-December Dad asked LaRee to buy Christmas cards for him to send. He made a gallant effort to sit at the table so he could instruct her on what to write on each one. For the past months Dad's handwriting had become as illegible as Mother's had before she died. Toward the end of their lives both my parents signed legal documents with a shaky X.

On December 17 Dad's leg became swollen and painful. Dr. Wilcken made a house call and diagnosed a blood clot. Dad was treated for six days at the Ashley Valley Hospital in Vernal.

Our family was shocked to learn that Dr. Madsen was now practicing medicine in Vernal instead of Roosevelt and was on staff at Ashley Valley.

"You can't get away from him," Orvin said. "After all our efforts to switch towns, doctors and hospitals, there he is."

Rumors were circulating in Roosevelt and Vernal that the two doctors who had been Madsen's associates at the Roosevelt Clinic were so upset over his handling of my parents' cases that they had asked him to leave.

Dad was taken home from the hospital two days before Christmas. That afternoon a man from Roosevelt, whom our family had never met, appeared at the door with a large basket of fruit. He was invited in and had a pleasant conversation with Dad and Orvin. It was after he left that Orvin noticed something hidden at the bottom of the basket and pulled out two $100 bills.

This is an example of the kindness that is frequently extended to AIDS sufferers by total strangers. Many people in the Denver area had shown compassion for Jonathan's family. And throughout the nation there is a noble effort made every day by thousands of AIDS caregivers, both paid and volunteer. They sacrifice much of themselves under the most depressive and relentless circumstances. Their dedication brings to mind the quote from *The Plague*, a book by Albert Camus. "For we learn in times of pestilence there is more to admire in men than to despise."

The last day of 1987 was one of Dad's better ones. He walked to the table and helped feed himself. Orvin, always an optimist where Dad was concerned, took this as a harbinger of a better year ahead. But LaRee was not as positive about the future and wished 1988 could be cancelled.

When LaRee called on the tenth of January, she was very upset. That day, Utah's leading newspaper, *The Deseret News*, had printed a full-page feature story about the world's first AIDS Alcatraz near Stockholm, Sweden. People infected with the AIDS virus were to be imprisoned on a bleak island so they could not infect others. The article quoted Dr. Lita Tibling from the Health University of Linkoping. "I would put all who test HIV-positive on the island for life so they can't spread the infection. As far as their families visiting; I would put them all on the island too. They are probably already infected."

Nearby inhabitants were said to be terrified that the AIDS-positive people might escape and infect them as they passed by their homes on the way to the ferry. The article was an uninformed writing and nearly all the major newspapers in the United States had chosen not to carry it.

"As if we haven't been harmed enough," LaRee said tearfully. "Now the church newspaper infers we all have the virus and anyone who passes us on the street will catch it. My kids will be scarred for life because of AIDS."

I, too, was very concerned for LaRee's children. Her youngest daughter had recently confided to her parents, "Many times my teacher has to send me out of the room while she talks to the kids and tells them not to say bad things about Grandma and Grandpa." The fourth-grader bravely added, "But don't worry. I'm getting used to it."

However, compared to the persecution experienced by AIDS patients in some of the rural areas in southern states, we fared well. Many people and health care providers in the Uintah Basin went out of their way to show compassion. There were others who were scared to death, but fear is easy to forgive. Self-righteous, moral judgment is not. Unfortunately, with AIDS, the two get confused and the former can be used to promote the latter.

In late 1987 Dr. Wilcken had contacted the LDS Blood Bank regarding Dad's AIDS. In January 1988 he received a letter from Dr. Myron Laub, director of the blood bank. Dr. Laub wrote, "After you reported to us that Mr. Orville Swain of Lapoint, Utah, had developed AIDS following his surgery at LDS Hospital in January of 1985, we began a look-back search to find and retest all the donors whose blood Mr. Swain received."

This was another example of how the blood bank continued to mislead all of Dad's physicians. The only look-back required had been a simple computer check to determine who had received the donor's prior donations after he tested positive for AIDS in 1985. That had taken place two and a half years before, instead of after, Wilcken's inquiry. Also, following Dad's hospitalization at the University Medical Center, Dr. Madsen and Dr. Ries had spoken with the blood bank—Madsen about the donor tracing the Health Department had suggested we request. But Dr. Laub was now, through a letter, establishing a recent date (late 1987) which he could legally claim as his first knowledge of Dad's HIV infection.

Dr. Laub did admit, however, that one of Dad's donors was found to be positive for AIDS. He said there was nothing more his bank could have done to prevent "this unfortunate occurrence" and they were being very generous to share this information.

When we saw the letter, we agreed with Laub. The LDS Blood Bank had generously shared a number of things with us, including hepatitis B and AIDS. But his statement that they had done everything possible to protect their blood supply infuriated us.

★　★　★

During January, Dad did not have any medical emergencies. But he was experiencing more pain and anxiety at night. Dr. Wilcken doubled his Xanax dose to help him relax. I thought back on all the trauma this drug had caused during the past year. I wondered if it had not been for Xanax would we have ever discovered that Dad had AIDS? Probably not. But a more significant question was how many patients are there who have died of transfusion AIDS without being told the cause of their illness?

Giving Dad his medications was a full-time job. Orvin had an elaborate schedule he adhered to in administering 33 doses of 10 prescription drugs during a 24-hour period. He tried to give just a few pills at a time with a small amount of food so they wouldn't be so hard on Dad's stomach. The AZT had to be given six times a day, exactly on schedule.

Our family was very appreciative of the excellent assistance given by Home Health Care. However, there was only one aide and one nurse besides the program director who would come into the house. The dedicated director, Edith Page, was giving a large amount of time herself, especially on weekends. She wrote, "Unable to get enough help in this home because of AIDS fear. Daughter is very tired and son is exhausted."

The caregivers of AIDS patients suffer physical and mental stress similar to battle fatigue. And the heavy care demands always promise to worsen as the disease progresses. The caregiver's exhaustion is coupled with a very slight, but nevertheless real, risk of catching the virus. Most of them have nightmares about getting AIDS. Anxiety over suspicious symptoms is common.

The *San Francisco Examiner* recently reported the suicide of a man who for two years cared for his wife and three-year-old daughter as they suffered with AIDS. The newspaper called the death of Doug Folsom of Duxbury, Vermont, an AIDS casualty—although he was not infected with the AIDS virus himself.

Throughout the first six weeks of 1988 Dad had a good appetite and enjoyed talking and joking with the caregivers. He was handling AZT well without serious anemia. However, his nights were becoming increasingly painful and anxious. He was having more nausea and running a low-grade temperature.

My father was the kind of loyal Republican who thought that to scratch on a voting ballot was a sin. One night he was watching TV when the news came on. The lead story was Vice President George Bush's surprisingly feeble showing in the Iowa caucuses. Political analysts said Bush's chance of winning the Republican nomination was slim. After the news, Dad drifted off to sleep. Suddenly he awakened and started climbing out of his bed. Orvin grabbed him to prevent a fall.

"Bring me my pants," Dad ordered.

"Why do you want your pants? You haven't had your pants on in months."

"I've got to help him," Dad said.

"Help who?" Orvin asked.

"I've got to go help George Bush. He's in trouble."

One Friday evening LaRee stayed over so Orvin could get some rest.

"I want to listen to the basketball game on the radio," Dad told her.

LaRee was surprised when he sat up in his wheelchair throughout the entire BYU vs. San Diego State game. But he was unhappy that his favorite team lost. "BYU should have won that game," he grumbled.

"Dad, when do you ever think BYU should lose a game?" LaRee asked. She was grateful that he could still be distracted by sports.

However, by morning LaRee was worried that Dad was coming down with a cold. The caregivers often wore masks around Dad but it was difficult to protect him from germs during the winter months.

The cold developed into pneumonia and he was taken to Salt Lake City and hospitalized at Holy Cross where his infection proved not to be

PCP. Again Dad responded very rapidly to treatment and on February 28 Dr. Ries released him to return home.

Dad was tethered to an oxygen tank by tubing attached in his nose. As they left the hospital, LaRee pushed his wheelchair toward the exit while Orvin walked behind carrying the oxygen tank. Unfortunately, when they came to the end of the hallway LaRee turned left and Orvin turned right which brought a loud yelp from Dad. "Stop! You're ripping my nose off."

After LaRee hurriedly checked Dad and found the nose damage to be slight, she and Orvin burst out laughing. But that day Dad did not have his famous sense of humor. He was furious. "What kind of dummies would rip an old man's nose off his face and then laugh?" he asked.

Dad was only home a few days before his condition deteriorated and he had severe difficulty swallowing. All he could get down were liquids and ice cream. His medications had to be mashed, mixed with water and given in a syringe. It was decided he should be returned to Salt Lake City and evaluated by Dr. Ries.

Testing at Holy Cross Hospital revealed Dad had significant neuro-muscular impairment of the tongue and pharynx causing "incomplete swallowing." The family was instructed to feed him only blended food as he sat upright and to encourage dry swallows during the meal to keep his throat clear. All liquids were to be given by a straw or syringe.

Dad returned home and a suctioning machine was kept by his bed to extract mucous and yeast infection from his throat. Orvin became very adept at this procedure. He found if he could get Dad to cough a few times he could remove a large amount of secretions which allowed Dad to get some restful sleep.

However, the feeding techniques and suctioning were making home care all the more demanding. Edith Page was spending more time at the house. One day she arrived with a large bowl of blended chicken, potatoes and carrots which the cook at the hospital in Roosevelt had prepared. To her astonishment Dad ate the entire amount as he sat watching a TV program. She found his ability to rebound from one crisis after another remarkable.

Dr. Wilcken shared her amazement. "Your father is the toughest old Uintah Basin greasewood I've ever seen," he told Orvin. "He just keeps coming back."

★   ★   ★

For six months the Colorado media had carried the heated controversy over Jonathan's acceptance into school.

Shiela said, "Every time we meet with the school board there is a new delay or they haven't lived up to a promise. They are stalling—waiting for Jonathan to die."

The publicity had been picked up by the national media and the family was besieged with calls from promoters of "AIDS cures" which they wanted Jonathan to try.

Some of the offers of "cures" spilled over to me. A doctor from a neighboring state became very irate with my reluctance to let him experiment on Dad with a toxic drug. "It's never been given to AIDS patients but I know it will work," he said.

"How do you know?"

"I'm a doctor and I know."

When I refused he said, "You won't even try to save your poor father. What kind of a daughter are you?"

After Dad's last stay at the Holy Cross Hospital his condition gradually worsened and became unmanageable. During the nights and weekends the strain on Orvin was horrendous. The days became so difficult that one afternoon Orvin and LaRee wrapped Dad in a blanket and took him to the emergency room in Vernal.

Dr. Wilcken admitted him to the hospital and treated him for pneumonia. After a week Dad had improved enough for the family to take him back home. But Dr. Wilcken warned that within a short time another opportunistic infection would advance upon his weakened body.

Unfortunately the doctor's prognosis was accurate and within a few days Dad started going downhill. Wilcken ordered phenobarbital as a sedative but it barely took the edge off his misery. Soon Dad was in the hospital again with another pneumonia.

Although it appeared to be the appropriate time to quit fighting, Dad struggled instinctively to survive. He had now reached the point where his undefeatable determination worked against him and prolonged his suffering. He would not surrender to AIDS and neither would his oldest son.

Orvin had never been neutral in anything he did or believed. He had strong moral convictions against contributing to the death of a human being and never doubted his staunch stand on this issue. Orvin had fought AIDS with all the commitment that was part of his character, with his love for Dad transcending any concern for his own health.

Nearly a year before, Orvin had agreed not to put Dad on a respirator and not to resuscitate him in case of cardiac arrest. But he believed that as long as his father's heart beat and he could breathe on his own, he should receive antibiotics for treatment of infections. Orvin, like Dad, who fed the starving animals of his impoverished neighbors, had never been able to watch suffering without trying to alleviate it. And he knew antibiotics brought Dad relief from pain.

"When they want to stop treatment and just give pain medication they are splitting hairs," he fumed. "Antibiotics take a fever of 105° down better than Tylenol. Damnit, they treat pain."

I consulted with Dr. Ries. "We were pressured last summer to stop treatment," I said. "But after Dad was put under your care he had some lengthy periods of quality time."

"That's true, but I fear more good days are unlikely," Dr. Ries said. "It would probably be wise to consider discontinuing antibiotics."

"Well, we all lean toward that approach except for Orvin and he's been the primary caretaker."

"I realize you're in a difficult position. Without a living will, a physician must treat until the family can agree to stop."

I had no opinions of my own on how long AIDS patients should be treated. All I knew was I wanted an end to Dad's suffering and between his strong constitution and Orvin's strong convictions I saw a lingering death ahead.

One of the hospital nurses complained to Orvin that Dad was terminal and should not be on antibiotics.

"What do you mean by terminal?" Orvin asked.

"That he is bound to die no matter what we do."

"Well, what about yourself? Do you think you aren't ever going to die—that you'll live forever?"

"Of course not."

"Then that makes you terminal, doesn't it?" Orvin turned to another nurse and said. "Don't let this woman have any lunch. She's terminal."

★   ★   ★

It was nearly the last of April before Jonathan got into the classroom. The press was on hand as his teacher introduced him to the children.

Unexpectedly, Jonathan spoke up. "I have something to tell them." He faced the kids. "I have a disease," he said. "My bad blood could kill you."

The children stared at him, unimpressed. Then one asked, "Want to play with the blocks?"

The school district had been pressured into accepting Jonathan because of community opinion. Numerous letters had been written to the editors of the two major Denver newspapers criticizing the district's delay tactics.

To reduce parental concern the district assigned a nurse to be in the classroom at all times to assist Jonathan with his oxygen and handle any problems. Some parents had feared he would bite their children. However, during the few remaining weeks before school closed for the summer,

Jonathan convinced the school that he was a friendly, outgoing little boy who did not have aggressive tendencies toward other kids.

"Our battle to get Jonathan his little space in the world has been worth it," Shiela said. "He's stopped asking when Jesus is going to come get him and now talks about his new school friends."

Dee, Jonathan's father told me, "I always felt that he would live a long time. If the psychologists had spent less time preparing him to die and more time preparing him to live we would be further ahead."

"That sounds like something Orvin would say," I responded. "The attitude must be genetic—something in the Swain genes."

★   ★   ★

The late May sun laid a shoulder of warmth against the window of Dad's hospital room. He had been there for nearly a month. The only sound in the room was the gurgle of the machine as Orvin sucked out mucous from Dad's throat. The nurses were afraid of the task, fearful of becoming infected with AIDS or the other germs AIDS patients carry.

Orvin turned off the machine. "You should be able to breathe better now."

For a brief moment Dad's eyes made contact with Orvin's—seeing but not understanding. When he did comprehend, he was not able to speak because he couldn't move his swollen tongue. Dad was unable to swallow at all now and was receiving nourishment and medication through tubes.

Orvin had been at the hospital for three straight days and nights. Every muscle ached and deep fatigue had settled into dark pockets under his eyes. Yet he worked around the clock trying to take away some of his father's agony. Dad would point to painful spots on his body and Orvin would rub him gently and ask for more pain medication or packs.

A man came to the door and motioned to Orvin. "Do you remember me?" he asked. "I used to buy hay from your dad."

"Yes, I remember. How are you?"

"Good compared to you. What happened is terrible. I think a lot of Orville. Are you here with him all the time?"

"Either I or my sister try to be here."

The man looked over at Dad while keeping at a safe distance. "I have a blood disorder," he confessed. "I have to have a transfusion at least every month."

"That could be trouble."

"I don't worry about it because I go to the LDS Hospital in Salt Lake and they give me blood from the LDS Blood Bank. I know it's safe."

"How do you know that?"

"The doctors there have told me the blood from LDS is the cleanest blood in the country."

"Well, that's where Dad got AIDS—from the clean blood at the LDS bank."

The man's face turned ashen and he made a hasty exit down the hall.

On the morning of Memorial Day, LaRee called me from the hospital. "Joleen, Dad's had a horrible hemorrhage. Dr. Wilcken says he's lost a large amount of blood."

"Where's he bleeding from?"

"Internally, but the doctors aren't sure where. He vomited pan after pan of bright red blood. It also came out of his nose, the corners of his eyes and his rectum."

I felt my knees weaken as the dreadful images built in my mind. Poor LaRee. From the sound of her voice I knew she was hanging on by a thread.

"It appears to have stopped now. Dr. Wilcken needs to know if we want him transfused."

"No, we don't. How long can he live without?"

"Wilcken says he couldn't last through the night."

"Does Orvin know about the bleeding?"

"Yes, but he hasn't left to come to the hospital yet."

"I'll try my best to convince him that Dad shouldn't be transfused. I'll persuade him to stay at home so you can take care of it."

"Dad's barely conscious. He isn't aware of anything."

As LaRee was returning to his room, a nurse stopped her and said, "I hope you're not going to order a transfusion for him. When are you going to just let him die?"

LaRee's anger erupted like a volcano. "For your information, no member of our family has ever asked for him to have a transfusion. The last year he's been on 'no code' status. He's never been on a respirator. The staff is afraid of getting AIDS and I'm tired of being blamed because he isn't dead. It was the damned medical profession that gave him AIDS. Go bitch at the blood bank."

LaRee burst into tears and ran to the waiting area. Convulsive sobs shook her body. Dr. Wilcken sat with my sister and tried to comfort her. "I'm so sorry you had to see this," he said. "You won't have to watch much more. It will soon be over."

LaRee shook her head. "For my family this will never be over."

Tears rolled down Dr. Wilcken's face as he shared a box of tissues with my sister.

Although it was like asking an old soldier to lay down his arms on the battlefield, Orvin did not oppose the transfusion decision. By now a part of him realized there was nothing more that could be done. It was the suffering that he couldn't stand to passively watch. He agreed to wait a day before returning to the hospital.

I was relieved, expecting that by then Dad would be gone. But again he defied all odds and lived. Dad was indeed as resilient as a scraggly greasewood being beaten down by continual storm.

"The doctors can't understand it," LaRee said. "They didn't think he could possibly live without a large transfusion of blood."

However, we were grateful that after the hemorrhage Dad was more peaceful with few outward signs of pain. The doctor said he was semi-comatose, usually in a deep stupor and unaware of his surroundings. For some weeks Dad had not been given any heart medication and his pulse was between 120 and 140.

"Doctor Wilcken can't understand how his heart keeps on pumping," Orvin said. "Wilcken says Dad has the strongest cardiovascular system he's ever seen and if we inherit it, we'll live to be 100."

I thought of how Dad had lived through one AIDS-related pneumonia after another without suffering heart failure or a heart attack. "It's hard to believe that we've gone through all this hell because of surgery on a heart that strong," I said.

"Dr. Ries says bypass rarely helps patients live longer. It just reduces chest pain," Orvin said.

By this time I had read the medical studies and was all too aware of that fact. It was one more example of something we had learned too late. Had we been told of the limited benefits of coronary bypass surgery, Dad would probably not have had it at that time. And if surgery were done, his own blood would have been recycled, had we known of that option, and our family would have arranged for one platelet donor. There's nothing more tragic than knowledge that comes too late. Our only comfort is that others may learn from our experience.

Shortly after Dad had surgery, his brother, Hank, was told by Dad's group of doctors that he was also in dire need of bypass surgery. However, Hank had the good sense to get a second opinion. He refused surgery and after six years is alive and doing moderately well on drug therapy. He recently celebrated his 80th birthday with a large party in his honor.

★　　★　　★

It was July and Dad had lived 34 days in the foggy twilight between life and death. He was getting morphine for pain. His heart rate stayed around 136, his blood pressure was often dangerously low and his fever raged between 102° and 105°. Yet he continued to hang on.

At three in the afternoon LaRee parked her car and entered the hospital. As she walked down the hall toward Dad's room she could hear his labored, gurgly breathing caused by the fluids that were building up in his chest. He was obviously worse and LaRee had witnessed too many painful scenes. The sound sent a chill through her.

"How long has he been breathing like that?" she asked Orvin.

"It just got worse a half hour ago."

"Have you eaten today?"

"No, I hated to leave him."

Orvin went out to eat and returned to the hospital. Dad's condition was unchanged and at 9:00 he left for Lapoint to get some sleep.

A nurse came in and took vital signs.

"I think the end might be near," LaRee said.

But the nurse was dubious. "His blood pressure has gone back up in the normal range," she said. "We've thought he was dying so many times. I'm beginning to think he never will."

LaRee prepared for a long night—the kind of night she and Orvin knew so well. Sometimes the depression from seeing Dad like this day after day overwhelmed her. He had not responded to her voice or touch for weeks.

Twice during the night LaRee rang the nurses' station to ask for assistance in cleaning Dad up and changing his bed. By 4:30 a.m. she was exhausted and lay down on a cot, trying to block out the rattling gasps Dad made as he struggled to breathe.

She did not want to remember her father in this distorted way. Her mind fled to the past in an effort to keep alive the memory of his former vitality, his humorous view of life. She recalled how hard he had worked 30 years before as Chairman of the Uintah County Commission to build the new administration building and public library. She was certain all that had been forgotten and Dad would merely be remembered as Uintah County's first AIDS case. It was as if this disease blotted out all that had gone before, overshadowing a lifetime of accomplishment.

Suddenly LaRee sat up. A welcome silence had filled the room after Dad's loud breathing stopped. My sister rang the nurse. "My father just died," she said.

It was the fourth of July.

★　　★　　★

Dad had wished to be buried in a casket of yellow pine. Several months before his death he asked if one could be made for him. Orvin placed the order and was later pleased with the finished casket. He described to Dad the exquisite workmanship and simple beauty of the wood grain.

After Dad's death LaRee made the funeral arrangements and returned to her home. Later that evening the phone rang. It was the mortician.

"I'm sorry to have to tell you this," he said. "Your father's long, difficult death left his body so contorted we can't get him into the custom casket."

"Can't you take out some of the padding?" LaRee asked.

"I'm afraid not. We already tried. The only way we can get him in would be to break his legs."

"I'll call you back," my sister said.

LaRee made the decision alone without upsetting the rest of the family.

After Dad's funeral, the procession circled the block by the church and stopped in front of the Swain home. The house and yards looked unchanged. The manicured lawns were still circled by artistic rock fences and planter boxes laden with vibrant flowers. I thought of how Dad and Orvin had meticulously chosen and placed each rock after arguing over which one would be just the right shape, color and size.

I recalled Mother's nurturing care of her flowers and the endless hours she had spent in the orchard picking fruit for canning. How we often picked a bushel of peas from the garden and sat under the pine tree while we shelled them. That tree was now enormous. I had grown up with it. When I was four feet tall, it was only three. But this home which had been an anchor for our family for so many bygone years was not the same. It was now branded as "the house of AIDS."

The hearse started to move forward. On both sides of the road were green, purple-tinged fields of hay. The fields where Dad had sweat and toiled for five decades to turn his land into one of the top producing farms in the Uintah Basin. Now his work was done. After 78 years he was leaving Lapoint.

Our procession passed Ft. Duchesne. Established before the turn of the century, it later became reservation headquarters for the Ute Indians. At one time government troops were stationed there to quell uprisings.

We continued on our way through Roosevelt, turned into the cemetery and stopped. The doors of the hearse swung open and the afternoon sun cast a reflection off Dad's casket of sleek steel. His two sons and four grandsons carried him to the prepared place beside Mother's grave. On Dad's right was the small grave of Rocky, the grandson he had loved so much. In the distance stood the silhouettes of a few surviving greasewood.

And it was there, surrounded by the dusty, wind-swept hills, that Orville Hatch Swain was laid to rest.

Chapter 10

A Boy Named Jonathan

Jonathan made up for his delayed classroom admission by attending summer school. At five years of age he was one of the youngest children in the nation to go to school with diagnosed AIDS. Colorado health officials hoped his case would serve as a model to encourage other school districts to accept children who also have the disease.

The small boy had decided that he wanted to be a policeman when he grew up because they "helped people." Although he was still sensitive to any signs of rejection, he was resigned to it. "Why don't they understand that I'm not going to give them my AIDS?" he sighed.

In the fall Jonathan was excited when the school district allowed him to attend a regular kindergarten. He would be going to the same school as his brother, Josh, who was two years older than him. "Josh is my best friend ever," he said. "He pulls my oxygen tank for me."

Jonathan had an obsessive interest in sharks. He loved them. Almost everyone he knew looked for shark toys to buy for him.

"Are there sharks in heaven?" he asked.

"Yes."

"Are they nice?"

"Everything is nice in heaven," his mother said.

By Christmas vacation Jonathan seemed more fatigued. His mother worried that the minor infections he had caught during the previous eight months of school had worn him down. "And at times his mind doesn't seem as sharp," she said.

However, he had enough pep to give out his want list for Santa—helicopters and sharks—and to participate in decorating the tree. Christmas was a magical time for Jonathan but the tree did not meet with his approval. "It's too blue," he complained. "It's not green enough."

He had a new puppy named Bojangles who ran around chewing on his toes and eating tree ornaments.

It was a normal Christmas-with-kids scene except that Jonathan had to be reminded to hook himself back into his oxygen. Though he seldom complained, the tube could get tangled in the wheels of the cart and trip him. When that happened, he would get up and either untangle it or disconnect it for a few minutes so he could be more active. Usually he was responsible about hooking it up again without a reminder.

Eventually Bojangles had to be given away because the neighbors feared he could carry the AIDS virus and would bite their children.

In early 1989 it was evident to Jonathan's doctors that his AIDS-related lung disease was worsening. Nevertheless, Jonathan persuaded them to let him stop using his oxygen. The doctors felt he had only a short time left to live and knew the quality of his life would improve if it were discontinued. They were impressed with the child's courage in coping with the adversity he had been given.

Shortly after being freed from the oxygen tubes, Jonathan was one of 15 children in the nation chosen to receive dideoxyenosine (DDI) in a trial study to determine its effectiveness against HIV. The drug was in the same family as AZT and would prove to be less toxic. However, it was necessary for Jonathan and Shiela to take a weekly flight from Denver to the National Institutes of Health in Bethesda, Maryland, for treatment.

Jonathan's condition soon improved significantly and he was mentally sharper. DDI counteracted the effects of the AIDS virus on his brain. He had more energy and less infections.

A year later, at Jonathan's birthday party in March 1990, there were few signs of outward illness as he took charge and bounced around the room with his friends. The weekly visits to the NIH had been cut down to once a month and Denver doctors were now monitoring his progress.

Jonathan's first grade teacher was at his party. Much to his mother's dismay, she gave him a water gun. Confetti littered the floor and leftover ice cream puddled on soggy paper plates but none of the adults cared about the mess. Jonathan had lived to see his seventh birthday—an achievement his doctors had not thought possible when they diagnosed AIDS four and a half years before.

During 1990, the book *My Name is Jonathan (and I Have AIDS)* was published. It was written by Jonathan and author Sharon Schilling for the purpose of educating students in kindergarten through sixth grade on the subject of AIDS. The book does much more. It is a tribute to a small boy's invincible spirit and the loving support of his family, friends and community.

Throughout, Jonathan shines as a loving, giving child with great compassion for those who hurt. He sees a dead robin and wishes it could be alive. He finds a dying duck at the lake and takes it home but is unable to save it. He understands his own disease and that it ends in death. He accepts it with sadness. "It's too bad I got AIDS," he says.

Dr. Franklyn Judson, Director of Denver Public Health, describes the book as "touching, personal, and scientifically accurate." It is currently used in schools to educate children about AIDS.

During the summer of 1990, Jonathan moved to a small community in another state with his mother, maternal grandparents, and brother, Josh. Several years before, his mother and father had divorced. Jonathan's entrance into school in the area where he now lives was without incident. Although the community knew he had AIDS, he was generally well accepted by the other children and their parents.

It was gratifying to Shiela that the past few years had brought progress in public understanding of AIDS. "I like to think that Jonathan played a small part in educating others about this disease," she said. "But much remains to be done."

Both the intravenous gamma globulin he received to slow serious bacterial infections and the DDI have contributed to Jonathan's longevity. He has handled the DDI well with few problems from side effects. His father said, "We're lucky that he can take DDI because it's the only drug out there for children and there's nothing new on the horizon."

In March 1991, Jonathan's grandmother had tears in her eyes as she watched him open his presents. "He's eight years old," she marveled. "He's so precious. Every birthday is a blessing."

During the summer, Jonathan's doctors took him off DDI because they were concerned that it was damaging his liver. However, by the time school started in the fall he was back on the drug and had gained a little weight. The small boy was delighted to be in school again. "I just love my teacher," he said.

He was also excited because he had been asked to talk at some of the local schools and tell the students about AIDS and how it cannot be contracted by casual contact. All his life Jonathan has been upset and hurt that some children aren't allowed to play with him. However, after he spoke at the high school he was exhilarated. "The kids sure asked me a lot of questions," he said. "But I told them everything they wanted to know about AIDS."

★　　　★　　　★

Jonathan dragged himself into the house after playing with his brother, Josh. Shiela poured a glass of juice and took it over to the couch where her son was curled into an exhausted ball. There was always an unsettled uneasiness at the bottom of her heart from the tragic memories of the past and the grim prognosis of the future.

"I love to play so much," Jonathan said. "But I can only do it for a little while 'cuz I get so tired. That's why I play real hard."

"If you would take it easier you could play longer."

"No, Mom," he sighed wearily. "I tried doing that—it doesn't work."

The pervasive fatigue is a part of his illness that forces Jonathan to face the reality of his condition. But he struggles to conceal it because he feels guilty that his death will bring others so much pain.

He asked his Grandmother Swain, "You know, don't you, that I'm going to die?" Then seeing her eyes fill with tears he quickly added, "No, I'm not—just kidding." He anxiously searched her face. "Do you feel better now, Grandma?"

However, all who know him are impressed with how much Jonathan enjoys and appreciates every minute of his life. Despite what he's been through he is usually a very happy child. Jonathan Swain has lived seven years since being diagnosed with full-blown AIDS in 1985—longer than any other child with the disease. His is one of the "happy" AIDS stories.

Part II

Exposé—
The Truth About
Blood Safety

Chapter 11

All Swain Family AIDS Infections Were Avoidable

For the past decade, most of America has considered the spread of AIDS to be the sole result of sexual excesses and drug abuse. But other causes should be added to the list. Deceiving past and future transfusion recipients ranks near the top, as should policies shaped by self interest and regulatory agencies who shirk their mandated duty to protect the public health. It's time to drop the double standard of blame. Sex and drugs aren't the only cause of AIDS.

Jonathan Swain

On March 20, 1983, the neonatologist informed Jonathan Swain's parents that their newborn infant needed a transfusion. The baby's father, my cousin Dee Swain, requested directed donation. Dee wished to have family members donate all blood necessary for his son.

Directed donation has been a controversial issue since the beginning of the AIDS epidemic. In the early 1980s blood banks generally opposed and discouraged its use. They, along with doctors and hospitals, frequently refused the requests of patients and families. Transfusion recipients were told that the blood of relatives and friends was no safer than regular banked blood.

A 1986 study concluded blood banks had additional reasons for their lack of cooperation on the directed donation issue. One reason was that the donations of relatives and friends were inconvenient for blood banks to process and took extra staff time. But more importantly, the blood industry feared that an acceptance of directed donation programs would be perceived by the public as a lack of confidence in the regular blood supply. Policies against directed donation were shaped by blood banking interests.

Dr. Daniel Hall and the Lutheran Medical Center in Denver refused the request for directed donation and Jonathan was transfused with AIDS-tainted blood.

Almost a decade has passed since Jonathan received the blood supplied from the Belle Bonfils Memorial Blood Center. One of the donors was infected with HIV. Yet all of the directed donors Dee had lined up to give blood for his baby remain free of the viral infection. Jonathan's life-long illness, his eventual death from AIDS and his family's devastation could have easily been avoided. The honoring of my cousin's simple request for directed donation would have eliminated all the heartache.

Orville Swain

There were three ways my father's AIDS infection could have been avoided:

1. The HIV-positive donor should have been provided educational information on AIDS and been verbally screened to determine if he was at risk.

2. The infected donor's blood should have been eliminated by use of the hepatitis B core antibody test.

3. A combination of directed donation and IAT should have been used for my father's blood replacement which would have eliminated all exposure to regular banked blood.

Donor Education and Screening

In a deposition taken seven years after my father's surgery, the HIV-positive donor described how he was not given any information on AIDS or asked any questions to determine risk or symptoms of AIDS. The donor first gave blood in 1984. He made a donation in June and another in December which was the one Dad received. He said the subject of AIDS was totally ignored by LDS Blood Bank personnel at the time of both donations. The FDA had required AIDS educational materials to be provided and some verbal screening since March 1983.

The Hepatitis B Core Test

My father got both AIDS and hepatitis B from his transfusion. If the LDS Blood Bank had used the long-disputed core antibody test for hepatitis B, it would have eliminated the infected donor's blood.

In early 1985 the LDS Blood Bank was using just one test for hepatitis. That test was a measurement of surface protein which is *usually* produced in excess and is detectable in the blood of an infectious hepatitis B donor. However, it is possible for the surface protein test to be negative even though the blood is capable of transmitting hepatitis B. According to the book *Blood, Blood Products and AIDS*, "if this does happen, the antibody to the core of the 'e' protein of HBV is detectable in the donation." The core test, so strongly resisted by blood bankers, detects the antibody to this core protein. If the LDS Blood Bank had used the core test in addition to the surface protein test, my father would not have been infected.

Transfusion Options

Prior to surgery, the LDS Hospital should have offered my father options to regular banked blood and a combination of directed donation and IAT should have been used. The family could have chosen one donor to provide the number of platelets Dad got from eight donors. And using IAT procedures, blood lost during surgery would have been collected for later reinfusion. IAT technology had been available for 10 years and large Utah hospitals already had the capability.

However, not one word was said to Dad or our family about transfusion alternatives. We weren't even told of the risk of AIDS and hepatitis. When discussing his surgery, doctors and hospital staff never brought up the subject of transfusion. It was not an informed consent item.

Ora Swain

My mother's AIDS infection would have been avoided if the LDS Blood Bank and Hospital had called Dad in for AIDS testing and counseling when they first learned in June 1985 that one of his donors was positive. Elderly people in their 70's do not use condoms unless instructed to do so and abstinence should have been advised.

By 1985 it was well known that transfusion recipients who received AIDS-infected blood became infected and could pass the infection to their sexual partners. Evidence of HIV transmission from male to female was well established. A blood bank does not have the ability to determine if an older couple will be celibate.

Under federal law, hospitals are required to keep transfusion records listing recipients' donors for at least five years. Blood banks keep registries on donors who test positive for AIDS, hepatitis and other blood-borne illnesses so that these donors can be excluded from future donation.

After HIV testing began it was not unusual for some donors from a blood bank's regular donor pool to test positive for HIV. These AIDS-positive donors were added to the bank's dangerous donor registry. A look back program, such as the one in use for hepatitis, then traced the recipients who had been given the prior donations of these positive donors. If the donor had donated blood regularly for years, a large number of people could have been infused with it before the AIDS test was available. The question was: how long had the donor been infected with AIDS? Those who had most recently received the infected donor's blood were at highest risk.

When Dad's donor was found to be HIV-positive in June 1985, it was almost certain that he would have been infectious when he gave the donation Dad received five months earlier. It can take six months before the body produces antibodies for the test to detect. But during that time the infection can be given to others.

However, after my father was identified from hospital records as the recipient of that prior suspect donation, he was not notified, tested or counseled. Neither was he informed in April of 1986 when the AABB, of which the LDS Blood Bank is a member, the Council of Community Blood Centers and the American Red Cross recommended that all prior transfusion recipients of HIV-positive donors be notified and tested for the AIDS infection.

Dad had been impotent for a considerable time after his heart surgery, well after the blood bank had found his positive donor and knew he was almost certain to be infected with AIDS. Mother's sexual infection was a result of the blood bank's concealment of life-saving information from my father.

Chapter 12

Safe Blood Crock-Talk

For decades the public was incorrectly led to believe the blood supply was safe. When that safety image was tarnished by AIDS, public health officials and blood bankers formulated a more convincing language. Our family called the verbiage "crock-talk" because it consisted of a barrage of meaningless statistics, ambiguous half-truths and a few blatant lies. For transfusion and clotting factor recipients, safe blood crock-talk became the language of death.

A Meaningless Statistic: *"The risk of getting AIDS from a blood transfusion is less than one in a million."*

On August 2, 1983, Dr. Joseph Bove appeared before the House Subcommittee on AIDS. Dr. Bove was chairman of the FDA's Blood Products Advisory Committee and of the American Association of Blood Banks' (AABB) Committee on Transfusion Transmitted Diseases.

At the hearings, the doctor presented his charts and tables of the following meaningless statistics which did not have the support of evidence:

1. The risk of getting AIDS from a blood transfusion was less than one in a million.

2. The average American had twice the chance of dying in a flood than from AIDS contracted through a transfusion.

3. A Californian should be twice as concerned about dying in an earthquake as from transfused AIDS.

4. Anyone having an appendicitis operation would have 20 times the chance of death.

Dr. Bove did not discuss the chances of a newborn baby and an elderly man from the Swain family both contracting AIDS from transfusions. If asked, I'm sure he would have said the chance was infinitesimal, almost beyond the ability of statisticians to compute.

Dr. Bove continued to churn out his creative statistical risks for some time, but by the spring of 1984 his concern had shifted to the danger of bees. Bove told the *Wall Street Journal* that bee stings kill more people than transfusion AIDS.

Orvin is not a statistician but he observed, "There weren't two million Swains in Utah and Colorado." Orvin doubts that there are ten thousand Swains in America.

Until testing for AIDS began in early 1985, the one-in-a-million risk was continually parroted by health officials and blood bankers. There were an estimated four million transfusions given in the United States each year with an average of 5.4 component units used for each transfusion. With a one-in-a-million risk, the total HIV (AIDS) infections from the four million transfusions would be four per year. The AIDS virus is believed to have been in the blood supply since 1978. If the one-in-a-million theory were valid, there would have been only 28 transfused AIDS infections given in the seven years before 1985.

Instead, a Centers of Disease Control (CDC) study states, "We estimate that 29,000 transfusion recipients of all ages from these years (1978-1984) received a unit of blood infected by HIV." At four million per year, the number of transfusions given during the seven-year period was 28 million from which 29,000 people received infected units. Therefore, according to the CDC study, the risk of getting HIV from a transfusion during these combined years was not one in a million but one in 965! In 1983, during which the CDC estimates 8,400 infections were given, the risk was one in 476. And studies have found that in high-risk cities like Los Angeles it was as high as one in 100.

A Misleading Truth: *"Less than half the people who receive HIV-infected blood transfusions will get AIDS."*

This misleading statement is still occasionally heard from health officials and blood bankers. The public is led to believe there is more than a 50/50 chance of surviving a tainted transfusion. That is untrue.

Almost everyone who receives a transfusion containing HIV will become infected with the AIDS virus, but approximately 60% will die from their original illnesses within a year. Therefore, over half of those infected will not live long enough to develop AIDS. Yet the public should not be misled into believing that an HIV-contaminated transfusion is inefficient in transmitting AIDS. Dr. Elizabeth Donegan, the lead author of a 1990 medical study, told Associated Press, "It's important not to have any illusions about how infectious HIV is. If it's there in the transfusion, you'll get it." How many patients considering elective surgery would be willing to die early from their illness to avoid getting AIDS from a contaminated transfusion?

A Misleading Half Truth: *"Concern about the safety of the blood supply is unwarranted except for hemophiliacs and those requiring large amounts of blood."*

This is an earlier quote of health officials which was often used in the media. Actually there was reason for concern for patients receiving *any* amount of blood, large or small. But the risk multiplied with each unit received. By leaving much unsaid, the above statement was effective in diverting attention away from prospective surgery patients who were not medically sophisticated enough to recognize the danger they were in. Most Americans are not knowledgeable about the types of surgical procedures that require "large amounts of blood." Our family was not aware that bypass surgery could necessitate the transfusing of up to 50 component units of blood.

An Untruth: *"I want to assure the American people that the blood supply is 100% safe."*

This is probably the biggest blood lie of all time, spoken in July 1983 by the country's number one health official, Margaret Heckler, Secretary of the Department of Health and Human Services. Compare this to the following statement made by Brian McDonough, President of the Irwin Blood Bank in San Francisco, appearing on ABC TV's "20/20": "The blood supply has never been safe. The public is being told it is safe. This is just not true. Blood is a very dangerous drug."

The book *Blood, Blood Products and AIDS* published by John Hopkins Press lists the known types of infectious agents (germs) that can be given to a patient through transfusion. The viral category includes hepatitis A; hepatitis B; hepatitis non-A, non-B; cytomegalovirus and Epstein-Barr virus. Parasitic diseases that can be spread through the blood supply include: malaria, filariasis, trypanosomiasis, toxoplasmosis and babesiosis. Syphilis is yet another type of infection that can be transmitted through blood transfusion, as can many different disease-causing bacterial organisms.

There have been millions of hepatitis infections given by transfusion in the United States during the past two decades. The danger of viral infection escalated with the appearance of retroviruses, and HIV became the most deadly organism in the history of blood banking. There is some concern that another new or "improved" virus could bring the next future disease and repeat the AIDS crisis. It's possible that could be happening in the 1990's. A few patients with an AIDS-like illness are not testing positive for HIV.

Is it possible for the blood supply to be 100% safe? No. In fact some experts feel blood transfusions are the biggest obstacle to a safe recovery after surgery.

Another Untruth: *"The blood supply is safe both for the hemophiliac and for the average citizen who might need it for surgery,"*

Secretary Heckler told the press. Hemophilia is an inherited bleeding disorder which is passed in genetic code from mother to son. A family with hemophilia can have several boys who use Factor VIII, a substance that when injected helps their blood to clot normally. Without treatment, cuts may bleed for days and bleeding into joints can cause crippling deformities.

Factor VIII is made from the pooled blood plasma of up to 48,000 donors per batch. Before the clotting factors were pasteurized in 1985, the hemophiliac risk for getting AIDS was horrendous. Such was the tragic fate of the three young Ray boys in Florida who are all infected with HIV.

In the *Saturday Evening Post*, Dr. Theresa Crenshaw, member of the Presidential AIDS Commission assigned to safety in the blood supply, wrote, "Up to 90% of hemophiliacs requiring blood products have become infected with AIDS, and most were infected while the blood industry delayed taking precautionary measures."

The CDC has a category for reporting AIDS cases resulting from hemophilia products and a separate category for reporting cases resulting from transfusions. The cases from both categories must be added to determine the number of AIDS cases from banked blood and clotting factors. The *HIV/AIDS Surveillance Report* with statistics through June 1992 lists 2,054 hemophilia cases and 4,959 transfusion cases for a total of 7,013 AIDS cases from contaminated blood or clotting factors. This number is extremely low compared to the CDC estimate of 29,000 AIDS infections given via banked blood and another 10,000 given by clotting factors. It's obvious the number of reported AIDS cases do not reflect the magnitude of HIV infection through these routes.

A Half Truth: *"We did all we could," say the blood bankers. "We didn't have a test for AIDS."*

This statement can be refuted by the fact that they did not use surrogate tests for AIDS and they did not defer gay men from their donor pools at an earlier date. Steps were not taken during the late '70s to implement all available tests for hepatitis. Red Cross experts now admit that had the blood banks been using additional laboratory tests for hepatitis in the early 1980s, half of the AIDS contamination in the blood supply would have been removed even before the presence of the disease was known. Other experts feel considerably *more* than half would have been removed as AIDS and hepatitis frequented the same high risk groups.

In January 1983, the CDC requested a meeting with representatives from the FDA, National Institutes of Health (NIH), American Red Cross, AABB, CCBC and the Pharmaceutical Manufacturers Association. CDC researchers and epidemiologists were alarmed at the mounting evidence that AIDS was contaminating the nation's blood supply. However, they had no authority to take action that would protect transfusion recipients; the blood supply is under the jurisdiction of the FDA.

At the meeting, one of the CDC's top virologists, Dr. Thomas Spira, presented evidence to support the CDC's plea for the testing of all blood and blood products with surrogate tests to eliminate donors who were at risk for AIDS. At the time, there was no AIDS-specific test because the virus had not yet been identified. However, the hepatitis B core antibody test could detect donors who had a prior history of hepatitis B. Most gay men and intravenous drug users had such a history. Dr. Spira's test results indicated that the core test could identify 80% to 95% of the patients with AIDS and could be used to eliminate two-thirds of the donors whose behavior put them at high risk for the new disease.

The CDC doctors hoped that the blood industry would agree to test all blood or, at the very least, would adopt strict guidelines to prevent people in high-risk groups from donating. As it turned out, neither of these objectives was achieved and the meeting erupted into a fracas.

Each group represented had its interests to protect. The FDA group was annoyed because it felt the CDC was trying to usurp its authority over blood policy. At first, the blood bankers chose to deny the existence of an AIDS epidemic and attempted to argue down the CDC evidence. But eventually they focused on the cost of the core test and the loss of what they knew would be 6% of their free product—those donations that would test positive. Blood bankers also insisted that adoption of the test would do nothing to improve blood safety.

The refusal to use the core test was not a result of pressure from the gay movement. There were leaders from gay groups present at the Atlanta meeting. They did not object to the testing of blood but strongly opposed the screening of donors. Surrogate testing could have discreetly begun with little opposition from gay groups.

The assembly adjourned with no plan of action. Donald Francis, a retrovirologist who directed the CDC's research laboratory on AIDS, was both angry and vocal during the day's discussions. At one point, he pounded the table with his fist and shouted, "How many people have to die? How many deaths do you need?"

Nine years later, after he left the employ of the CDC, Dr. Francis talked of the frustration he had felt in early 1983. During testimony before a jury in Denver he said, "It was frustration I had in their inability to accept the reality that AIDS could be transmitted through transfusions. It was something like having a bend in the train track and sitting there, and you hear the whistles and the signals are blinking, and the tracks are beginning to shake, and they're saying, 'There's no train coming.'"

But there is evidence that suggests blood leaders *did* realize a train was coming. Three weeks after the Atlanta meeting, Dr. Joseph Bove, whose public stand was that the blood supply was safe with less than a one-in-a-million risk of AIDS, sent his Committee on Transfusion Transmitted Diseases a memo. In his memo Dr. Bove stated that he was certain there would soon be more cases of AIDS contracted from transfusions and he believed that the most blood bankers could do was "buy time." He wrote, "We do not want anything that we do now to be interpreted by society (or by the legal authorities) as agreeing with the concept—as yet unproven—that AIDS can be spread by blood." Dr. Bove's colleagues were urged, "I hope that we are equipped psychologically to continue to act together."

Before the memo was written, CDC doctors had informed the blood industry that AIDS was an exploding epidemic and that the virus was transmitted through transfusions and clotting factors. The American Association of Blood Banks' Committee on Transfusion Disease believed transfusion AIDS cases would continue to mount. Yet instead of protecting the public, blood leaders chose to stall while they debated and studied the issue to death. Unfortunately, transfusion and clotting factor recipients could not "buy time." Dr. Francis testified that "tens of thousands of Americans" died because of the blood industry's slow response.

In their exposé, "Inside the Billion-Dollar Business of Blood," *Money* magazine concluded: "The problem is that building an ever-increasing supply of blood feeds the industry's revenues, while taking steps to make blood safer, or to reduce unnecessary transfusions does not. Blood suppliers are looking at the bottom line."

Ross D. Eckert is an economics professor who has studied the blood industry and serves on the FDA Blood and Blood Products Committee. In the *Reader's Digest* special report titled "How Safe is the Blood Supply?" Mr. Eckert is quoted as follows: "Blood banks are portrayed as heroic, altruistic organizations. But in most communities they have been either monopolies or cartels. Tight screening forces them to discard more product which means lost revenues, and to solicit even more donors. That's why they were slow to respond to the AIDS threat."

However, the failure of blood banks to use surrogate tests for hepatitis and AIDS before 1987 was also partly due to medical differences of opinion over the seriousness of the two diseases and the cause of AIDS. But probably more significant was the mindset of blood banking leaders forged by 40 years of blood monopoly—a tendency for complacency and an unhealthy resistance to change or criticism.

The HIV-specific test for screening out donors infected with AIDS was implemented in March 1985. Two years later, in 1987 the hepatitis B core test was also implemented. Suddenly the test that would do nothing to improve transfusion safety in 1983 was credible. The AIDS crisis had focused public attention on the blood supply. The extremely high post-transfusion hepatitis risk which had been downplayed by the blood industry during the 1970s was attracting media attention. And despite the exemption of blood from product liability, hepatitis and AIDS lawsuits were mounting. Because of increased consumer concern and the threat of litigation, blood banks finally adopted the hepatitis B core test.

A Lame Excuse: *"But," say the blood bankers, "we didn't know how bad the AIDS threat was. We were dealing with an unknown virus."*

To a lay person it is inconceivable that doctors and scientists, faced with a killer virus they didn't understand, would have chosen to err on the side of risk rather than on the side of caution. But at the very beginning of the AIDS epidemic, many doctors in the blood industry believed the new disease among gay men and hemophiliacs was an immune disorder caused by frequent exposure to foreign human protein. Some scientists were further confused by the long, variable incubation period between infection and the time AIDS symptoms appeared. They doubted that the illness was caused by a virus.

At the beginning of the epidemic these were honest, understandable mistakes. However, the CDC is considered to be the world's most expert organization in combating epidemics. Trained to take swift action, CDC doctors soon became convinced that a virus was the cause of AIDS and that it was transmitted in the same ways as hepatitis B. The CDC scientists presented an urgent warning to blood leaders, accompanied by a plea for adoption of the hepatitis B core test. Blood banking leaders chose to ignore the warning.

While initial scientific disagreement is understandable, the lengthy foot-dragging of the blood industry in protecting the blood supply is indefensible. There was a delay of over two years without any testing whatsoever to identify suspect donors—despite a constantly growing mountain of evidence which proved the blood supply was contaminated. The plea by CDC doctors for use of the core test was made on January 4, 1983.

Exactly two years to the day later—January 4, 1985—my father was transfused with blood containing both the hepatitis B and AIDS viruses. The core test would have prevented his AIDS death and the HIV infections of many thousands of other transfusion recipients between 1983 and March 1985. The central question is: how much time did blood banking leadership need to buy before changing their "scientific" opinion? A non-expert, responding with common sense instead of the arrogant indifference displayed by the blood monopoly, would have heeded the CDC doctors' warning and traveled the road of caution in early 1983.

A Dangerous Exaggeration: *"The AIDS antibody test has virtually eliminated any risk of AIDS from the blood supply."*

This assurance is constantly heard at the present time. Although the risk of getting AIDS in a blood transfusion is significantly reduced, it can still happen. The present antibody test can miss some donors who are positive because there is a "window" between the moment of infection and the time antibodies are developed. During the window period the test will be negative but the donor will be infected and contagious. Usually this window is from two weeks to three months, but in a significant number of cases, it can be up to six months. And a few people may never develop antibodies to the AIDS virus. As a result of some AIDS-positive donors not being detected, health authorities estimate as many as 460 blood recipients a year can be infected with HIV.

But the risk from the test's inadequacy must be added to yet another risk: the increasing problems blood banks are having with human and computer error. A medical textbook published by John Hopkins Press reports: "The experience of blood transfusion services over many years is that serious failures in the release of infected donations are more often the result of human error than of an intrinsic inadequacy of laboratory tests."

Human error may occur at every stage of testing, particularly in transferring specimens, adding reagents (substances that chemically react to detect other substances) and recording results. When testing for hepatitis and AIDS, the reagents must be of the highest quality and be checked each day to ensure accuracy.

The complex computer systems used to track blood from collection to transfusion and to permanently defer infected donors are crucial to blood safety. Any failure in these systems or any data entry errors can cost the lives of blood recipients. Blood banking is a complex business requiring meticulous labeling of blood and safe storage at exact temperatures.

Gilbert Gaul, the *Philadelphia Inquirer*'s Pulitzer Prize-winning reporter on the blood industry, studied FDA records between March 1988 and March 1989. During that year the FDA ordered blood banks and plasma centers to recall nearly 100,000 blood components and medicines because they had been mistakenly released.

In April 1990 the FDA ordered Belle Bonfils Blood Center in Denver to recall 11,000 units of blood for retesting. The FDA was afraid the blood might contain either AIDS or hepatitis as a result of incorrect testing. The center's staff had followed the wrong procedures for mixing test chemicals for a period of seven weeks. By the time of recall, 10,670 units (97% of 11,000) had already been transfused into patients at 55 Colorado hospitals. Sample vials of each unit had been kept, but most of them had been discarded before retesting began.

Dr. Joel Levine, president of Denver's University Hospital medical board, said the "statistical risk" was that one of the 11,000 pints of blood drawn would be infected with the AIDS virus. Dr. Levine did not explain that if one HIV-infected pint were drawn, it would be divided into at least three component units and given to a minimum of three patients. Neither was the press told that there was a high risk of getting hepatitis from a transfusion of the incorrectly tested blood.

For over a week I recorded the meaningless statistics and reassuring half truths that were fed to the Colorado media. Panic was avoided. But our family knows the absence of public panic will be of small comfort to those who will suffer from the blood-borne illnesses resulting from this fiasco in human error.

This latest incident was not the first for Belle Bonfils. In 1988 the FDA had reprimanded the center for distributing 22 units of blood despite initial test results showing them to be contaminated. These units were transfused into 45 people.

In 1989 a jury ordered Belle Bonfils to pay $5.5 million to a woman who got AIDS from blood supplied in 1985. The center had not tested the blood although it was equipped to do so.

Today there is still a risk of getting AIDS from a blood transfusion. The window period allows a few infected units to slip through the test undetected. Furthermore, computers and personnel are prone to make mistakes. Therefore, "virtually every unit" of HIV tainted blood has *not* been eliminated from the blood supply.

A Pressure Tactic: *"The media has a responsibility to report on the blood supply in a manner that will not erode public confidence or induce panic."*

This message was given to reporters covering the House Subcommittee Hearing on Blood Supply Safety in July 1990 and is a major reason why consumers have been so slow to understand that blood can be a dangerous medical product. For the last decade blood centers and public health officials have implied that the public is better served if problems in blood safety are played down or left unreported.

The media is often admonished to "report the facts." However, public relations releases from blood banks are not always limited to facts and are usually misleading. A TV reporter affiliated with one of the major networks told me, "Reporting on the blood supply is the most frustrating assignment I can have. Last week the local blood bank lied to me three times." Statements by blood banks must be carefully studied for bias and self interest.

A Fear Stratagem: *"Nothing can be allowed to impair the availability of blood and we will do whatever is necessary to make sure nothing does."*

A blood banker made this statement to the *San Francisco Chronicle* in 1989. This type of statement implies there is a danger of running out of blood and endangering patient care. The possibility of blood shortages was one of the arguments used against adoption of the core antibody test. It is not unusual for reporters to be reminded that the viability of the entire health care delivery system depends on an adequate blood supply.

As the health care industry had revenues of $672 billion in 1990 and accounted for 12.2% of the gross national product, any talk of disruption also causes big-dollar concern.

However, the shortages that blood leaders said would occur if surrogate tests were implemented for hepatitis and AIDS, never materialized. After those and other tests were eventually adopted, a medical study concluded there was an *absence* of nationwide blood shortages during the 1980s. Actually, blood banks can always recruit new donors to replace the ones who are deferred or they can purchase blood from other areas. But these measures are likely to increase the cost of blood to local hospitals.

Another reason shortages were avoided is that during most of the 1980s it was unnecessary to collect and transfuse so much homologous (regular donor) blood. In 1986, Dr. Dennis Donahue, former director of the FDA's Blood and Blood Products Laboratory told ABC TV's "20/20," "Much of the blood transfused is unnecessary. All blood products are overused. Doctors order too much blood."

It has been recognized in blood banking circles for well over a decade that the use of banked blood could be dramatically reduced by practicing blood conservation and by implementing autologous blood programs in which patients are reinfused with their own blood. The book *Autologous and Directed Blood Programs* published in 1987 by the AABB estimated that up to 50% of all surgical procedures could be performed with autologous programs alone.

Both health establishments and patients would benefit if options to traditional transfusion were universally encouraged by doctors, hospitals, and blood banks. The Presidential AIDS Commission concluded: "Some regional blood centers have been hesitant to promote strategies that minimize the use of transfusion therapies since their operating income is derived from the sale of blood and blood products." Although the use of IAT is growing, there are still some hospitals and doctors who prefer to reassure patients that their local blood supply is safe and continue to provide transfusion therapy in the old way.

However, a growing number of patients are predonating their own blood before surgery. Hospitals and blood banks discouraged predonation in the early 1980s because it is cumbersome to administer but they now willingly provide the service to those having major surgery. Unfortunately, not all surgeons encourage eligible major surgery patients to donate their own blood. And patients having minor surgery are usually discouraged or talked out of making donations.

Until the AIDS crisis there was little patient interest in donating several pints of blood before surgery because the public had been kept in the dark about the risks of being transfused with someone else's blood. Before that time, doing whatever was necessary to maintain the availability of blood rarely included promotion of the concept that patients can often give themselves a transfusion and avoid the risk of viral infections.

A Simple Truth: *"AIDS is political. You must weigh the political orientation of any statement made by the medical establishment."*

This statement was made by an epidemiologist who worked for a health department counseling and testing people for HIV. Sadly, it appears to be true. Once a position is taken on an AIDS issue, all health professionals are expected to fall into line. When the FDA allowed blood banks to avoid using surrogate tests for AIDS, those few who did test came under severe criticism.

The break from rank brought vilification. This was the experience of Dr. Edgar Engleman, medical director of the blood bank at Stanford University Hospital. He couldn't agree with the downplayed position of blood leaders on the spread of AIDS through transfusions. Neither did Dr. Engleman agree that surrogate testing for AIDS was "of no value." In May 1983 Dr. Engleman began using not the core test, but another test measuring helper-suppressor ratios of T-cells—a test indicating status of the immune system. The doctor believed it would reject donors with severe immune abnormalities of the type seen in AIDS patients.

Dr. Engleman was firm in his resolve to not use any untested blood at Stanford. Other blood bankers were furious that he had taken contrary action at a time when lack of unity was embarrassing to their position. They said Dr. Engleman's use of screening tests for AIDS was a gimmick—an advertising ploy to pull patients away from other hospitals.

The efforts of some doctors to get screening tests implemented for blood donations were ignored. Shortly after the Atlanta meeting, a group of California doctors issued a public appeal for blood banks to use the hepatitis core test on the nation's unprotected blood supply. Their appeal went unheeded. In early May 1983, Dr. Dale Lawrence of the CDC met with blood banking leaders and presented 10 additional cases of AIDS that had been transmitted by blood transfusion or hemophilia clotting factors. During June, CDC experts in infectious disease again presented growing evidence of blood supply contamination and warned leaders that blood banks could face negligence suits if they refused to use the core test and continued to dispense blood suspected of being tainted with AIDS. But unfortunately, blood leaders viewed their concerned critics as a mother cat does a kitten playing with her tail—a mere nuisance.

However, the leaders intensified their efforts to reassure the public the blood supply was safe. The AABB, the American Red Cross and the

Counsel of Community Blood Centers issued a joint statement condemning irrational fears about transfusions being a vehicle of AIDS death. The statement asserted that even if there was any link between AIDS and transfusions, the risk was less than one in a million.

It was in early July that Secretary of Health, Margaret Heckler, donated blood at the Red Cross blood center in Washington, DC, and told the press the blood supply was "100% safe." There was not a physician or a scientist in the entire Red Cross blood organization who believed the blood supply was anywhere near 100% free of hepatitis and other viral infections. Yet the well-intended Heckler was duped into telling America that it was. And both Assistant Secretary for Health Dr. Edward Brandt and the FDA went along with the exaggerated claim of a one-in-a-million risk which was not based on any scientific proof. It's ironic that while blood leaders were quoting their *unfounded* one-in-a-million, they were refusing to take action to test blood because there wasn't enough scientific proof that they should do so.

The evidence points to a conspiracy of the Red Cross, the two major blood trade organizations and public health authorities to mislead the public on the issue of blood safety and keep the danger of transfusions downplayed. Silence on those dangers predated the arrival of AIDS with the downplaying of astronomical numbers of hepatitis infections given to transfusion recipients during the 1970s. It will be argued that the blood conspiracy is well intended—that it is benign. The malignant consequences suggest otherwise.

Also disturbing is the public discrediting of doctors who question the safety of the blood supply. On March 9, 1988, Surgeon General C. Everett Koop was interviewed on ABC TV's "Good Morning America" and attacked the conclusions of authors Dr. William Masters, Dr. Virginia Johnson, and Dr. Robert Kolody of the book, *Crisis: Heterosexual Behavior in the Age of AIDS*. Dr. Koop accused the authors of using scare tactics and being irresponsible and unscientific. He was referring to the doctors' warning of the growing danger of heterosexual spread of AIDS and also to their conclusion that the blood supply, after three years of testing for HIV, was still far from safe. Koop said he feared the book would cause "hysteria" and pleaded with Americans to "stick to their usual habit of listening to the facts, sorting them out and doing what's right." In the ensuing weeks, Dr. Koop was joined by other health officials and researchers, all voicing extremely strong criticism of the book.

On March 22, 1988, a response to the criticism was written by syndicated columnist Thomas Sowell. Mr. Sowell pointed out that *Crisis* is unique because its orientation is toward protecting the general public against AIDS—in contrast to the orientation of most other medical authorities, public health officials and politicians who protect their own political interests. Sowell pointed out that many lives had already been lost because the public health establishment had delayed testing the blood supply and called the criticism of the book hysterical and distorted.

He concluded, "This is a book by qualified and responsible researchers writing about matters of life and death. It deserves serious analysis, not the politicized, knee-jerk responses all too common among those whose policies and party line have been challenged."

It is vital that past public statements on blood safety be analyzed under the harsh light of reality. Otherwise health consumers listening to the present assurances of a safe blood supply may believe that problems do not still exist. Uninformed consumers are not motivated to donate their own blood or to demand the many available options for safe transfusion therapy.

The blood conspiracy has been vast in its scope, long in its duration and devastating in its results. It will not be broken without consumer involvement. Several years ago I was told by a member of the Presidential Commission on AIDS, "The victims are the only ones who can tell the story of unsafe blood." Perhaps this is true—dissenting doctors have to work within the system.

Chapter 13

Scientific Intrigue, Politics and the AIDS Blood Test

For the U.S. Public Health Service, AIDS made its presence known at the worst possible time. Beginning during the Carter Administration, the FDA experienced cutbacks in personnel which continued throughout the early years of the AIDS crisis. Between 1977 and 1984 the agency's number of inspectors dropped by 22%. Because the FDA monitors several huge industries in addition to blood and plasma centers, inspectors were spread very thin.

All the public health agencies were adjusting to reduced funding. Sandra Panem reports in *The AIDS Bureaucracy* that in fiscal year 1982 the "CDC alone reduced its personnel approximately 30%." The health agencies did not have the resources to track and research a new disease of the AIDS magnitude. Moreover, at the first of the epidemic, the Reagan Administration failed to recognize the seriousness of the deadly viral threat and did not provide leadership for a coordinated AIDS response.

Tight funding slowed AIDS research and fueled intra-agency rivalries within the public health system. Some agencies felt the CDC had "invented" the AIDS epidemic to get a larger share of money. Turf struggles surfaced between the FDA and CDC over blood policy. There was competition between the National Cancer Institute (NCI), the National Institute of Allergy and Infectious Diseases (NIAID) and the CDC over the sharing of blood and tissue samples from AIDS patients. The CDC found it easier to work with the Pasteur Institute in France than with Dr. Robert Gallo at the NCI in Bethesda, Maryland. Specimens and samples were flown across the Atlantic Ocean between France and the CDC in Atlanta, Georgia.

Much of the scientific competition centered on efforts to discover the virus that caused AIDS. The top contenders in the race were researchers at the National Cancer Institute and the Pasteur Institute. Dr. Robert Gallo was chief of the NCI's laboratory of Tumor Cell Biology. Gallo had isolated the first human retrovirus in 1980, the T-cell leukemia virus HTLV-1. In 1982 a Gallo co-worker isolated a second retrovirus in the same family. It was called HTLV-2. By February 1983 Gallo was convinced that AIDS was caused by a variation of HTLV-1 or 2 but he had been unable to isolate it.

In May 1983 the Pasteur research team of Montagnier, Chermann and Barre-Sinoussi published their discovery of a different class of human retrovirus which they were certain was the cause of AIDS. The French virus became known as LAV.

After the Pasteur's work was published, Gallo became alarmed that the French would get credit for discovering the AIDS virus ahead of his laboratory. The stakes were high. Discovery would bring scientific prestige, an expected Nobel Prize and handsome profits from royalties on patented AIDS tests. Rumors were spread that the French discovery was not a virus but merely contaminants from other viruses that were in the Pasteur lab. When Gallo continued to insist that a virus of the HTLV family was the cause of AIDS, most scientists adopted a wait-and-see attitude regarding the Pasteur discovery. Everyone knew that the sophistication of America's vast governmental research facilities was unmatched. And Dr. Robert Gallo was the father of human retroviruses.

In September 1983 the Pasteur Institute sent samples of the LAV virus to Gallo in an attempt to prove to him that it was not a member of his HTLV viral family. Gallo had become frustrated with AIDS research because he still was unable to grow from the tissue samples of AIDS patients the virus that caused the disease.

The CDC was the one U.S. health agency that did not ignore the French discovery. In October 1983 the CDC sent 30 blood samples to the Pasteur Institute to be tested for the virus the French researchers claimed was the cause of AIDS. Twenty of the samples were from gay men who either had AIDS or early symptoms of AIDS, and 10 were from healthy heterosexuals. The samples were sent blind with only code numbers for identification. The CDC was elated when the Pasteur Institute correctly identified all of the samples from the gay men as positive for antibodies to LAV, and the 10 samples from the healthy control group as negative.

During the fall of 1983 the French were working on a standardized test to be used in blood banks. But they were having difficulty developing a method to grow the *large* amounts of virus that would be necessary for the test.

By late December 1983 Gallo told the director of the NCI that he had discovered the cause of AIDS. It was a virus. Had Gallo and the French each independently discovered the same virus? The two labs claimed their samples had been taken 17 months apart—one from a gay man in Europe and one from a gay man in America. Separate isolates of the same virus vary from each other by 6% to 20%. They are virtually unique. Yet comparisons of the French and American viruses showed their genetic deviation to be less than 1%. There was head shaking within scientific circles. Coming from separate AIDS patients, the isolates were far too alike. It would seem one lab had obtained its virus from the other, just as you could get a "start" of sourdough from your neighbor and grow it to make bread. Only in this case the neighbor was the Pasteur Institute and they had supplied the viral sample to Gallo the previous September.

The Gallo "breakthrough" was warmly embraced by the Reagan Administration. In a re-election year it was the perfect tool to deflect Democratic charges of administration ineptitude in dealing with the AIDS crisis. Announcement of the discovery of the cause of AIDS was delayed until April 23, 1984. On that day, Secretary of the Department of Health and Human Services, Margaret Heckler, called a gala press conference and gave lavish praise for the government's outstanding achievement in AIDS research. She said the virus that caused AIDS was called HTLV-3. Heckler continued, "We now have a blood test for AIDS which we hope will be widely available within about six months." But it would be another 11 months before testing kits got into the blood banks. During that time, 10 million more units of untested blood were collected, divided into two or three components and infused into the veins of unsuspecting patients.

There were considerable research steps leading to the development of an AIDS blood test. The first hurdle was isolating the virus. Then the virus had to be established as the disease-causing agent by finding it in numerous AIDS patients. It had to be cultured from the patients' tissue samples and antibodies had to be detected in their blood. Chimpanzees were then injected with the virus and their T-4 cells compared to the immune irregularities seen in people with AIDS. Finally a way had to be found to mass produce the virus in large quantities. The AIDS test, an ELISA, presented a lesser challenge. ELISA-type tests had been in use since the mid-1970s and detected antibodies which the body produces in response to infections. However, a small amount of the AIDS virus would be required for each ELISA AIDS test.

The victims of transfusion AIDS have speculated on how many months could have been shaved off the time it took to make the blood test available if the Gallo lab had cooperated with the Pasteur Institute in early 1983. Gallo was hung up on the first step of isolating the virus and the French became stalled on the final step of growing it in quantities. Yet Gallo was able to mass produce the virus very quickly after he became involved. Clearly thousands of lives could have been saved if there had been collaboration instead of competition between America and France.

To their credit, the NCI lost no time in gearing up to produce the 750 gallons of AIDS virus that would be needed each month to test the blood collected at the nation's 2,300 blood banks and plasma centers. Months before Secretary Heckler's announcement of the AIDS discovery, a facility in suburban Maryland was being converted into a center for growing the AIDS virus. The P3 Containment Facility at the Frederick Cancer Complex was appropriate for this operation. At one time it had housed the nation's biological warfare research activities. But it is doubtful that, even when working with harmful agents of disease for use against a foreign enemy, the facility had encountered a more deadly carrier of death than the AIDS virus.

The federal government licensed five pharmaceutical companies to produce the ELISA kits. Costs were partially funded by taxpayer money. In May 1984 the NCI sent 25 liters of AIDS virus to the manufacturers of the antibody screening test. As the ELISA had been a standard test for 10 years it was not a new technology. Yet it took 10 months after receipt of the first supply of AIDS virus for the test kits to get into blood banks.

During the early years of the epidemic, Congress had routinely appropriated additional AIDS funding over the protests of the Reagan Administration. In the fall of 1984 Congress became concerned about the delay of the blood test and appropriated $8.25 million to be used for rushing the test to blood banks. The senators were upset when the administration released less than $.5 million to the FDA and let nearly $7.9 million go back to the treasury.

Within the AIDS bureaucracy, the agency most responsible for blood supply safety moved at a snail's pace with no sense of urgency. The FDA had for years taken the position that the risk of transfused AIDS was so small that regulation of blood was unnecessary. Unfortunately, it was the FDA that had to approve the AIDS antibody test—a lengthy and confidential process.

The administration and health agencies failed to anticipate the legal, ethical and social implications of the AIDS blood test. There was little advance planning or action taken to alleviate concerns of doctors and gay groups. The American Public Health Association and the U.S. Conference of Local Health Officers had requested the federal government to provide money for alternative blood testing sites. It was feared that many people at high risk for AIDS would donate blood just to determine if they had the AIDS infection. The government refused to provide funds for alternative testing sites. Finally on January 31, 1985, Dr. Mervyn Silverman made a statement to the press saying that government refusal to provide alternative testing sites would cause increased contamination in the blood supply. The administration quickly provided $12 million for the sites and delayed release of the blood test for two weeks so the program could be implemented. In her book *The AIDS Bureaucracy*, Sandra Panem commented on the confusion surrounding release of the AIDS test and the implementation of alternative testing sites, " . . . policy development followed rather than anticipated the needs."

Throughout February, gay groups threatened to block release of the blood test in court. They feared that if confidentiality of test results were not guaranteed by law, gay men would suffer severe discrimination. Many even feared that those with positive results would be quarantined in concentration camps as some far right groups had advocated. The federal government refused to ensure confidentiality of test results and gay legal groups filed a petition in federal court to stay the licensing of the blood test. More delay.

In early March 1985, FDA Commissioner Frank Young met with gay leaders. The FDA agreed to label the test for use in blood banks and laboratories only—inappropriate for screening groups at high risk for AIDS. The blood test was released and by evening of the same day ELISA kits began arriving at blood banks. Two months too late to save my father.

The AIDS virus was known as HTLV-3 for only a brief time. When the virus' genome structure was determined, it did not belong to Gallo's HTLV family but was in an entirely new viral class. However, it did show almost identical variant forms to the French LAV. Not only were LAV and HTLV-3 the same virus but there was strong evidence of shared origin. In an effort to avoid conflict between the Pasteur and NCI Institutes, an international scientific committee suggested the AIDS virus be called HIV (human immunodeficiency virus).

But renaming the virus did not satisfy France. In 1983 the French group had applied for a U.S. patent on a blood test to detect antibodies to LAV. The patent was never awarded. In 1984 the American group applied for a patent on the blood test and also on a method for growing the virus in culture. When the U.S. Patent and Trademark Office awarded the patent to the Americans, the French filed a lawsuit against the U.S. government. France accused the government of using the viable sample of the LAV virus which the Pasteur Institute supplied to Gallo in September 1983 to make the U.S. blood test. The patent office reversed its decision and ruled the French had discovered the virus first.

The dispute continued with appeals and revisions of decisions. It became apparent that a lawsuit would reveal details embarrassing to the U.S. government, including evidence of forged documents in Gallo's lab. The case was settled out of court in March 1987. The U.S. Department of Health and Human Services and the Pasteur Institute agreed to share rights and royalties to the AIDS virus.

The controversy between the Gallo and Pasteur labs surfaced again in 1990 when the National Institutes of Health announced it would investigate to determine if there had been misconduct on the part of Gallo and his researchers. In the fall of 1991 a preliminary report by the NIH Office of Scientific Integrity indicated it had been determined that Gallo's former chief virologist, Dr. Mikulas Popovic, had fabricated and falsified data and scientific reports relating to the lab's claim of discovering the AIDS virus. Although the report did not charge Gallo himself with formal scientific misconduct, it stated that his actions warranted significant censure. By then Gallo had conceded that the virus his lab used to make the AIDS blood test was the one received from the French. Popovic and Gallo have earned hundreds of thousands of dollars apiece in royalties from patents on the HIV blood test and their method for growing the virus. Additional tens of millions of dollars in licensing fees have gone into the federal treasury.

A scientific dispute of the Pasteur-Gallo magnitude has impact beyond academic interest. Gallo's insistence that AIDS was caused by an HTLV virus and his subsequent naming of the virus HTLV-3 left researchers groping in the wrong direction for a vaccine. And it slowed efforts to market an effective blood test. The CDC estimates 7,200 transfusion AIDS infections were given in 1984. According to that estimate, each month the blood test was delayed, 600 more transfusion recipients became infected with AIDS.

Equally as disturbing is evidence that the French-American dispute continued to impact negatively on blood supply safety even after testing for HIV began in 1985. Of the five companies chosen by the U.S. government to develop and sell the blood test, Abbott Laboratories was the first to receive FDA approval. The Abbott test quickly captured the blood bank market which, to a large extent, it retained after other tests became available.

Early in 1986 two new tests were released. One was by DuPont. The other was the French AIDS test manufactured in the United States by Genetic Systems Corporation of Seattle. Independent laboratories in California and at the National Institutes of Health soon determined that both the new tests were much better at screening out AIDS-positive blood donations than was the Abbott test used by most of the nation's blood banks. Laboratory comparisons showed that nearly all the known AIDS infected blood samples were identified by the new tests whereas the Abbott test *missed more than half.* The French test, which used a different method for producing the virus, got the highest rating. For blood supply safety, the test from the Pasteur Institute was the test of choice.

But in 1986 France was trying to take away the patent that had been granted to Gallo and the NIH and the Reagan Administration was preparing to bring patent infringement charges against Genetic Systems Corporation for manufacturing the French test. It was not a healthy climate for transfusion recipients on either side of the Atlantic Ocean. In France the testing of blood donations had been delayed for six months during 1985 to allow time for a French laboratory to market the Pasteur test rather than use the available Abbott test.

Unfortunately, after the flaw of the Abbott test was discovered, the FDA did not require blood banks to use either the available DuPont or French test until accuracy of the Abbott test was improved. A full 10 months elapsed before the false-negative problem was corrected—10 months during which time blood banks could have detected only half of the AIDS-positive blood donations. In January 1992 the U.S. House Energy and Commerce Committee asked Abbott Laboratories, the American Red Cross and the FDA to provide the committee with data, records and documents pertaining to the possible endangerment of the blood supply in 1986. The previous year France had filed criminal charges against four high-ranking French health officials for their delay in testing that country's blood supply and for their failure to warn consumers about contamination in the blood supply during 1984 and 1985.

I am indebted to the reporting of John Crewdson of the *Chicago Tribune* for information on the Abbott HIV blood test. Over the past several years Mr. Crewdson's in-depth writings on science issues has resulted in a number of government investigations, including probes into misconduct at the Gallo lab.

Chapter 14

The Multibillion Dollar Business of Blood

In the United States the collecting and selling of blood and plasma medicines is big business—an estimated $5 *billion* per year. The blood industry is made up of two parts: the nonprofit segment supported by unpaid blood donations and the commercial for-profit segment that pays for donated blood plasma.

Nonprofit Blood Banking

The nonprofit side of the blood industry supplies hospitals with the blood used for transfusions and in 1991 had over $1.5 billion in revenues. Blood banks or centers collect blood from volunteer donors in the communities they serve. They view their function as one of altruism—that of providing a product to save the lives of patients. But outsiders who have studied blood banking view it as a business which engages in classic competition for donors, market share and revenues.

Both of these views are correct. There is no doubt that the collecting, processing and distributing of blood saves lives—but it also offers an opportunity to engage in a high profit-generating business.

Nancy lives in a small midwestern city and has for years been a regular blood donor. The last time she donated was during a media appeal. The newspapers, TV and radio stations had carried the pleas of her local blood center. They said there was a crisis situation and blood supplies were dangerously low. Donors were urgently needed to avoid shortages at the two local hospitals. Nancy and others like her had responded to these crises before. They took pride in providing the gift of life for their community. It made them feel safer knowing that any blood their own families might need in the future would be donated by friends and neighbors and not by high-risk donors from larger cities.

The day after the media appeal, Nancy arranged to leave work early. Her boss didn't mind. The company encouraged its employees to participate. As her blood was being drawn, Nancy was glad she had donated. She was giving a precious gift to someone who needed it to survive and assumed the cost to the recipient would be small.

Three weeks later Nancy received an urgent phone call at work. Her daughter had been in a car accident. When Nancy arrived at the hospital, she was relieved to find her daughter's bleeding had been brought under control. She would be okay.

After her daughter was released, Nancy looked over the itemized hospital bill. She was outraged. How could the hospital charge nearly $800 for three units of blood that had been given by community donors for nothing? Nancy made inquiries and learned from a former employee of the blood bank that the center often sold a large amount of the blood it collected locally to metropolitan areas outside the state. She was told it was even possible the blood given to her daughter could have come from another part of the country and that the National Blood Exchange is located in San Francisco.

The concept of blood migration shocked Nancy. She'd always thought the blood she donated was kept for use in her own community. Now she was told that her blood could be sold and shipped around the country and that blood sent from San Francisco could be used in her local hospital. Nancy had learned one of the secrets of the business of blood.

When a local blood collection center has its periodic campaign for donors, the magnitude of the local need may be intentionally overstated. People like Nancy may be mislead. Blood banks are often motivated to sell, at a substantial profit, any surplus they can generate to other blood banks and hospitals anywhere in the country. The likelihood of hospitals running out of blood is remote. If they can't get blood from their local blood bank, they can buy it from others that have surpluses. Blood can even be bought on the spot market like the one where processors buy oil, sugar or wheat. The United States imports from western Europe up to 287,000 units of blood each year.

There has been little honesty with blood donors regarding the migration of blood. Blood bank personnel use vague phrases like "blood is a national resource." Few donors interpret that to mean there is a possibility of their donations being sold outside their communities.

"If you're going to do it, you have to tell people up-front, publicize the fact," Dr. Aaron Kellner, former president of the New York Blood Center told the *Philadelphia Inquirer*. "People are being fooled now. They don't know. It's unethical." The New York Blood Center buys 300,000 units of blood a year from all over the United States and Europe.

One of the reasons many blood centers in large urban areas must import blood is that people go there from other areas to have major surgeries. But because the trading or brokering of blood is largely unregulated, with little government control, centers with excess blood can charge whatever the market will bear. Those with shortages often pay excessive prices. Bidding wars can occur for scarce blood types with resultant escalating prices. A pint of blood can be bought and sold several times by sources anywhere in the world before it is ultimately used. Each source enjoys a profit.

Maximizing Profits

Beginning in 1990, Hearings on Blood Supply Safety have been held by the Subcommittee on Oversight and Investigations of the Committee of Energy and Commerce, House of Representatives (hereafter referred to as the House Subcommittee Hearing). During a Hearing in 1991 the House Subcommittee investigated the activities of one of the nation's recognized leaders in blood banking, the Gulf Coast Regional Blood Center of Houston, Texas. One of the most modern and well-equipped blood centers in the country, Gulf Coast serves the blood needs of four million people and over 80 hospitals in a 17-county area. In 1990 the nonprofit center collected 185,000 donations of whole blood. Since its founding in 1975, Gulf Coast has more than tripled its blood collections and aggressively markets blood components to other regions. It now exports approximately 25% of the blood it collects.

In blood banking, the selling of blood to hospitals or other blood banks outside the local area is known as resource sharing. But according to testimony on the Gulf Coast operations, "sharing" may be a misleading term. Nationally there is always a surplus of type A positive blood and a short supply of both O negative and O positive red blood cell units. Red cells cannot be stored longer than 45 days and if not used within that time must be discarded and the sale revenues lost.

When a blood center's inventory of O red cell units gets dangerously low it must purchase them from another blood center. But the seller might also require the buyer to take short dated As which the buyer does not need, as a condition of the sale. The seller then reaps revenue from both the Os and As and the buyer takes the loss on the As. Blood package sales arrangements are called "tying" and are used by a *few* blood centers that aggressively promote the sale of blood. The opportunity to unload A units that are nearing expiration in a package with desperately needed O units is an incentive for blood centers to collect more blood than local need requires.

Hard-headed economics may influence the objectives of nonprofit blood banking. There is concern that blood inventories in local areas may be sold down to very low levels to close a deal. Examples were given at the House Subcommittee Hearing where hospitals had to import blood from out of state or accept newly drawn blood labeled "test pending" which had not been determined to be free of AIDS or hepatitis. Former employees of Gulf Coast felt this was due to large amounts of blood being shipped outside the area. There was also concern that the hasty collection, processing and shipping of blood pushed out in assembly line fashion increased the risk of testing and labeling errors. There was evidence of units reaching hospitals with the wrong ABO or Rh factor labels. If the hospitals don't catch these errors, patients receiving blood with an incorrect blood type label on it could die. As the distribution network becomes more complex and as more blood testing is required, opportunities for errors grow. In the past decade blood bank errors have multiplied dramatically. Former FDA Commissioner Frank E. Young told Gilbert Gaul of the *Philadelphia Inquirer*, "The potential for fatal mistakes is a ticking time bomb."

From the consumer viewpoint, I am not disturbed by blood banks making a profit (excesses over expenses) as long as safety is not sacrificed or the patient overcharged for blood. In fact, profits are necessary to buy new equipment and upgrade operations to meet the demands of modern blood banking. And some cash reserves are needed to act as a cushion against future blood bank losses. However, if blood banks accumulate *large* reserve funds in excess of their costs it is doubtful that blood prices have been kept low enough to deserve the generosity of donors or the banks' tax-exempt status. It would be more appropriate if people were not led to believe that blood is a gift and it were called what it really is—a purchase that requires involved consumer input.

But, blood bankers get upset when their function is called a business that "sells" blood because most states have statutes which require the provision of blood to be a service. They can't charge for blood—merely for the service of collecting and processing it. The nonprofit designation of blood banks appears inconsistent with an industry that collects such huge "service" revenues. And it is not unusual for some blood banks to make profits of over 10% on those revenues—much higher than the profits made by the nation's leading corporations.

The top executive of a large blood center may earn over $200,000 a year. The compensation of the president of Gulf Coast is tied to bonuses and varies from year to year. In 1987, 1989 and 1990 his compensation was $230,837, $195,106 and $203,542, respectively. Salaries vary widely. The majority of blood bankers make considerably under $200,000. It should also be recognized that many smaller blood banks have dedicated executives and staffs who work long hours for low salaries.

During the last two decades, profits became a major objective of nonprofit blood banks. Before that time the collection and distribution of blood for transfusions was largely a humanitarian service with minimal profitability. That changed dramatically in the late 1960s when the practice of component therapy was initiated. A pint of whole blood could be subdivided into two or more components (e.g. red cells, platelets and plasma). No longer was it necessary to transfuse a pint of whole blood into a patient. That pint could be divided and given to two or more patients, which enabled high profits to be made from a single donation of blood. At the present time, up to four different component units can be produced from each blood donation. Few people realize that by splitting whole blood into various parts, a single pint of donated blood can generate up to $900 in revenues.

Blood Prices Vary

A 1989 *Philadelphia Inquirer* survey found that charges for blood and blood services varied widely throughout the country. In Waco, Texas, a hospital paid $33 for a unit of red blood cells. In San Jose, California, it cost $79—a 139% difference. Prices varied 60% within the state of California. Prices for cryoprecipitate, a blood component used for bleeding disorders, varied a whopping 290% nationwide.

These prices are what blood banks charge hospitals. Prices that hospitals charge patients also range widely and are influenced by various factors such as blood bank charges, geographical areas, hospital operating costs and most importantly—hospital profit margins. Profit margins are influenced by hospital philosophy—whether they view their mission as one of service at minimum cost to the patient or one of profit maximization where prices are placed as high as patients and insurance companies will bear. For example, hospital costs for typing and cross matching vary from as little as $15 to well over $100 per unit. Transfusion fees may be $125 or more.

Today hospitals may charge patients up to $250 or more for just one component unit of blood. Costs of a transfusion, requiring 5.4 component units, are significant. Costs to organ transplant patients, who can require over 100 units, are staggering! Large amounts of blood are also needed to treat some illnesses. An extreme example is that of a four-year-old girl in Utah who during a five-month period in 1988 received 634 units of blood.

Blood banks incur equipment and staff costs for donor recruitment, testing, separating the blood, storage and delivery. Hospitals must pay for the blood bought from the blood banks, for tests to crossmatch the blood and for transfusing it into the patient. But after costs and salaries are paid, there is an attractive profit left over for both blood banks and hospitals. Blood revenues help to defray hospital losses in other areas. It's understandable why there was little motivation to reduce blood usage.

The Red Cross

The American Red Cross dominates the collection and distribution of blood. Each year its 54 regional centers collect over 50% of this country's 13.5 million pints of blood and sell it to 3,300 hospitals. The balance of the blood is supplied by the members of two organizations—the AABB which has about 2,400 hospitals and community blood centers, and the Council of Community Blood Centers with 31 regional blood banks.

In 1991 the Red Cross generated $780 million in revenues from its blood operation. This would have placed it 407th on the Fortune 500 list of America's largest corporations. The Red Cross blood program averaged profits of $38 million a year from 1980 through 1987. In 1987 its high 8.7% profit margin (profits shown as a percentage of revenues) would have ranked 98th in the Fortune 500 and much higher than America's three largest corporations. General Motors, the largest, had a profit margin of only 3.5%. Exxon had 6.3%, and Ford was at 6.5%. Red Cross profits, or "excesses over expenses" as they prefer to call them, were nearly $307 million for the 1980-1988 period. Sidney Shainwald, a CPA and former chief financial officer of Consumers Union, told *Money* magazine, "This is a very rich organization. If it were public, I'd love to own stock in it."

The Red Cross is not the only nonprofit blood banking operation to amass huge profits. In 1987 Blood Systems of Scottsdale, Arizona, earned an annual profit of $1.85 million while Gulf Coast Regional Blood Center in Houston, Texas, netted $1.80 million on revenues of $15.5 million (11.6%). The Central Blood Bank of Pittsburgh serves only two counties. Yet for the fiscal year ending June 30, 1987, it generated a profit of $2.1 million—an impressive 11.9% as a percentage of revenues. This was much higher than most Fortune 500 corporations which averaged 4.6% that year. The Pittsburgh center had a net worth of $17.7 million of which $11.9 million was in savings and short-term cash investments—an example of how excess earnings grow in nonprofit organizations.

To be successful, most business owners must be as good or better than their competitors. They must be efficient, have top employee performance and make few or no mistakes. If they maximize revenues and minimize costs they might make a modest profit. If they don't do these things, they're out of business. This scenario does not apply, however, if they are in the nonprofit blood business. That business will be profitable regardless of their management practices. If costs become excessive, management simply raises prices. The ultimate user, the patient, will have to pay for it. The nonprofit blood business does not have to offer the safest product at the lowest price because in most geographical areas there is no real competition.

Blood banks were granted exclusive rights to collect blood in specified geographical areas through a government-industry agreement worked out in the early 1970s. This essentially eliminated competition for the source of blood. The sum of these regional monopolies has *given* the Red Cross over 50% of America's blood supply. Public utilities also have protected geographical territories but unlike the blood industry, their charges to customers are controlled by public utility commissions. If blood banks choose to raise their prices they can do so without any government oversight.

Finally, nonprofit blood banks are granted tax-exempt status despite exceptionally high profit margins. They are not obligated to pay federal or state income tax on most of their operations. Blood banks get free publicity for donor recruitment and enjoy the service of volunteers. Without stockholder dividends to pay, any revenues collected on the sale of blood, less operating costs, go directly into the company's reserves.

With these large profit margins and excess reserves, blood banks have the financial resources to make blood safety a top concern. When human lives are at stake, accumulating profits should not be the primary goal of a blood banking organization. Enough money should be spent on equipment and well-trained personnel to ensure that consumers are getting the purest possible product at a reasonable cost. Unfortunately, with the focus on the bottom line, this has not always been true.

The combined charitable programs of the Red Cross are dwarfed by the scope of its blood operations. In 1988 the organization spent 59% of its expenditures to operate its blood program. Only 9% was spent on disaster relief while 22% was spent on various other services to the community and the Armed Forces. The remaining 10% went for management and fund raising. The Red Cross received $315 million in public contributions in 1988 to support its disaster relief efforts and other community services. Their blood business generated $536 million in revenues that year. The blood business is self-supporting and requires no public money contributions.

Critics complain that the organization downplays how big its blood operation is while promoting disaster relief. This strategy, coupled with approximately $90 million of free media advertising a year, has been very effective. When the Red Cross made an appeal for contributions after the 1989 San Francisco earthquake, Americans generously gave $55 million. The public is equally generous with service and blood donations. The Red Cross has the services of 1.4 million volunteers and 4.3 million blood donors.

However, all the business advantages the Red Cross enjoys have not ensured safer blood for transfusion recipients. During the past few years the Red Cross has been besieged with operating problems in its blood business:

- Almost 2/3 of its blood centers have been cited by FDA and Red Cross inspectors for blood safety deficiencies.

- An FDA quarantine forced it to shut down its $75 million-a-year plasma operation for six months in 1988 because of blood safety concerns.

- In mid-1988 the Red Cross shut down testing laboratories in Washington, Nashville and St. Louis because they had released blood that had initially tested positive for AIDS and hepatitis.

- Its multi-million dollar computer system was declared a "dismal failure" by a Red Cross study. FDA inspection reports said that the computer program could not ensure that only safe blood was released and that the system had no reliable way of identifying dangerous donors.

- In July 1990 the FDA released a critical report on the Red Cross system of reporting, investigating and following up on accidents and errors that occurred in Red Cross blood banks. One FDA disclosure was that the Washington, DC, Region had been notified by doctors that 228 patients had been diagnosed with AIDS after receiving transfused blood which the region had supplied. The Washington Region reported just four of the cases to Red Cross headquarters and none to the FDA as required.

For some time the continuous problems and bad publicity caused internal finger-pointing and a top management shakeup within the Red

Cross organization. A number of senior executives resigned or were replaced, including the head of computer operations. Several top regional blood center administrators were demoted or terminated and the top blood program staff at national headquarters was reorganized. Finally, in August 1990, the Red Cross, in an effort to bring its local blood service programs under national control, announced dozens of new positions and tighter supervision of its blood services.

In an effort to bolster tarnished image, Elizabeth Dole, the former Secretary of Labor and Transportation, was placed at the helm of the American Red Cross in early 1991. With 2,200 active chapters, 23,000 paid employees and over half the nation's transfused blood supply in her hands, health consumers have more than a passing interest in Mrs. Dole's administrative skills.

★　　★　　★

Operational problems aren't peculiar to just the Red Cross, as evidenced by the April 1990 recall of 11,000 units of blood by Denver's Belle Bonfils Blood Center discussed previously. The center had implemented a new automated testing system and, for seven weeks, had used the wrong procedures to mix chemicals. The result was inadequate testing of all blood donations for both hepatitis and AIDS. By the time the suspect blood had been recalled, 97% had already been given to patients.

Competent management would have run the new procedure simultaneously with the proven method until the new approach had been thoroughly debugged and proven to be failsafe. Why did it take seven long weeks to discover that the new procedure wasn't working? It is inconceivable that 11,000 units of potentially dangerous blood can be shipped to hospitals before an error is discovered!

For-Profit Blood Industry

The for-profit side of the industry is comprised primarily of companies that manufacture medicines from blood plasma. Unlike blood banking, these businesses:

1. Are highly competitive in a worldwide free market which limits the prices they can charge for their products

2. Pay for their raw material (plasma)

3. Get no territorial protection for their share of donors

4. Pay taxes

5. Must be efficient to be successful

Like the nonprofit segment, this part of the blood business is also very large with estimated revenues of $3 billion per year.

The manufacturers collect plasma from paid donors at collection centers and transport it to pharmaceutical laboratories where it is made into medicines. The plasma derivatives are sold on a global scale wherever the most money can be made. It is not unusual for a fully processed unit of blood plasma to eventually yield over $1,000 worth of pharmaceutical products.

Both plasma and the medicines made from it are bought and sold like other commodities with events in one country causing sharp price changes or shortages in another. Plasma can change hands several times in the international market. Brokers make profits by bringing together those who have plasma with those who need it. This worldwide exchange is shrouded in secrecy. There is no regulation of the activities of blood plasma brokers or of their operations.

As the top producer of the international plasma industry, the United States has been called "the vampire of the world." The nation collects 60% of the world plasma and exports aproximately two-thirds of it. Japan, by contrast, collects only 5% of the world plasma but uses an astounding 44%. There are 400 commercial centers in the United States that pay between $8 and $15 or more for a donation of plasma.

The plasma sold at commercial centers should not be confused with the blood donated for free by volunteer donors at nonprofit blood banks. It is very rare for hospitals to transfuse blood from paid donors because of concern that they would have an incentive to conceal vital health information. Any blood from paid donors must be marked as such on the bag according to FDA requirements.

America has the most liberal standards in the world for how often a person can sell his or her plasma. Federal regulations allow a donor to give plasma twice a week, 104 times a year. This is four times as often as the World Health Organization recommends as safe for a donor's health. Unfortunately, the majority of plasma is sold by disadvantaged people who are the least likely to have the high-quality diet needed to build back the protein lost with each donation. A string of plasma centers operate along the Mexican border which attract thousands of poor Mexicans who sell their plasma each week.

Plasma is a yellow intravascular fluid containing water, minerals, chemicals and protein. It takes one hour for an individual to make a plasma donation. A procedure called plasmapheresis is used to separate plasma from red cells and other solid components of blood. During the process a couple of bags of whole blood are drawn from the donor and spun in a centrifuge machine. The separated plasma is kept and the red cells are transfused back into the donor.

The FDA inspects the plasma centers only once a year. Centers have had their license suspended because of "overbleeding"—taking too much blood during a donation, accepting donors too often, drawing off plasma from donors who have a hematocrit (percentage of red cells in blood) test result of less than 38 and falsifying the donor's records. These centers maximize their profits on the volume of plasma collected and sold. Overdraws are difficult for the FDA to catch unless they are tipped off by an employee informant.

Placentas as a Source of Plasma

A little-known source of plasma protein used to make medicines is placentas. If a woman gives birth at a hospital which sells placentas, that previous part of her womb will be bagged and frozen without her knowledge. Later it will be sent to a manufacturing company which uses the rich maternal blood to make plasma derivatives.

Most of the placentas formerly sold in the United States were purchased by Institut Merieux of France. In the late 1980s Merieux was buying 15 tons of placentas a day—five million placentas a year from all over the globe. They processed the placenta blood into products sold in 100 countries including the United States. Today the market for placentas has decreased and they are rarely sold by American hospitals.

A placenta, or any other part of the human body, carries a risk of transmitting AIDS. Health consumers should be aware that all organs donated for transplant have the potential to transmit HIV and other viruses, as does sperm from a sperm bank. In this way transplants and donated sperm are no different from blood. Transfusions should be viewed as liquid transplants.

When products made from the worldwide collection of placenta blood are sold in 100 countries, it is obvious that the plasma industry is vast in geographical scope. It becomes impossible for doctors or patients to know the origin of the blood used in plasma medicines or the conditions under which they were collected and prepared.

Safety Obstacles

A 1989 medical study concluded that in some foreign countries appropriate infection-control practices are not being used when collecting plasma. It cited a plasma collection center in Mexico City where the same bottle of saline solution was routinely used for more than one donor. This caused AIDS to spread at an alarming rate among the center's regular paid donors. In poor countries the cost of disposable intravenous equipment becomes an obstacle to plasma safety.

When donors are paid, they have an incentive to falsify information about their health status. The majority of plasma donors are in severe need of money. A 1990 study of intravenous drug users in the U.S. found that 25% of them still sell their blood at plasma collection centers. The study's researchers at the John Hopkins School of Hygiene and Public Health expressed concern about inadequate protection of the nation's blood supply. They said, "The continued donation of plasma, and occasionally blood, by intravenous drug users . . . is troubling and warrants further attention."

The homeless, disadvantaged people who most often sell their blood plasma usually are in poor health and prone to carry disease. Obviously plasma collected at these commercial centers has a greater chance of being contaminated than does the blood donated at nonprofit blood banks. Because the fresh frozen plasma transfused in hospitals cannot be treated to kill viruses, it is almost always obtained from safer, nonprofit blood bank supplies.

Hopefully, the plasma collected at commercial centers will be manufactured into medical products. In the United States, plasma products are prepared by approved fractionation methods which have the capability of inactivating HIV to levels that carry no discernable risk of transmitting AIDS. The CDC states that "the margin of safety based on the removal of infectivity by the fractionation process is extremely high." But because much of the plasma is from high risk donors and the ELISA test does not detect all infected donations, safety depends on adequate preparation. Although plasma products are considered to be safe, no manufacturer can offer the consumer a 100% safety guarantee.

Three Groups of Plasma Products

Plasma is manufactured into three distinct types of medical products: albumin, immune serum globulins and clotting factors. Albumin replaces the vital fluids lost with serious trauma. It is often used for burn victims and surgery patients and acts as a sponge to keep fluids in the blood vessels so they won't collapse.

Immune serum globulins are used to supplement the body's natural immunity. This group includes some vaccines such as those used for rabies and hepatitis B. When consumers are treated with immune products, many are unaware of their connection to blood. My two oldest children had "gamma shots" for years because of frequent respiratory infections. I had no idea the serum came from the pooled plasma of over 1,000 donors who sold their blood at commercial centers. However, both albumin and the immune globulin preparations are prepared by a fractionation process that uses either heat or alcohol to kill infectious germs.

Unfortunately, the clotting factors used for the treatment of hemophilia were prepared without any steps that would inactivate infectious viruses. These clotting factors comprise the third group of plasma products and were responsible for the mass infection of the nation's hemophiliacs with hepatitis and AIDS.

Dashed Hopes for a Better Life

By 1975 America's 20,000 hemophiliacs were viewing their future with optimism. They expected that with the introduction of factor VIII and factor IX clotting concentrates they could live longer, more productive lives. These men and boys hoped they could participate in normal physical activities without the fear of a scratch or bump causing uncontrollable bleeding. Approximately 80% of them suffered from hemophilia A which can require the infusion of 50,000 or more units of factor VIII per year. Each infusion of factor VIII was made from the pooled plasma of up to 48,000 donors. Within a year's time, a hemophiliac could be exposed to hundreds of thousands of donors. Without a preparation method to inactivate infectious viruses, the clotting factors were a ticket to decimation.

A few months after receiving the new concentrates, hemophiliacs started showing signs of liver damage caused by hepatitis. It became well known in medical circles during the mid and later 1970s that hemophiliacs and recipients of blood transfusions were contracting both hepatitis B and hepatitis non-A, non-B at alarming rates. A study concluded, "The prevalence of abnormal liver tests in hemophiliacs increased rapidly with the widespread introduction of factor VIII and factor IX concentrates in the mid-1970s." Hemophiliacs did not want to discontinue the use of clotting factors because they made dramatic improvement in the quality of their lives. They had no way of knowing hepatitis was a prelude to a far more deadly virus.

An Escalating Infectious Threat

Unknown to the hemophiliacs, change had come earlier to another, far larger group of American men. This group was gay and would shape the destiny of hemophilia. The commercialization of gay sex had exploded in the late 1960s and 1970s with the opening of large numbers of bathhouses and sex clubs. Soon a tide of increasingly serious infections swept through the gay communities in urban areas. The problem was partially due to the growing popularity of oral-anal sex which made it difficult for participants to avoid contact with fecal matter.

At urban clinics, gay men were treated for sexually transmitted diseases (STDs) in ever increasing numbers. To the usual syphilis and gonorrhea were added all types of hepatitis and enteric parasitic diseases. The latter was referred to in medical journals as "Gay Bowel Syndrome". During the 1970s hepatitis B spread rapidly as a sexually transmitted disease. In some areas, gay men in their 30's experienced a 400% increase in hepatitis B infection during one four-year period.

The gay liberation movement also began in the 1970s and was fed by the financial support of the owners of bathhouses and sex clubs. These businesses grew into a $100 million industry throughout the U.S. and Canada and became fertile breeding grounds for the spread of infectious disease. The bathhouse owners were often leaders in the gay political movement. They promised their followers nirvana—but instead led them into an abyss of disease and death.

By the mid 1970s public health officials had documented the rampant sexual spread of hepatitis through the gay population. The CDC not only identified gay men as a high-risk group for hepatitis but by 1978 had enlisted several thousand of them as volunteers to assist in the development of a hepatitis B vaccine. Gay men were also recruited as plasma donors because their past hepatitis infections had caused antibodies to be present in their blood. These hepatitis antibodies were needed to manufacture the hepatitis B immune globulin.

The FDA and blood officials were aware of the research involving gay men and hepatitis B. During the mid and late 1970s they had observed the mounting cases of hepatitis among hemophiliacs and transfusion recipients. The chance of getting hepatitis from a transfusion became 1 in 10. Yet available surrogate tests for hepatitis were not adopted nor were gay men deferred from the donor pools.

Pasteurization of clotting factors which eliminated the risk of AIDS transmission began in 1985. But by then at least 50% of all America's hemophiliacs were infected with HIV. Of the 10,000 infected, 1,500 had died of AIDS by mid 1992. The Hemophilia Foundation estimates that approximately 30% of the sexual partners of HIV-positive hemophiliacs are also infected with the virus. This horrible tragedy was largely due to the blood industry's slow response in deferring the major high-risk group from donating blood and plasma.

Writing in the August 1984 issue of *The American Spectator*, Dr. Gordon Muir observed: "The question, usually met with thundering silence, is why was it only in 1983, after the AIDS scare, that homosexuals were discouraged from giving blood?"

Gene Antonio writes in his book, *The AIDS Coverup*: "Hard evidence reveals that the vast majority of hemophiliacs and other blood recipients

have fallen prey to liver disease and AIDS infection as a direct conse-
quence of blood donated by homosexuals. The contamination of the
nation's blood supply with AIDS is a problem which could largely have
been avoided if the medical establishment had appropriately restricted
male homosexuals from donating blood years before the AIDS epidemic
began, as they had good reason to do."

That "good reason" was hepatitis, and the time to have deferred gay
men from donating blood was in the late 1970s just as AIDS was
entering the blood supply. It should be recognized that these men were
donating blood with the best of intent—to save lives. The only relevant
issue is who had responsibility for blood safety. It was the mandated duty
of the FDA and the obligation of the blood industry to eliminate
contamination. The lives of consumers were in their hands, but it wasn't
until March 1983 that the United States Public Health Service issued the
first weak recommendations to defer fast-lane gay men from donating
blood. Far too late to save thousands of hemophiliacs and transfusion
recipients from contracting the AIDS virus.

Why wasn't action taken much earlier to defer gay men from donating
blood both at nonprofit banks and at plasma collection centers? The
reason is simple. Losing gay men as donors was a threat to the business
of blood, just as closure of gay bathhouses was a threat to the business
of sex. Traditionally a large percentage of the nation's blood supply was
donated by men between the ages of 25 and 45. Many of them were
single. It was not known what number of these men were gay but in
urban areas, civic-minded gay men donated a significant amount of
blood. Drives in their neighborhoods were extremely successful.
Therefore, the blood industry delayed as long as possible the loss of gay
men as a dependable source of their donated product. The Irwin Blood
Bank in San Francisco estimated the deferral of gay men cost them from
7% to 15% of their total donations. Recruitment costs for new donors
reduced blood industry revenues. Some banks had to purchase blood from
other areas, further cutting into their profits.

During the time the industry had stalled to avoid taking action, blood
bankers became supporters of gay civil rights, saying blood banks could
not discriminate against such a large number of men. They said they
could not deny gays the right to donate blood. Yet without troubled
conscience, blood bankers had previously refused intravenous drug users
the right to donate blood. But then drug users were not often inclined to
give their blood at nonprofit banks. When not faced with losing a large
number of donations, blood bankers could tolerate the loss of civil rights.

During the 1970s and 1980s little effort was made to educate doctors
or consumers on the conservation of homologous blood. Technology was

available to reduce the need for receiving someone else's blood during surgical procedures. Patients could have been told to donate their own blood before their surgery and IAT recycling procedures could have been used in operating rooms. These measures were sufficient to avoid any shortages caused from gay deferral or surrogate testing. But the blood banks had no incentive to promote blood conservation. Their revenues depended on the sale of blood.

The blood bankers' concern for the gay rights movement did not last. It ended in early 1983 as fears about AIDS grew and CDC doctors pushed for safety measures to protect the blood supply. There were two choices. The blood bankers could either use the core test for hepatitis B, which they knew would eliminate nearly all gay men from the donor pools, or they could restrict them from donating. The gay political movement supported using the test. From the viewpoint of public relations use of the core test would be less damaging to the gay movement than deferral. There was fear that if gay men were told not to donate blood the media attention would result in a backlash against their group.

However, the blood bankers resisted use of the core test more than gay deferral because it would cost $3 to test each donation of blood and all positive units would have to be discarded. They kept insisting the test would not improve blood safety though they knew it would exclude nearly all those in high risk groups. The doctor who headed the nation's largest blood center in New York City calculated the cost of using the core test at $100 million a year for the entire U.S. It would raise costs and lose more donors than deferral. The support for gay civil rights soon eroded and the first weak deferral of gay men began.

Lack of Government Regulation

The transfusion and hemophiliac tragedy could have been dramatically lessened if the government had acted quickly to curtail the spread of viral disease through blood and blood products. Unfortunately, national blood policy is formulated with a private sector approach rather than a government directed approach. The result? The government essentially allowed the blood industry to regulate itself!

Though the FDA has the responsibility of ensuring blood safety, policies are shaped by the FDA's Blood Products Advisory Committee which advises the FDA Commissioner on blood issues. Its members were from the blood industry. FDA insiders have called the committee an "Old Boy's Club" with members protecting the interests of blood sales. Don Francis describes the decision making of the FDA in 1983 as "inherently biased" toward blood banks. Dr. Francis believes the agency's attitude resulted in a "consensus of the status quo instead of a consensus for public health." A review by the *Philadelphia Inquirer* of the Blood Products Advisory Committee hearings showed that the Committee's recommendations were rarely ever rejected by the FDA. Actually the FDA rarely has any input from the consumers it is supposed to protect. In contrast, there is constant input from blood industry trade associations. And state legislatures have granted blood banks protection from product liability if they follow the minimal industry practices set by their trade associations. These practices are usually rubber stamped by the FDA. When public statements are issued on blood policy, they are made jointly by the American Red Cross, the AABB and the CCBC to establish a firm "standard of care" against liability.

Consequently, after it became known that AIDS had contaminated the blood supply, the FDA did not mandate the use of surrogate tests on blood or immediately call for strong policies to defer gay males. In 1983, the year the CDC estimated 8,400 people were infected with AIDS from infusion of tainted blood, the FDA *reduced* its inspections of blood banks from once a year to once every two years. In 1986 the FDA's Blood Products Advisory Committee finally recommended use of the disputed hepatitis B core antibody test as a surrogate test for non-A, non-B hepatitis—three years after the CDC had pleaded for its use for AIDS and 10 years after it first became available and could have reduced the spread of hepatitis!

Neither did the American Blood Commission (ABC) shape or influence any policy on AIDS contamination of the blood supply. This privately run commission receives funding from the federal government and was formed in 1975 to represent consumers. Unfortunately, it too became dominated by representatives from the blood banking industry and protected blood interests. In reality, the ABC has neither enforcement power nor statutory mandate for oversight of the national blood supply. In recent years the Commission has lost prestige among blood industry organizations and leaders. A consultant's study in 1989 criticized its inaction during the AIDS crisis. The study concluded that the American Blood Commission should either represent consumers or be dissolved.

Consumer Advocacy Is Effective

Without government protection, hemophiliacs suffered unnecessary carnage and over 8,000 still await an AIDS death. But there is good news for future generations of hemophiliacs. It's called consumerism. In 1982 and 1983 the National Hemophilia Foundation pressured the manufacturers of clotting factors for safer products. The Foundation insisted the concentrates be prepared in a way that would inactivate *all* viruses. Bacteria, protozoa and one-cell microbes can usually be removed from blood by filtering—but viruses are so small they pass through the filters. The Foundation knew there would always be some new unidentified virus waiting in the wings to contaminate the blood supply. The total viral threat had to be eliminated.

The manufacturers responded and by 1985 a pasteurized version of factor VIII was on the market. It was heated for 10 hours which usually killed the AIDS virus but was ineffective against hepatitis non-A, non-B. During the next two years, AIDS infections spread through the pasteurized product fell to 18. The Hemophilia Foundation pushed for additional safety measures and the manufacturers continued to make improvements. Today pasteurized-detergent versions are used along with more expensive monoclonal products. There have been no new AIDS infections from the new products and recently the risk of hepatitis was also eliminated.

Test trials have been run on a new recombinant factor VIII which is genetically engineered and does not use any human blood source. This product eliminates all infectious risk and was developed after researchers successfully isolated and cloned the gene for factor VIII. The down side of the various new clotting factors is their annual cost, which is between $50,000 and $100,000 or more per patient.

While consumer action has removed the threat of new AIDS infections for hemophiliacs, transfusion recipients still remain at risk. During an interview with Alan P. Brownstein, Executive Director of the National Hemophilia Foundation, I asked if throughout the 1980s any group had spoken on behalf of the four million people who have transfusions each year. "No, that never happened," he replied. "To my knowledge there was no consumer group other than the Hemophilia Foundation with an active interest in safety of the blood supply."

This is a dangerous situation. The nonprofit sector of the industry, which supplies the blood for transfusions, is a cartel and insular to a fault. It is monopolistic. It is essentially unregulated. It collects a free product, uses the free services of volunteers and enjoys an image of public service. It doesn't pay taxes, yet it accumulates large profits called "excesses." It operates as an untouchable island, protected by law against product liability. It must have consumer scrutiny.

Released in 1988, the report of the Presidential AIDS Commission stated: "The Commission strongly supports placing a high priority on the objective of a safe blood supply because it is achievable and *the transmission of this virus (AIDS) through blood products is preventable*." (Italics added) The Commission elaborated further, saying transfusion AIDS is preventable in the *absence* of a vaccine or cure. I question if it is preventable in the absence of consumer action. In the years since the

Commission wrote its report, the numbers of life-threatening errors made by blood banks have skyrocketed.

Blood safety should be a concern of every American because 95% of the U.S. population will require transfusion of blood or blood products by the time they are 72 years old. Consumers have the power to obtain safe transfusion therapy. If more elective surgery patients shopped around for the best autologous blood programs, operating rooms would rapidly become equipped with IAT equipment. Blood banks and doctors would be more willing to cooperate with patients requesting predonation of their own blood and other options.

Unfortunately, the track record of the blood industry does not inspire consumer confidence. The industry lauded the safety of products it knew were potentially dangerous to an unsuspecting public. Aware of the likelihood of litigation, the blood industry successfully lobbied for protective legislation against lawsuits. It refused to spend money to make its products safer and withheld promotion of alternatives to homologous transfusion.

However, there were a few blood banks that acted ethically and responsibly and their number continues to grow. Blood facilities now use many more tests to weed out infected donations. But it is impossible for consumers to evaluate the safety of their local blood supply. Migration of blood around the country further complicates the local picture.

There are proven steps consumers can take to protect their families from transfusion risks. They are covered in the next section of this book.

Chapter 15

A Self-Serving Blood Monopoly

A blood monopoly in an area having a low incidence of AIDS can make exaggerated claims of blood safety and never be challenged. Moreover, residents prefer to believe that AIDS is not a threat to their community and are uninformed about behaviors that put them at risk for HIV. If not countered by aggressive donor education measures, this ignorance presents a grave danger to the local blood supply.

On July 3, 1988, the day before my father died, *The Deseret News*, one of Utah's leading newspapers, carried an article on the superior safety of Utah's blood supply. The newspaper had interviewed Dr. Myron Laub, long-time director of the LDS Blood Bank and Intermountain Health Care (IHC) Blood Services. The LDS Blood Bank is IHC's largest blood collection and processing center and is located at the LDS Hospital. At least 80% of all blood used in Utah hospitals is supplied by IHC Blood Services. Dr. Laub talked to the press just a few hours before my father died from transfused AIDS—AIDS contracted from contaminated blood supplied by the very same LDS Blood Bank!

As he had done for years, Dr. Laub told the press that Utah had clean people donating clean blood. He said during all his years as the LDS Blood Bank's director he had only seen two donations of HIV-contaminated blood and in both cases the potential donors had disqualified themselves and their blood had not been used.

But Dr. Laub's statement was safe blood crock-talk. I have copies of an FDA inspection of the LDS Blood Bank in July 1985. The inspector was Edward M. Maticka of the FDA's Denver office. His report indicates that within a few months after AIDS testing of blood donations began in March 1985, there were six donors at the LDS Blood Bank who tested positive for the AIDS virus. The positive donors were confirmed by the Western Blot test.

Six confirmed AIDS-positive donors from a blood bank's regular donor pool has chilling implications. Laub said the average donor at the LDS Blood Bank donated blood three times a year. How many times during the *years* before testing began did each of the six infected donors give blood? What was the total number of people who received their tainted donations after *each one* was *divided* into three component units? And how many of those Utahns who received contaminated blood *know* they are infected with AIDS? From our family's experience with the Utah health care system, past blood recipients could have died from AIDS-related pneumonias, AIDS-related cancers and other AIDS-related illnesses and never been told they had the disease. As a result, how many of their sexual partners have been infected like my mother? The six HIV-positive donors were found within four months of testing. How many more were found later?

By 1988 blood bankers were saying the national risk for getting AIDS in a transfusion was one in 100,000. In the July news article, Dr. Laub said the chance of a person getting infected with the AIDS virus from a transfusion in Utah was one in one million compared to one in 100,000 nationally. At that time the national risk for getting hepatitis in a transfusion was one in 20. But in Utah the risk was a mere one in 10,000 according to the LDS Blood Bank director.

Dr. Laub said 100,000 Utahns get transfusions each year. If his one-in-a-million risk was valid, only one transfused AIDS case would have been contracted in Utah during a 10-year period. But by March 1992 the state had 16 documented transfusion AIDS cases and 7 HIV transfusion-acquired infections, which is remarkable considering the effort that the Utah blood monopoly has made to conceal them.

The LDS Blood Bank is perceived to have a safe blood supply because it carries the Mormon name and signs up many of its donors at Mormon Church meetings. People assume it is run by the LDS Church. That is incorrect. The LDS Blood Bank is under the umbrella of Intermountain Health Care. It is the lead receiving, storing and distributing center for IHC Blood Services.

IHC is headquartered in Salt Lake City—and owns 24 hospitals throughout Utah, Idaho and Wyoming. The organization also provides central lab services for 17 community hospitals in southern Utah and collects and processes blood for all Utah hospitals.

IHC employed over 16,000 people and generated over $1 billion in revenues in 1991. Its "nonprofit" status exempted it from paying federal and state income taxes and property taxes on most of its operations. It earned nearly $42 million in profits (earnings surplus) in 1991 after paying exceptionally high salaries and bonuses to top executives.

IHC's Blood Services is a classic example of a blood monopoly. The Red Cross stopped supplying blood in Utah in 1986 after IHC expanded its Blood Services, leaving the Red Cross with a mere 13% of the local blood market.

For many years the LDS Blood Bank and most of the IHC hospitals were owned by the Church of Jesus Christ of Latter Day Saints (Mormons). In 1975, the LDS Church made a decision to give its remaining 15 hospitals to the communities in the form of a trust. Community leaders were invited to serve as trustees of the various hospitals and IHC was formed to manage the operations. The LDS Church has never had any involvement in directing the activities of IHC.

IHC did not change the names of the former church hospitals. The largest is a 520-bed facility in Salt Lake City known as the LDS Hospital which houses the LDS Blood Bank. The name is misleading and enables IHC to solicit substantial donations of money, volunteer time and blood from the predominantly Mormon community. Other hospitals complain of the competitive advantage IHC obtains from using the LDS name. And the LDS name on the blood bank gives a false sense of security to Mormons who need transfusions.

The IHC mission is stated as one of noble dedication to patient care, reflecting the public trust placed in the organization. The treatment my father received from IHC stands in stark contrast to that affirmed mission. When, after two years of concealment, we finally forced disclosure of Dad's AIDS infection, the blood bank said his symptoms had appeared too soon for him to have gotten it from the transfusion. The LDS Blood Bank and Hospital slandered Dad by insisting: "We have no idea how he got AIDS. All we did was give the old man heart surgery. He got AIDS from his lifestyle." All my father's doctors were led to believe the blood bank had not previously known of his infection.

It was essential for Dad to know he was infected with AIDS. With early medical supervision, proper treatment could have slowed progression of the disease. Opportunistic infections could have been correctly diagnosed and treated. Lung damage from pneumocystis pneumonia could have been prevented or delayed. Dad would have had time to get his business affairs in order when his mind was clear—before AIDS dementia set in. But most of all my father needed to be informed that he was infected with the AIDS virus so he could protect his wife.

In addition, family care of two elderly parents who are dying from AIDS goes beyond casual contact. Some precautions are necessary to protect caretakers from HIV-infected blood and from the other diseases AIDS patients carry. But LDS Blood Bank officials kept their silence without concern for the danger they placed our family in.

For decades the U.S. medical establishment has recognized that important medical information cannot be concealed from a patient. A 1986 study concluded it may be viewed as unethical to withhold information of an AIDS infection from an individual. It became apparent soon after AIDS testing of blood began that recipients of earlier untested donations of HIV-positive donors must be told. By April 1986 all blood banking associations recommended notifying these recipients.

Doctors report the HIV infection of a prior transfusion recipient to the blood bank which supplied the blood. It would have appeared to the LDS Blood Bank and the University doctors that Dad would soon die. His prognosis was poor. He'd had bypass surgery and was suffering from hepatitis B, cytomegalovirus infection and AIDS-related conditions. Furthermore, his unsophisticated family was unlikely to suspect the major cause of his illness.

Dr. Norwood Hill, a physician-scientist and blood banker testified at the House Subcommittee Hearing on May 15, 1991. Dr. Hill made the following statement regarding the failure of blood banks and doctors to inform patients of the probability that a unit of infected blood has been transfused: "Why would any physician who took the Oath of Hippocrates to 'first do no harm' withhold important medical information from his patient or the patient of another physician, especially when withholding that information can harm the patient? One of the principal reasons appears to be fear, especially fear of litigation. Fear drives irrational behavior and can cause some physicians and administrators, among others, to become confused about their duty to patients."

Each time one of Dad's doctors talked with the LDS Blood Bank about my father's AIDS, the blood bank pretended not to have known about it previously. Dad's last doctor received a letter to that effect in early 1988, long after several other doctors had discussed my father's case with the blood bank. It was not until after my father died that we learned the blood bank had known about his HIV-infected donor since June 1985—something his doctors probably never knew.

Unfortunately, our experience with the concealment of HIV infection given via transfusion is not unique. For many months doctors in San Francisco had repeatedly assured the frantic family of Francis Borchelt that she had no indications of the AIDS syndrome. The doctors suggested to the family that the feisty grandmother had picked up a disease from her parakeet. Mrs. Borchelt finally died of AIDS contracted from contaminated blood transfused at the time of her hip surgery.

Mary Johnstone, another San Francisco woman, discovered the reason for her debilitated health when she obtained copies of her voluminous medical records. As she sifted through the pages she found a letter which was exchanged between doctors stating that one of her blood donors was an AIDS patient. At that moment Mrs. Johnstone realized she had AIDS and her doctors had known for a long time.

When blood donors develop AIDS or test positive for the disease, the persons who received their past donations can be discreetly monitored by their doctors for years without their knowledge. Some are lucky and will have received blood donated prior to the time the donor became infected. But the others will have their failing immunity tracked with a chilling intensity.

In 1987 an elderly couple went to a public testing site in San Diego to get tested for AIDS. They felt strangely out of place among the younger people who waited with them to have the test. But since his heart surgery William Polikoff had suffered from devastating health problems. Although his doctors had insisted that he didn't have AIDS, the couple had the unusual common sense to get tested on their own.

The news was much worse than they had feared. Both of them were infected with HIV. The husband had been transfused with AIDS-tainted blood and had unknowingly infected his wife. But after their positive HIV tests the retired couple was subjected to degrading insinuations. Mr. Polikoff's doctors tried to convince him that his wife had been unfaithful, gotten infected by a lover and given AIDS to him.

A safe blood supply depends on two measures: screening the donors who supply it and testing the blood itself. Under the Freedom of Information Act, I obtained FDA inspection records of the LDS Blood Bank for an 8-year period. Throughout those years, Dr. Myron Laub was the blood bank's director. All FDA inspections cited the LDS Bank for deviations from FDA safety regulations.

Beginning in January 1980, inspections of the LDS Blood Bank cited inadequate quality control of reagents which continued for a six-year period. A reagent is a substance that takes part in a chemical reaction to detect the presence of other substances. The reagents used in the testing of blood must be of the highest quality and the FDA requires them to be tested every day to check their reactivity and specificity. An inspection in August 1981 found the LDS Blood Bank was performing quality control checks on reagents only once every 15 days—just two quality control checks per month instead of the required daily tests. On every pint of blood donated at the LDS Blood Bank the chance of inaccurate test results was increased by this deficiency.

Problems of poor reagent quality control continued at the LDS Blood Bank. A 1983 inspection found improvement in the number of quality control checks, but performance was still below FDA standards. There was not another inspection performed for two years prior to 1985 because the FDA had reduced inspections during the most critical years of the AIDS crisis. But in the mid-1985 inspection of the blood bank, citations were again given on the quality control of reagents. At that time there was also a problem with reagent storage. Outdated, unmarked reagents were not segregated and were kept in a refrigerator with the reagents used for blood testing.

That same FDA inspection found deficiencies in the calibration of hepatitis test equipment. When a follow-up inspection was performed five months later, the LDS Blood bank had still not corrected the problem. Although calibration was required on hepatitis equipment every month, none was accomplished for over four months, leaving blood recipients at increased risk for getting hepatitis B. Neither had deficiencies in reagent quality control been corrected. In a three-month period, checks were not done on 26 days. Reagent deficiency had been cited in all five inspections between January 1980 and December 1985.

In the July 1985 inspection, the FDA cited LDS Blood Bank with a total of nine deviations from safe blood handling practices. Persistent low-grade fever is a symptom of AIDS. Yet electronic thermometers used to take donor temperatures were not calibrated. The blood bank also lacked adequate Standard Operating Procedures for AIDS testing. The FDA inspector expressed concern over inadequate AIDS information on donor educational material and donor suitability forms.

On March 24, 1983, the FDA sent regulations to all blood banks for reducing AIDS contamination in the blood supply. From that time on donor information was to identify those groups at increased risk of AIDS and to instruct them to not donate blood. The FDA required the donor medical history card to include questions which elicit a history of AIDS symptoms. I have copies of the donor cards the LDS Blood Bank used between 1979 and mid-1985. During those years only one AIDS symptom (shortness of breath) was added to the blood bank's donor card under the category of heart disease. For over two years the following AIDS symptoms, which the FDA required to be covered, never appeared on the LDS donor card or educational material: night sweats, unexplained fever, persistent diarrhea, persistent cough, swollen lymph nodes and symptoms and signs of Kaposi sarcoma. FDA regulation 21CFR640.3 stated, "The donor's response to these questions should be recorded." How can a response be recorded if the questions weren't listed on the donor card?

My father's HIV-positive donor eventually revealed that he was not given any educational materials explaining which groups were at risk for AIDS. Nor was he asked about symptoms of AIDS, even though the lethal donation was made 21 months after the FDA required donors to be educated and screened. Neither had the subject of AIDS been mentioned during a prior donation made in June 1984.

Effective donor screening is the first line of defense against contamination of the blood supply. All the blood my father received in his transfusion was collected by the LDS Blood Bank. Those donors needed adequate educational materials before they could recognize risks in their lifestyle. The religious orientation of the Salt Lake City community necessitated strong AIDS education to counter the lack of sophistication regarding sexually transmitted disease. Any culture will have closet homosexuals and bisexuals and prior intravenous drug users. When many of the donors are recruited at church meetings, great pressure exists to protect image. The Utah cultural climate required forceful, printed information to convince those donors in high risk groups that their blood could kill others.

In July 1985, FDA inspector Maticka asked Dr. Laub why the AIDS symptoms in the FDA guidelines were not mentioned in the LDS Blood Bank's educational brochure or on the donor suitability form. Dr. Laub said they asked some verbal questions but he had no intention of adding the AIDS symptoms to his donor cards because it wasn't necessary.

The FDA inspector asked Laub why the six confirmed AIDS-positive donors which the blood bank had found were not deferred, even temporarily. FDA guidelines indicated these donors should be deferred after routine testing was being done. The LDS Blood Bank was doing routine AIDS testing but Dr. Laub said he doubted the test's reliability and considered the six AIDS-positive donors in a "phase-in" category. The attitude of the blood bank's director was one of indifferent noncompliance.

Even more incredible, during an interview with reporter Jess Gomez in summer 1990, Dr. Laub stated that the LDS Blood Bank did not begin interviewing donors to determine if they were at risk for AIDS until late 1989!

When the CDC confirmed the first 15 transfusion AIDS cases acquired from HIV-tested blood, approximately half the patients had received their tainted transfusions in smaller cities having a low incidence of AIDS. Some researchers believe the risk of getting AIDS in a transfusion is directly related to "the incidence of newly acquired HIV infection in a community and the awareness in that community that persons with risk factors for HIV infection should not donate blood." My father's case proved that health consumers in areas with conservative lifestyles should not blindly believe their blood supply is safe. If the local blood banks are lax in educating and screening donors in communities having few AIDS cases, there could be a higher chance of HIV contamination in the blood supply than in a city such as Los Angeles.

Chapter 16

Blood Safety in the 1990s

A Changing Scene

As of March 1992, 141,273 people in the United States have died of AIDS—more than the combined battle deaths the nation suffered in the Korean, Vietnam and Gulf wars. It is estimated that another one million Americans could die of the disease by the end of the century. On a national level the spread of HIV infection is shifting toward women and children. Although the number of AIDS cases in men remains high, the rate of new HIV infections is increasing faster in women than men.

While IV drug use or sex with an IV drug user are the major causes of infection in women, contaminated transfusions and sex with hemophilia clotting factor recipients have also been contributors. According to the CDC *Morbidity and Mortality Weekly Report*, by January 1989 11% of all women with AIDS had contracted the disease through blood transfusion. It was reported in March 1991 that blood transfusion had been responsible for the infection of 27% of the HIV-positive women in the state of California.

Heterosexual transmission of HIV is becoming more common. In 1990 the nation's number of heterosexual AIDS cases was at 3,100. In early 1992 they were at 12,510. It is estimated that 100,000 Americans may have already been heterosexually infected with HIV. As the current epidemic spreads among heterosexuals it presents additional challenges for ensuring a safe blood supply. Merely asking blood donors if they are homosexual or IV drug users does not weed out heterosexuals who are infected with AIDS. As the epidemic expands into different groups, donors may not recognize behaviors that place them at risk for HIV infection.

The *potential* for AIDS contamination in the blood supply goes up as the incidence of HIV infection increases in the population. During a House Subcommittee Hearing the FDA estimated the number of AIDS infections being given via transfusion in the months immediately before HIV testing began was at a yearly rate of 8,400. The agency stated that *without* intervention such as donor deferral and blood testing that, by 1991, the number would have ballooned to 72,000 transfusion AIDS infections per year. Although the blood industry deserves credit for safety measures implemented since early 1985, the *potential* for donors to be HIV-positive increases as more people become infected with AIDS.

The Tip of the Iceberg

The nation's AIDS cases are compiled and reported by the CDC. Statistics include only full-blown AIDS cases—those patients who are HIV-positive and have specific AIDS-related illnesses that have been diagnosed by their doctors. The "indicator diseases" the CDC requires for reporting include certain cancers and opportunistic infections that attack patients whose immune systems have been weakened by the AIDS virus. Individuals who are just infected with HIV are *not* reported to the CDC. From the beginning of the epidemic through June 1992 there were 230,179 full-blown AIDS cases tabulated by the agency.

It may take as long as 12 years before a person who is infected with HIV develops symptoms of AIDS, and another two years before the case is diagnosed and reported. Because of the lengthy lag time between infection and reporting, AIDS *cases* are extremely slow to reflect the extent of AIDS *infections*. Nationally, the number of people estimated to be infected with HIV is between 1 and 1½ million.

There is no national law requiring doctors to report AIDS cases. However, they are *supposed* to be reported to state or local health departments for forwarding to the CDC. But a two-year study by the General Accounting Office concluded that *33% of all AIDS cases and fatal HIV-related illnesses never get into the CDC data*! Doctors may treat private patients discreetly and not report them as AIDS cases to protect the patient from questions and social stigma. Or, after a patient's illness progresses to the reportable stage, busy doctors may purposely avoid doing the paperwork required to get an AIDS case into the CDC statistics. In addition, there are patients who die from AIDS-related illnesses without ever being diagnosed. Amazingly, many doctors do not test for HIV unless patients *look* like they are from high risk groups.

When AIDS cases are reported to the CDC, the reporting doctor has questioned the patient and indicates how it is believed that individual contracted HIV, or if there was more than one risk factor for exposure. There are five major exposure categories and they are ranked in the following order: gay men, IV drug abusers, hemophiliacs, heterosexual contact and lastly, blood transfusion recipients. The ranking order forms a *hierarchy* of exposures which means patients who possibly had more than one type of exposure are placed in the category listed first in the report. With a few rare exceptions, the CDC does not require *proof* of how patients contracted HIV. Therefore, the number of cases in the various categories cannot be considered accurate.

We have been discussing *all* AIDS cases. But the transfusion and hemophiliac exposure categories each have a set of unique factors which influence how well the reported cases indicate the extent of HIV infection through those routes. Ironically, the two blood categories differ widely as to how many infections will end up in the CDC report as cases. While only a small percentage of those infected via blood transfusion will *ever* get into the report, hemophilia AIDS cases should eventually be a meaningful accounting of HIV exposure through clotting factors.

The hemophilia group is unusual because a high percentage of its members were exposed to AIDS between 1977 and 1985. High-risk clotting factors made from the pooled plasma of tens of thousands of donors infected at least 50% of all America's hemophiliacs. These patients are painfully aware of their fate and are well monitored by their doctors for AIDS. By early 1992 less than 2,000 were in the CDC report as AIDS cases although 10,000 hemophiliacs became infected 7 to 15 years before. This is an example of how long it takes for AIDS *infections* to get reported as AIDS *cases* even when their HIV infection is known.

But in the transfusion category most of the HIV infections given are unknown and never show up as AIDS cases. Even after an incubating and reporting period of 12 years, only around 20% of the AIDS infections acquired through the transfusion route will be reported. There are sound reasons for this conclusion:

- According to medical studies 60% of those who contracted HIV infection by *transfusion* will die within a year from their underlying medical condition. These patients do not have *time* to develop AIDS and get diagnosed before they die.

- An unknown number of those who develop AIDS from transfusion have their cases listed in other exposure categories because transfusion is placed at the bottom of the hierarchy. By April 1992 there were 4,833 AIDS cases listed under transfusion. But *another* 4,741 transfusion recipients also had full-blown AIDS and were counted in other categories because they had more than one exposure risk.

  Sadly, tainted transfusion is the most efficient mode of HIV transmission; it is at least 95% certain to infect the recipient! Blood is 1,000 times more infectious than sperm. Yet 510 transfusion recipients are counted as acquiring AIDS heterosexually! The CDC never puts a patient with any other type of possible exposure into the transfusion category.

- Remember that according to the GAO study, 33% who do develop AIDS and *die* from AIDS-related illnesses do not get into the CDC data. There are two reasons this percentage is higher for those who acquire AIDS from transfusions. Patients who have the majority of the nation's blood transfusions are over 50. And the AIDS diagnosis is easy to miss in elderly patients. Their AIDS-related symptoms are dead ringers for those that frequently accompany old age: forgetfulness, confusion, depression, anxiety, motor dysfunction, even incontinence and stroke. Many doctors do not look for AIDS in older patients or test for it. New York City Health Department records indicate that during the 1980s, 78% of the city's dentists and doctors never ordered an AIDS test for a single patient!

  The other reason some fatal AIDS illnesses in prior transfusion recipients do not get reported is because these cases are political. Doctors may be under pressure to preserve the local area's safe-blood image and keep them out of the state health department statistics. And should the AIDS diagnosis be concealed from the patient, as it was from my father, it certainly won't be reported to government agencies.

Thus, a combination of unique factors keep approximately 80% of the HIV infections given from tainted transfusions from *ever* being reported to the CDC as AIDS cases. Nevertheless, there are now nearly 5,000 AIDS cases from contaminated transfusions. It can be concluded that for that number to surface, approximately 25,000 infections would have been transmitted. (This number does not include cases still in incubation.) In 1987 the CDC estimated that 29,000 HIV infections were given via transfusion before testing of donations began in 1985. The CDC also estimated that 12,000 of the recipients were still alive and unaware of their plight. If that many did survive the illness they were transfused for, we can expect transfusion cases from *un*tested blood to continue to rise for years, just as hemophilia cases will.

The Iceberg Tip is Now Submerged

Up to this point we have discussed AIDS cases given from untested blood. But are there cases that were acquired from blood donations that *were* tested for HIV? It is essential that health consumers understand the answer to this question.

If we listen to blood bankers and public health officials the problem has been solved. "Virtually every unit of HIV infected blood is removed by the test." "A safe product (blood) has been made even safer." But the public has *always* been told the blood supply was safe—even while millions of hepatitis infections and tens of thousands of HIV infections were being transfused into the veins of innocent victims. The CDC presently tells the media there are just 20 cases of AIDS linked to transfusion from tested blood. However, an examination of how that number is obtained suggests that the tip of the iceberg could still be there. It is just statistically submerged.

It was in April 1989 that I noticed a footnote at the bottom of the CDC's monthly surveillance report on AIDS. The transfusion category included two recipients who had come down with AIDS after getting blood that had tested negative for HIV. It was not surprising that the test failed to detect evidence of AIDS infection because it allows tainted units of blood to slip through if the donors have just recently been infected. Blood facilities had also been experiencing growing problems with the release of potentially tainted blood because of testing and computer errors. After four years of HIV testing, I was puzzled that the number of AIDS cases from tested blood was so low.

In the spring of 1990 the House Subcommittee on Blood Supply Safety wrote to Dr. William Roper, Director of the CDC, for an explanation of the handful of AIDS cases from blood tested for HIV. Dr. Roper answered in a letter and described the cases, which then numbered 11, as a "meaningful statistic." He wrote, "These are confirmed AIDS cases for whom a seropositive donor was identified upon repeat donation or testing."

When I read the Roper letter a light blinked on. I realized the CDC was handling transfusion cases given after the spring of 1985 differently than those given before testing began. Cases from *un*tested blood had to be reported and have no other known exposure risk than transfusion. But cases from *tested* blood had to also be confirmed. One of the requirements for confirmation was the formidable task of finding an HIV-positive donor. Between the time testing began and the writing of Roper's letter, there had been 3,500 transfusion AIDS cases added to the CDC report. I wanted to know the total number of reported—not confirmed—cases from tested blood to compare against the early cases from untested blood.

I wrote to the CDC and under the Freedom of Information Act requested a breakdown of the reported cases from untested and tested blood. After an extremely lengthy delay my request was answered by the CDC on July 31, 1991. The agency wrote, "A search of our records reveals no documents responsive to this question." Crock-talk! If the agency didn't keep before-and-after testing records, how did it know which cases to confirm?

Ten Months Later

The CDC broke its silence. The May 28, 1992, issue of the *New England Journal of Medicine* published a letter to the editor written by Dr. Scott Holmberg and Lois Conley of the CDC. This letter revealed that during the *first five years* of HIV testing, 158 cases were reported to the CDC of patients who had purportedly acquired AIDS from blood that had been tested.

By comparison, after the first seven years of the AIDS epidemic (1978 to April 1985) just 145 transfusion AIDS cases had been reported from *un*tested blood. And those 145 cases proved to be a harbinger of the 5,000 transfusion AIDS cases which would be reported by spring 1992—almost all of them from blood that had *not* been tested for the AIDS virus. It is worrisome that there were 13 more cases reported from tested blood during the first five years of HIV testing than were reported in the seven years prior to testing. Could history be repeating itself and those 158 cases also be a harbinger of what is to come?

My exception to the information the CDC provides the media is that apples are being compared to oranges. At this early date, the few *confirmed* cases from tested blood cannot be compared to the large number of *reported* cases from untested blood as proof of a safe blood supply. Yet they are being used for that purpose by the media and health establishment.

Transfusion AIDS Cases Are Difficult To Confirm

The CDC has not disclosed how many AIDS cases from HIV-tested blood have been reported since 1990. But the 158 cases between 1985 and 1990 would have represented less than 20% of the *infections* given during the first five years of testing. (As discussed, this is due to unique problems in reporting *any* transfusion AIDS cases and because 60% of the recipients die soon from underlying illnesses.) In addition, most of these cases would still be in incubation. It is significant that of the 158 cases that were reported from tested blood just 15 were confirmed—less than 10%. The CDC letter to the editor detailed the protocol for confirmation.

When a transfusion AIDS case from tested blood is reported to the CDC, the agency will not consider it for confirmation if the report lists any other risk factor for acquiring AIDS. If the sole risk is transfusion, the CDC contacts the state or local health department that sent in the report. The department is asked to verify when a transfusion was received. They are also asked to make further investigation of additional risk factors. If the patient has already died, the *case* is closed. This can prevent confirmation of valid cases because some patients do not live long after diagnosis. The greatest obstacle to confirmation is finding a donor who is HIV-positive but the CDC merely requests that health departments investigate the HIV status of the donors "when feasible." Thus the donor investigation, on which confirmation depends, can be discontinued after a token effort.

Tracing and testing donors is both difficult and political. The blood bank's cooperation is required because it alone knows the identity of the donors. Some transfusion recipients can have 20 or more donors and letters have to be sent to each one so they can be tested again for HIV. After as many as 10 years it is often impossible to locate all of them. Those infected with the AIDS virus may have left the area to be cared for by their families or have already died. And donors who suspect they may be positive may prefer to avoid testing or questions about their lifestyle.

More importantly, there is no incentive for blood banks to find positive donors! The longer blood banks can stall, the less chance there is of confirmation or lawsuit. Under the law, hospitals and blood banks are only required to keep a transfusion recipient's donor records for *five years*, after which the records are usually promptly destroyed so donors can't be traced. And the average time before AIDS symptoms appear in transfusion AIDS victims is *seven years*. Therefore, before most transfusion recipients know they have contracted HIV infection, their records have been destroyed. Without records there is no way a transfusion AIDS case from blood which was tested for HIV can be confirmed.

The reluctance of blood banks to cooperate with regulatory agencies was discussed at a House Subcommittee Hearing in July 1990. Testimony was given by Mary T. Carden, the FDA's National Expert Investigator for Biologics, who had recently inspected the blood operations at Red Cross National Headquarters. The American Red Cross supplies approximately half of the nation's blood supply. House Subcommittee concern centered around the Red Cross' failure to report transfusion-associated AIDS to the FDA. The Washington, DC, blood center received reports from the doctors of 228 transfusion recipients who had come down with AIDS-related illnesses after getting blood from that one Red Cross Region.

FDA regulations which are issued pursuant to statutory authority of the Food and Drug Administration require that accident/error reports be filed on each case. The blood regions of the Red Cross are required to send a report to Red Cross headquarters for investigation and forwarding to the FDA. However, only four of the 228 cases were reported to Red Cross headquarters and none to the FDA. And without being informed the agency cannot ensure that unsafe blood-handling practices are corrected.

In a written response to the House Subcommittee, Ms. Carden commented on the non-compliance of blood banks in providing information to the FDA on probable transmission of AIDS from the blood they have supplied. She wrote, "The blood banking industry, sensitive to the potential for litigation in these cases, is very unwilling to share this information with the agency." Blood banks have every reason not to provide incriminating information that might be obtained under the Freedom of Information Act.

Inspector Carden wrote of how difficult it is to conduct donor investigations because of the unavailability of donor records, "In some instances because of record discrepancies, proper investigations cannot be conducted . . . since all records relevant to some donors are not available." For example, the FDA inspection of Red Cross National Headquarters in summer of 1991 revealed there were 4,500 donor history records missing for blood collected at the Washington, DC, Region having the 228 reported transfusion AIDS cases. The "missing" records meant there could not be any donor tracing or confirmation of AIDS cases from the blood given by those 4,500 donors. And those donors had all given blood *after* donations were being tested for AIDS.

The earlier FDA inspection in 1990 revealed that investigations of many of the reported AIDS cases in the Washington Region had not been performed. Some of the cases had been reported over *four years before* but donors of the AIDS-infected recipients had not been notified so that tracing could begin. Blood facilities have strong incentive to postpone these investigations until it is too late to find positive donors. It isn't difficult to understand why the CDC's number of confirmed transfusion AIDS cases from tested blood is so low.

Mary Carden referred to a magazine article which asserted that transfusion AIDS infections were essentially eliminated when HIV testing was added in March 1985. Ms. Carden replied with classic understatement, *"I believe it is underreported."* (Italics added) She further explained the FDA had determined that 16 of the 228 AIDS cases in question had been given after testing of blood began. She noted, "Also of importance is the fact the 228 cases in the Washington Region represent transfusion-associated AIDS cases from that region alone. FDA has not examined cases from the other 53 regions of the American Red Cross." Unfortunately the FDA does not conduct investigations of that depth until safety conditions in either Red Cross or other blood collection centers become critical.

In Summation

The CDC admits a small number of AIDS cases have been acquired through transfused blood that was tested for HIV. These few cases do not project the present risk of getting HIV infection in a transfusion for the following reasons:

* No more than 20% of any transfusion AIDS infections (from untested *or* tested blood) are reported to the CDC.

* The first AIDS cases contracted from HIV tested blood are from the small group of recipients who develop AIDS rapidly after infection. It's too soon for the majority to be diagnosed with AIDS and get reported.

* Reported AIDS cases from tested blood must be *confirmed*. Ninety percent of those reported are not being confirmed. Some of the reasons are legitimate; others are due to the following roadblocks:

    —An HIV-positive donor must be found for each case. But records linking recipients to donors are destroyed after five years—long before most of the cases surface. Also, blood banks can stonewall in providing information and tracing donors because of fear of litigation.

    —If the patient dies the case is not investigated and confirmed.

    —The placing of transfusion recipients at the bottom of the exposure hierarchy prevents some infections contracted through transfusion from being counted in the proper category.

The confirmed transfusion AIDS cases given since testing began are meaningless as an indicator of blood supply safety. Nevertheless, the media accepts and reports them without question.

On May 22, 1991, the lead editorial in the *Gazette Telegraph*, Colorado Springs' daily newspaper, maintained that there have been only "a few well-publicized cases" of transfusion AIDS which were given in the early 1980s. The editorial lamented that those "few" early cases had left the false impression that recipients of donated blood run a risk of contracting the AIDS virus and explained that any risk virtually ended in 1985 after blood banks began testing donations for HIV. Referring to the May 1991 statistics, the editor wrote, "Of the 174,893 AIDS cases reported since 1985 only 15 are linked to medical blood transfusions."

When the editorial was written, 4,023 transfusion AIDS cases had been *reported* since blood banks started testing. But the editor was confused by the CDC's 15 *confirmed* cases from tested blood. Considering the CDC shaping of statistics released to the media, the editor's mistake (off by 4,008) is forgivable. Nevertheless, this type of reporting is very misleading.

However, it isn't just the lay public that is subjected to a barrage of misinformation. The last issue of *AIDS Alert*, a monthly update for doctors and other health care professionals, contained the following paragraph on blood safety:

> Prior to testing, more than 4,700 people became infected with HIV as the result of blood transfusions, says Liz Hall, spokeswoman for the American Red Cross. Since testing began in 1985, only 20 cases of HIV infection due to blood transfusions have been reported.

Few doctors reading that message would have realized that the 20 cases were *confirmed* ones for whom a positive donor was found and that an *undisclosed* number of cases have been *reported* from tested blood. By 1990 that number was 158—more than the number of cases from *un*tested blood reported in the first seven years of the epidemic. Nor would many professionals realize the 4,700 reported adult cases were but a fraction of the approximately 29,000 HIV infections given from untested blood. Doctors are not immune to safe-blood propaganda.

The Good News

AIDS forced public attention on the blood supply and blood banks had no choice but to make long overdue improvements in blood safety. Between 1985 and early 1992, seven additional tests to detect infectious diseases were added to the processing of each donation of blood. Education of donors was expanded and deferment of high risk groups tightened. As a result, the number of AIDS-infected donors volunteering to give blood has decreased.

There were also improvements in consumer services. The outcry over transfusion AIDS cases put pressure on blood banks to offer improved autologous predonation services. There was increased cooperation with patients wishing to donate their own blood before surgery and some blood banks now provide IAT equipment and trained operators to hospitals not having their own IAT capability. This makes it possible for more patients to have their blood recycled during surgery, thus giving themselves a transfusion.

Armed with knowledge and a firm resolve to obtain the best in transfusion medicine, health consumers now have a better chance of avoiding the pitfalls of transfusion-transmitted disease and the serious reactions that may occur because of incompatibilities between the donor's and recipient's blood. It's called consumerism. Progress is being made.

There are positive indications that the FDA is making a serious effort to gain control of the nonprofit blood industry, and in 1991 it was given more power to enforce regulations. More money has been allocated to the agency for oversight of blood safety. Additional employees have been hired and field inspectors and compliance personnel are both dedicated and better trained. Efforts are now being made to reduce bureaucratic delays. In the past it could take the FDA up to three years to publish new regulations for the blood industry.

Historically, the FDA allowed the blood industry's trade associations to shape the guidelines for safety procedures with emphasis on industry interests rather than consumer protection. Worse yet, after the agency inspected blood banks and found deficiencies, strong action was often not taken to enforce correction of unsafe practices. The LDS Blood Bank in Salt Lake City ignored deficiencies in the quality control of reagents for six years with each successive FDA inspection citing the same problem. After reviewing these inspections our family could not understand why the FDA bothered to inspect if it could not compel blood banks to make corrections of unsafe procedures. We discovered that the FDA can *choose* not to take regulatory action even though a law has been violated.

However, there is evidence that the FDA is beginning to take a tougher stand. Prodded by the House Subcommittee the agency recently took the American Red Cross by the scruff of the neck and forced a major reorganization of its Blood Services.

Problems in the 54 Red Cross blood regions had been growing for years. Nationwide, the regions were using 10 different computer systems which the FDA found were not properly maintained, up-to-date or upgraded. Computer demands of modern blood banking are astronomical because the nine blood tests for infectious disease require burdensome and exacting recordkeeping. A glitch in a computer system can cause quarantined blood which has tested positive for hepatitis or AIDS to be mistakenly released before confirming tests can determine if it must be destroyed. When human or computer errors cause quarantined units to be released only a portion of them will be infected—the rest will be false positives. However, the ones that are truly positive for AIDS carry a death sentence. Even more worrisome are the false negative units—those that test negative but are actually HIV-positive.

Problems with Red Cross computer systems continued to grow. In 1988 the FDA asked the Red Cross to sign a Voluntary Agreement pledging closer monitoring of its blood regions and a major overhaul of its computer systems. The agreement also addressed poor laboratory practices and inadequate screening of blood donors in Red Cross blood centers.

However, when the FDA inspected Red Cross national headquarters in 1990, it was determined that the conditions of the 1988 agreement were being violated. The computer systems were still judged to be inadequate, some blood *known* to be infected had been released and infected donors had not been deferred. There was also evidence of mixed up records and violated testing procedures since the agreement was signed. More disturbing was the nonchalant attitude at Red Cross headquarters and a lack of willingness to correct problems.

During the last half of 1990 the FDA worked with the American Red Cross in structuring a sweeping reorganization of the way it collects and handles blood. The extent of those changes are unprecedented in the history of blood banking and will cost a projected $120 million.

Red Cross Blood Services was placed under the centralized control of Red Cross headquarters with full accountability and authority given to Dr. Jeffery McCullough, the new Senior Vice President, brought in to reform the blood program. The Red Cross' patchwork recordkeeping system will eventually be handled by one computer system which will take two and a half years or more to bring on line. The testing of blood will be limited to 10 regional centers with highly trained personnel. New and nationally uniform procedures will be established and there are noteworthy plans for more Red Cross involvement in IAT surgical procedures.

I have studied Dr. McCullough's statement of June 18, 1991, to the House Subcommittee and found it impressive, refreshingly honest and devoid of the usual crock-talk. But the Red Cross faces a horrendous task in getting a collection of idiosyncratic blood regions to bow to central authority. As recently as May 1991, the Red Cross Pacific Northwest

Regional Blood Center in Portland had been cited with *51 deviations* from FDA safe-blood handling procedures. The director was put on probation for a year. The FDA will no longer allow the center to test blood for hepatitis and AIDS. Samples of each unit collected are flown daily to St. Paul, Minnesota, for testing and the results faxed back to Portland.

Dr. Marcus Simpson, head of the blood bank at George Washington Medical Center told Associated Press, "Only time will tell if the new measures will increase the level of (Red Cross) blood safety." But it is certain that, in the increasingly complex business of blood banking, a bandaid approach would not fix the Red Cross' blood woes. Hopefully $120 million will buy a good start.

The Bad News

Conditions in the Red Cross Blood Services were so unsafe they necessitated a major reorganization. The bad news is that the performance of the other half of the blood industry not under the Red Cross is *worse*. Those blood establishments are cited more frequently during FDA inspections for non-compliance violations than the Red Cross Centers. Information presented to the House Subcommittee by the FDA indicate the following:

A Comparison of Violative Rates for the Red Cross and Non-Red Cross Blood Establishment Inspections

Year	*Red Cross*	*Non-Red Cross*	
1989	6.1%	11.9%	
1990	9.2%	11.8%	
1991	12.8%	13.8%	10-1-90 to 3-31-91

The blood banks and centers that collect the half of the nation's blood supply not under the Red Cross are members of the AABB and CCBC. These two organizations have *not* announced plans for major changes that would improve blood safety. With violations in the non-Red Cross establishments now running substantially higher than the Red Cross, it would appear improvements are overdue in these blood banks as well.

To prevent infusing patients with blood that may cause life-threatening illness, units must be meticulously labeled. The nation's largest blood facility is the New York Blood Center which is not part of the American Red Cross blood network. The New York Blood Center's FDA inspection in 1991 determined that unit labels were not being adequately examined for accuracy and, as a result, numerous inventory control errors were occurring. Each month hospitals were returning between 55 and 70 units to the blood center because of incorrect labeling or outdated blood. These errors included units that were ABO mistyped, had the wrong expiration dates, were already outdated, were without any expiration dates or identifying numbers and units with no labels at all. When hospitals return up to 70 such units per month one wonders how many other questionable units get transfused to patients.

In June 1991, Dr. Gerald Quinnan, acting director of the FDA's Center for Biologics, told the House Subcommittee " . . . infectious diseases continue to be transmitted by blood and blood products. In addition, blood establishments continue to have problems maintaining compliance with good blood banking practices and an increasing number of error and accident reports are being submitted to the agency." More disturbing are the unknown numbers of accidents and errors that are concealed from the agency.

Recalls of suspect blood are growing. This includes blood that has been improperly tested, quarantined blood that was mistakenly released or blood from dangerous or potentially dangerous donors. Nearly all of the "recalled" blood will have already been infused into patients but investigation is necessary to prevent future errors and to get infected donors on the dangerous donor registry. In 1987 the FDA ordered just 21 recalls of suspect blood and blood products. In 1989 there were 252 recalls ordered and during the first six months of 1991 there were 202 with a projection of over 400 for the year. It is difficult to know how much of the growth in recalls is due to increased problems in blood banks and how much is because of tighter FDA surveillance.

There is no question that with the backing of the House Subcommittee the FDA is doing a better job of policing the industry. However, the agency's performance rating for protecting consumers of blood and blood products between 1982 and 1985, during the height of the AIDS blood banking crisis, was zero minus one. There was no place for FDA surveillance to go but up.

The agency points to its 1988 change from inspecting blood banks every two years to once a year as a major accomplishment. But my copies of FDA inspections indicate the agency had inspected on a yearly schedule until 1983. Six months *after* the Atlanta meeting in January 1983, the agency *decreased* inspections to once every two years. FDA inspectors did not go into the LDS Blood Bank in Salt Lake City between June 1983 and July 1985—the 25-month period when the majority of the nation's AIDS-tainted blood was transfused. My father received his viral cocktail of hepatitis B, cytomegalovirus and AIDS during the 19th month of non-surveillance. Our family had depended on the FDA to protect us. The relevant question today is can consumers rely on the FDA to protect them during the next blood contamination crisis?

In May 1991, a blue ribbon advisory committee on the FDA reported that the agency needs more money, more staff and more enforcement powers. In Senate testimony, former FDA Commissioner Charles Edwards, who chaired the panel, called the FDA "vulnerable to fraud and blunder" and "living on borrowed time." In addition to more funding, Dr. Edwards recommended the FDA be made independent of the Public Health Service bureaucracy. When asked if the agency is capable of carrying out its public health mission, Dr. Edwards answered "It's a close call." My concern is that the present improvements in FDA blood surveillance might not last after the agency's next budget cut.

The Present Infectious Risk

There will always be a risk of transfusion transmitted disease. A public that before AIDS believed the blood supply was safe is just beginning to realize that being transfused with someone else's blood is risky business. Any germ present in donated blood may be given to the person who receives it, including the next *new* disease that may be going around the block. Depending on the germ or germs in the transfusion, the recipient can become acutely ill soon after infusion or not until years later. For most of the past two decades, the infectious risk of blood transfusions was generally ignored by doctors and downplayed to their patients. Consequently, a large number of people suffered disability and, in many cases, death without understanding the origin of their illnesses.

However, by 1992 the blood industry was using nine tests to screen out infectious diseases. Although these tests all have a margin for error, they have brought a remarkable decrease in blood supply contamination. The extent of that contamination has been one of medicine's best kept secrets.

Hepatitis

Hepatitis has presented by far the most serious viral threat to transfusion recipients. The FDA estimates that prior to testing and donor screening there were 900,000 non-A, non-B hepatitis infections a year given by transfusions plus 360,000 hepatitis B infections—a total of 1.26 *million* hepatitis infections a year.

Types of Hepatitis

Hepatitis A   Rarely transmitted by transfusion. Blood banks do not test for it.

Hepatitis B   Two hepatitis B specific tests (HBsAg and HBc) are done on every blood donation.

Hepatitis C   Formerly called non-A, non-B. Blood banks are using a new test (HCV) which detects antibodies to the hepatitis C strain. Researchers have found there are other unidentified strains that also cause non-A, non-B hepatitis, but the vast majority of cases appear to be from hepatitis C.

Hepatitis D   Known as delta hepatitis. Infects in a piggyback style along with hepatitis B. Donations are not tested for hepatitis D because only some of the units infected with hepatitis B carry it. Hopefully those units will test positive for hepatitis B and be discarded.

Note: Blood banks also use the ALT test to detect signs of liver damage which is an indicator of hepatitis.

The threat of post-transfusion hepatitis has been extremely difficult to solve. During House Subcommittee testimony, Dr. Edgar Engleman, director of the Stanford blood bank, stated that before the two 1986 hepatitis tests were added, up to 10% of those transfused got hepatitis non-A, non-B. Ross Eckert, who sits on the FDA's Blood Products Advisory Committee, estimated the number of non-A, non-B infections given during the three years *after* the tests were adopted at 200,000 per year, with 4,000 dying of cirrhosis of the liver within 10 years. Mr. Eckert said, "Losing 4,000 people per year is about like losing a fully loaded DC-10 each month. I doubt that Congress would tolerate in airline travel the rate of casualties we have had in blood banking."

In 1991, a year after the hepatitis C test was implemented to reduce non-A, non-B hepatitis, the FDA estimated that there were still 54,000 hepatitis C (non-A, non-B) infections being given yearly.

The HBc test implemented in 1986 was the disputed hepatitis B core antibody test which had been available since 1976. Dr. Edgar Engleman told the House Subcommittee that because the core antibody test identifies past hepatitis B infection, it is a surrogate test for both hepatitis non-A, non-B and AIDS. Those viruses are frequently carried by people who have previously had hepatitis B. In addition, before the core test was used, many transfusion recipients like my father got hepatitis B from infected blood that the HBsAg test had not detected. That number is now thought to have plummeted.

The blood industry has never admitted that one of the present benefits of the core test is that it provides a backup for eliminating AIDS infected blood which the HIV test does not detect. To save face, the industry insists the core antibody test is merely a surrogate test for hepatitis non-A, non-B and has nothing to do with AIDS. But regardless of why the blood industry claims to use the test, consumers have benefited from the extra protection it gives the blood supply.

AIDS

The HIV-1 antibody test that was implemented in blood banks in 1985 is considered to be 99% effective in excluding AIDS-infected donors. The test does not detect the virus—just antibodies to it. Unfortunately, it takes some time after becoming infected for the body to produce those antibodies—from three weeks to six months. During this window period the donor's blood is infected and will infect anyone who is transfused with it. A few other donors could be silently infected and *never* produce antibodies. In rare cases, antibodies are produced but after awhile drop sharply and are no longer picked up by the test currently in use.

A CDC medical study concluded that 460 Americans who are transfused with properly tested blood could be infected with AIDS each year due to the *window period*. This estimate is from the test's inadequacy only and does not include infections given because of improper testing or other errors which occur in blood banks. There are approximately 3.6 million transfusions given yearly in the United States which places the risk of getting AIDS in a transfusion, according to the above study, at one in 7,840. However, other studies have concluded the risk is lower. The findings of two recent ones report rates of AIDS transmission from blood that has been tested for HIV at about one in 60,000 for *each* component of blood transfused. If the average transfusion requires 5.4 component units, according to those studies the present risk for getting AIDS in a transfusion is one in 11,111.

But statistics mean very little. At least the old one-in-a-million risk meant nothing in 1983. If we compare today's lowest estimated risk of one in 11,111 with the previous one-in-a-million risk, the chance of getting AIDS in a transfusion is now *90 times higher* than it was in 1983 and 1984 when *no* testing was being done. It's presently known that the one-in-a-million risk had no creditability but what is known about today's risk? The answer to that question will be available in about ten years.

Donor Screening—The First Line of Defense

Many experts in blood banking feel that meticulous donor screening and exclusion of those at high risk for AIDS is the major defense against contamination of the blood supply. Although at the present time the majority of high-risk donors are not going to blood banks to donate blood, there are still some who do.

In most of the world AIDS is spread primarily through heterosexual sex and in the United States that transmission route is growing. Studies reported at the June 1991 Conference on AIDS help explain heterosexual transmission. Researchers have found HIV in mucosal cells in the lining of the genitals, anus and mouth which indicates the virus can be spread in the absence of broken skin. The studies indicate how AIDS can be transmitted through oral sex and have disturbing implications for donor screening. It will become increasingly difficult to identify high-risk donors by groups and defer them from donor pools.

In December 1990 the FDA sent revised donor screening guidelines to blood establishments which were implemented in July 1991. Questions are slanted toward specific, risky behaviors but there is a lot of denial in that area. Some donors won't admit even to themselves that they engage in high-risk behavior—it's too frightening. Donors are currently asked if they have had sex with a prostitute or sold sex for drugs or money and if they have been treated for sexually transmitted diseases. The blood industry is between a rock and a hard place when screening blood donors. While those with more conservative lifestyles have less infections in their blood they are also the ones most likely to be offended by frank questioning.

In the past, transfusion recipients had been excluded from donating blood for a period of six months after transfusion. That restriction is extended to a year under the new guidelines so the body has more time to produce antibodies. But there is no 100% assurance that present blood tests will detect infections after a year or even longer and transfused blood can carry a variety of viruses that blood banks do not test for. Donors from high-risk groups such as gays and IV drug users are excluded. Transfusion recipients are also in a high-risk group for an assortment of viruses but they are only excluded for a year.

Ross Eckert told the House Subcommittee, "I think it is very important that we reform blood donor screening practices to remove from the donor pool anyone who has been transfused since 1977." Mr. Eckert maintains that the deferment of prior transfusion recipients would not only reduce the risk of transmitting AIDS but also reduce post-transfusion hepatitis—which kills more people annually than transfused AIDS.

At Irwin Memorial Blood Bank in San Francisco, risk factors of AIDS-positive donors were compared for the years 1984 and 1985. (The blood bank had kept frozen samples of the blood drawn in 1984 and tested them after the HIV test became available.) Irwin found that by far the largest number of AIDS-infected donors were in the homosexual risk group. However, the next highest category of AIDS-positive donors was *prior transfusion recipients—double the number of IV drug users.* The study supports the argument that transfusion recipients should not be allowed to donate blood and refutes the theory that prior recipients are in poor health and rarely donate.

There is another deficiency in present donor screening policy—again in the sensitive area of health care. Dr. Marcus Conant, a professor at the University of California Medical Center, expressed concern to the House Subcommittee over the collection of blood from people whose lifestyles are socially acceptable but whose work puts them at risk for disease. "I am not sure we should be taking blood from physicians who stick themselves with needles all the time and are being exposed to a whole variety of agents (germs)."

A June 1991 study found that 55% of the residents and interns in internal medicine at the University of California's three hospitals had, during the year, stuck themselves with needles containing the blood of patients known to be HIV-positive or at high risk for being so.

Accidental needle pricks are common among nurses and doctors even when all precautions are being adhered to. Health care workers at highest risk for contracting AIDS on the job are:

1. Those in areas where AIDS is prevalent

2. Those who work in emergency centers and come in frequent contact with patients' blood

3. Surgeons, especially those who perform "probing" surgeries

This last group is another well-kept secret.

Health officials have known since the beginning of the epidemic that AIDS is transmitted in the same ways as hepatitis B. It is well documented in the medical literature that hepatitis B can be given to patients by their surgeons and that surgeons can contract it from their patients. All that is needed is an exchange of blood from an infected surgeon or patient. It is also well known which procedures are the most hazardous for this exchange—those operations requiring blind probing with sharp instruments into patients' body cavities. Unable to see, surgeons are more likely to puncture their gloves and cut their hands on sharp, broken bone. A mix of the surgeon's and patient's blood can result in the transfer of disease. Some of the surgeries requiring blind probing are vaginal hysterectomy, pelvic surgery and dental surgery. Other invasive procedures of concern are abdominal surgery, heart surgery and root canals.

Blood drives among hospital personnel are common. But health care workers at highest risk for contracting AIDS should be excluded from donating. They are not aware of every exposure and could have a silent infection which the blood test would miss.

★　　★　　★

Dr. Joseph Feldschuh, an assistant professor at Cornell Medical School, has recently written a book on the blood supply. Dr. Feldschuh fears that the many transfusion AIDS infections transmitted in the early 1980s by contaminated blood may now be in the process of being repeated. He questions the inconsistency between FDA safety regulations for banked sperm and banked blood. The FDA requires sperm to be kept frozen, after donation, until the donor is tested again six months later and found negative the second time. The backup test reduces the chance of the donor having an AIDS infection which was undetectable by the first test. Feldschuh is astounded that this responsible precaution is taken for those undergoing artificial insemination while blood, which is 1,000 times more infectious than sperm, is transfused to nearly four million people a year without a waiting period. If blood were given the same safety precautions as sperm, it too would be frozen until the donor tested negative again at a later date.

There is a test for the AIDS virus itself—the HIV antigen test which does not have the problem of a window period like the ELISA test does. Blood banking leaders have taken the position that using the antigen test would *not* improve blood supply safety. Consequently, very few blood banks use it. But transfusion recipients could have greater confidence in blood safety if a second or more efficient method were used to test blood donations.

There is also a second AIDS virus, HIV-2, which, since early 1992, blood banks are required to test donations for. The disease caused by HIV-2 is identical to the AIDS caused by HIV-1 but in the United States the infection is considered to be rare. (This form of the virus spreads more slowly and is usually confined to Africa.)

Is There A New AIDS Virus?

At the 1992 international AIDS conference in Amsterdam there were reports of patients in Europe and the United States who had AIDS-like illness without evidence of HIV infection. None of the current tests could detect a trace of HIV, including sophisticated genetic probes capable of detecting minute quantities of the virus. Yet these patients were sick or dying, had collapsed immune systems and some were in high risk groups for AIDS.

The cases caused a storm of concern at the conference among both scientists and the press. Are the mysterious cases caused by an altered strain of HIV that eludes tests? Or is it an entirely different infectious agent? Some doctors doubted it was caused by an infectious agent. Perhaps it was some other type of immune dysfunction.

At a conference meeting one doctor after another stood up and reported similar cases—patients without evidence of HIV who appear to have AIDS-related symptoms. As the participants sat down, others got up and criticized the CDC for not reporting the cases the agency had identified during the past three years and for not making an early request for doctors to report similar cases. The doctors were concerned because if the illness is a new virus, there is no test to track it in the population or to remove infected donations from the blood supply.

Dr. Jeffrey Laurence, an immunologist at Cornell University Medical Center, has five patients with the AIDS-like illness. He told the *Wall Street Journal*, "We have to look back to 1981 at the start of the AIDS epidemic. People should bank their own blood."

A week after the AIDS conference, the CDC published its first formal report of the puzzling disease. Three of the six patients had received blood transfusions and two of them were transfused with blood that had tested negative for HIV. A later report out of Atlanta placed the number of U.S. patients with the AIDS-like disease at 26. But 16 of the 26 had none of the risk factors for AIDS. Of the remaining 10 patients, five were homosexuals and five had received blood transfusions. This means that present blood bank screening to determine lifestyle risks would have only eliminated five of the 26 as blood donors—those who were homosexual. Transfusion recipients are allowed to donate blood after one year.

It is too soon to know if the blood supply is becoming contaminated with a new virus but the recent scare illustrates how vulnerable the supply is. When viruses having lengthy incubation periods infiltrate the population, they may not be detected for years. Thus, the safety status of the present blood supply is always unknown.

Other Diseases Blood Banks Test For

Donated blood is tested for two other infectious diseases in addition to hepatitis and AIDS. One is syphilis, which is now almost never transmitted by transfusion because today's numerous tests require blood to be refrigerated for 36 to 48 hours before infusion. After that period of time, the infectious organism which causes syphilis dies, but blood banks still test each donation for it.

In 1988 testing was instituted for the retrovirus HTLV-1 (Human T-cell leukemia virus, type 1) which can cause adult T-cell leukemia. This cancer virus was discovered by Dr. Robert Gallo in 1980 at the National

Institutes of Health and, later, another strain, HTLV-2, was isolated. It is believed that testing blood donations for HTLV-1 has also had the secondary benefit of reducing the spread of HTLV-2 by transfusion. A new test is now available for blood-bank use which detects both HTLV-1 and HTLV-2.

Studies in the United States donor population have found that six out of 10,000 donors test positive for HTLV-1 and the infection is usually associated with drug use. Since testing began, the FDA places the number of HTLV-1 and 2 infections given yearly by transfusion at less than 150. However, because the incubation for T-cell leukemia/lymphoma can be 30 years, it is difficult to prove how much HTLV infection has been eliminated by testing the blood supply for these viruses. Despite the screening of donors and added number of tests, infection transmitted by transfusion can never be totally prevented.

Stanford's Dr. Edgar Engleman, who became a maverick blood banker in 1983 by taking a stand on the side of blood safety rather than conforming to industry politics, is worried that after the public concern diminishes the industry will slip back into complacency. He told the House Subcommittee, "While the safety of today's blood supply is much improved over past years, one of the reasons why we are using so many more tests is public pressure and perhaps fear of litigation on the part of blood banking institutions rather than industry insight into the real needs of the blood industry."

Laws Needed to Protect Transfusion Recipients

The maze of issues influencing blood supply safety are complex and political. Those who contracted AIDS through transfusion have not had any organized groups to speak in their behalf. The majority have concealed their infection and become voiceless victims. They have died betrayed, leaving behind shattered and disillusioned families.

For over a decade, the tragic consequences of the public health establishment's failure to protect transfusion recipients from hepatitis and later AIDS were not addressed. Today the needs of those suffering from transfusion diseases are still ignored. With the emphasis on downplaying risks, public health policy is seldom shaped from the viewpoint of those who have contracted, or could contract, AIDS and other infections through transfusions.

After receiving *two* AIDS-tainted transfusions, my family would like to feel that telling our experience might focus attention on some neglected issues. We suggest that national and state legislators consider the following to reduce the primary and secondary spread of transfusion AIDS:

1. A national law requiring blood transfusions to be an informed consent item before surgery with adequate explanation of the risks and alternatives to homologous blood. (California and New Jersey now have such a law.)

2. A national law requiring hospitals to keep donor records for 15 years. That is how long it may take before some HIV infections pass through incubation and get diagnosed. The present five-year law makes it almost impossible to "confirm" transfusion AIDS cases from HIV tested blood because records have been discarded and donors can't be traced.

3. Repeal of state laws which protect blood banks from product liability. Present laws permit blood bank officials to make untrue claims of blood safety because the statements can't be used against them in court.

4. A national education campaign to encourage all prior transfusion recipients from 1977 on to request testing for AIDS. Hospital notification by letter would be expensive and many recipients would have died or moved. It is more sensible to make a media appeal for testing.

5. A national law requiring blood banks to *immediately* call in for HIV testing any prior blood recipient thought to have received suspect blood. Some banks do this but the practice is still not universal.

6. A national law requiring that any person who tests HIV-positive must be told the accurate test result without delay. Today doctors are still not required to tell HIV-positive patients they are infected with AIDS! The physician may decide if any purpose would be served by informing the patient. Not to have the infected recipient's sexual partner die of AIDS should be reason enough.

The Credibility Gap

The blood industry and the media persist in insulting the public's intelligence. The American Red Cross has 300 public relations specialists who portrayed the unsafe conditions in the organization's blood centers as achievements. Few reporters asked the obvious question: Then why is the American Red Cross spending $120 million to improve safety? Those who did were told the organization was spending a large amount of money to make "a safe product even safer."

"No diseased blood has been released," said Red Cross officials. When questioned further, they explained the Red Cross had "often come close to shipping contaminated blood." In reality, the American Red Cross has supplied approximately half of the many *millions* of hepatitis-infected blood units transfused during the past two decades and half of the many thousands of AIDS-infected units. But according to the Red Cross, "No patient has been put at risk."

The *Washington Post* wrote that deficiencies in Red Cross reporting "were not in any way responsible for the (228 Washington) HIV infections." However, at that time the cases had not been investigated or the causes determined. Said FDA Inspector Carden, "There is no basis for the statement that American Red Cross procedures were in no way responsible for the 228 HIV infections." The House Subcommittee concluded that Red Cross statements downplaying the seriousness of their blood safety problems were "simply inaccurate."

In the summer of 1992, public health authorities stepped up safe-blood assurances to dispel fears about the new AIDS-like illnesses. Said Dr. James Allen, director of the National AIDS Program Office in Washington, "There is no evidence that these cases are caused by a new virus and you can rest assured that the blood supply is safe." Granted, there wasn't evidence proving the cases were caused by a new virus—but neither was there any evidence proving they weren't. The last time my family "rested assured" that a new virus had not endangered the blood supply it turned out to be HIV and two Swains got transfusions that were contaminated with it.

I am concerned that those considering surgeries or therapies requiring blood still do not have adequate information. Consumers who do not understand the risks of regular banked blood will not be motivated to donate their own blood and insist on IAT or other procedures. And without knowledge of how to arrange for safer transfusions using homologous blood, patients may be exposed to four or five times as many donors as is necessary.

Sound solutions to the transfusion dilemma will not be implemented as long as unpleasant truths are withheld from consumers. Public health authorities should promote educational programs instead of downplaying problems. Recently I received a letter from a doctor who has spent decades in blood banking. The doctor admitted that "homologous transfusion is akin to playing Russian roulette."

Part III

For Consumers—
Steps That Can Save
Your Life

Medical Alert

This book does *not* advocate refusing a transfusion of someone else's blood if doctors say it is necessary. If blood is needed to save the life of a patient who is ineligible for autologous procedures, regular banked blood or directed donor blood should be accepted. In this situation the risks of refusing homologous blood far exceed the risks of accepting it.

A careful reading of this entire section, however, will help consumers understand how to reduce the risks of homologous blood when it cannot be avoided. Consumers will also learn how to receive transfusions with their own safe blood.

An Appeal to Blood Donors

Please do not stop donating blood. The national blood supply is dependent upon the continued generosity of volunteers.

There is a misconception that AIDS can be caught by donating blood. This concern is unfounded. In the United States a new disposable needle is used to draw blood. Then it is destroyed. Blood donors are not at risk of getting AIDS or other diseases.

If you have never donated blood, are healthy and have a conservative lifestyle—please consider becoming a donor. There is a great need for platelet monodonors. Ask your local blood bank about becoming one.

Chapter 17

Testing of Prior Transfusion Recipients

Health consumers should beware that in 1992 there is still no law requiring blood banks, hospitals or doctors to inform a person if it is known that he or she has received an AIDS-contaminated transfusion or has tested HIV-positive. According to a FDA spokeswoman, if a doctor is notified that a patient was probably transfused with AIDS-tainted blood—and later testing finds the patient is infected with HIV—the doctor does not have to reveal the accurate test results. A doctor may use "professional judgement" to determine if the patient should be told and decides if there is a risk of the patient infecting sexual partners.

One might wonder if doctors use tarot cards or crystal balls to determine if AIDS-infected patients will have sex. Does the crystal ball also indicate the likelihood that condoms will be used even if the woman is well past her childbearing years? The numbers of sexual partners infected with AIDS by transfusion recipients of tainted blood are growing. Many are the direct result of information that was withheld by a doctor with a faulty crystal ball.

Anyone who had transfusions between 1977 and 1986 should be tested for HIV. So should their sexual partners. The Presidential Commission on AIDS recommended in its 1988 report that hospitals call all prior transfusion recipients in for AIDS testing. It is now also recommended that those who have had transfusions since 1970 consider being tested for hepatitis C. Inform any members of your extended family who have had surgery that many surgery patients never know they have received blood transfusions. And children may be transfused without their parents knowledge.

Those Transfused Since 1977 Should Be Tested for AIDS

In 1988 the Presidential Commission on AIDS wrote in its report to the President, "Both public health practice and case law make it clear that persons put at risk of exposure to an infectious disease should be alerted to their exposure." The Commission firmly believed in an individual's right to be notified of their possible exposure so that they can seek prompt medical attention and avoid potentially exposing others. The Commission strongly recommended that hospitals notify all recipients of blood and blood products since 1977 of their possible exposure to AIDS and encourage them to be tested for HIV. (This would have required sending notices to over 25 million Americans.)

Although the recommendation was sound, the cost was high and only a small minority of recipients could have been found. Consequently, prior transfusion recipients were not notified and must assume the testing responsibility themselves. Nearly 4 million people a year have had transfusions. Few realize that a single medical procedure put them in a group which is at risk for AIDS. The public is warned of other high risk behaviors, but if the subject of transfusion surfaces, the health establishment breaks into the safe-blood shuffle. It's little wonder that those who've received blood do not realize they should be tested for AIDS.

However, an amazing number of people who had transfusions don't know they got them! Doctors do not normally reveal details of operating room procedures unless the patient or family specifically asks. The parents of many children who are given blood do not know it. "Transfusion" is hidden in the fine print of most treatment-permission forms signed when a patient is admitted to the hospital. Transfusion has rarely been an informed consent item where risks are clearly explained to patients. Unless you know for sure that blood was *not* given at the time of surgery it is perhaps better to assume that it was and be tested for AIDS.

The other option is to obtain your surgical records from the hospital. This is a good solution if it hasn't been over five years since the surgery. If it has, there is a possibility that any clue to transfusion might have been destroyed with the donor records, which can be discarded after the five-year law requirement has expired. This policy varies from hospital to hospital. I recently obtained records for a family member who had surgery 12 years ago and the transfusion records were intact with donor numbers. The hospital or blood bank probably had destroyed information linking the patient to specific donors, but in this case the transfusion record told me all I needed to know. The patient had received blood.

If you wish to obtain your surgical records, call the hospital and ask to talk with the medical records department. Most hospitals will require the patient to make a request in writing and will charge $10 or $15 for the copies. When you receive your records, read through them carefully. If there is a transfusion record, study it to determine if the donor blood that was crossmatched to the patient was actually transfused. Frequently it isn't needed and will be sent back to the blood bank. Look for mention of red cells, platelets and plasma—blood products that are transfused more often than whole blood. If the records indicate three "units" were given, the patient would have received three component units of blood products, from three separate donors.

If you find it probable that you or members of your family have received a transfusion since 1977 it is wise to be tested for AIDS. The chance of being infected is very slight but nevertheless real.

AIDS Contamination in the Blood Supply During the Early 1980s

It is impossible to know the extent of AIDS contamination in the blood supply in the early 1980s. But a revealing study was done at Irwin Memorial Blood Bank in San Francisco. Between 1982 and 1988 the blood bank obtained the patient names of AIDS cases that were reported to the health departments in the Bay Area. The names of those known AIDS patients were compared to blood donor rolls at Irwin Memorial and it was found that 199 had donated blood at that bank.

Those 199 donors had given 634 prior donations at Irwin. The study does not indicate how many component units were transfused from these 634 donations but it was usually two or three per donation. The study states, "Approximately half of the prior recipients of components from these donors were themselves infected." Using a low average of two components per donation, 1,268 people would have received the blood of these AIDS patients. Half, or 634 people, would have contracted the AIDS infection. (The other half would have received blood from the donors before the donors became infected.) Without the confidential patient information, only 10% of the infected donors would have been known to Irwin if their names had not been provided by the health departments.

Over 600 transfused AIDS infections is a staggering amount from a single blood bank. Yet it was just a fraction of the total. A larger number of unknown HIV-positive donors who had not yet developed AIDS were left uncounted. Although Irwin no doubt had one of the highest rates of AIDS contamination in the nation, the study gives a frightening insight into the extent of the contamination. A lookback study at Cedar-Sinai Medical Center in Los Angeles found that between 1979 and 1985 the actual risk of acquiring HIV infection from a transfusion at that hospital was between one in 100 and one in 200. In 1987, some California transfusion recipients of untested blood were called in and tested for HIV. One in 56 tested positive for the AIDS virus.

Knowledge Is Your Most Effective Weapon

Although knowing you are HIV-positive is bad, not knowing is worse. If patients suffer from AIDS-related illnesses without HIV infection being identified, there is a risk of infecting others and proper treatment is unlikely. Pneumocystis pneumonia is difficult for doctors to diagnose if they are not familiar with the disease. Unrecognized, it may simmer for some time and cause serious lung damage. The first attack of pneumocystis can be delayed by routine inhaling of a Pentamidine mist into the lungs or by taking other drugs. And many doctors recommend the use of AZT or DDI in the earlier stage of HIV infection. My parents' health care is a good example of what can happen when you don't know the name of the disease you are fighting. Doctors rarely look for AIDS in the elderly and often not in younger people either.

Arthur Ashe, one of the most gifted and respected figures in tennis, had two heart surgeries when he was still a young man. His first cardiac bypass was in 1979, shortly after the AIDS virus infiltrated the nation's blood supply. His second operation in 1983 was at the zenith of blood supply contamination when blood bank leaders were refusing to use surrogate tests to reduce the risk. Both of Mr. Ashe's surgeries would have likely exposed him to the blood of large numbers of donors from the New York City area which had an extremely high incidence of AIDS.

In 1988, five years after his last surgery, Mr. Ashe's right hand became paralyzed. His doctors were well aware of their famous patient's heart surgeries but *they did not test him for HIV*. Instead, they performed exploratory surgery on his brain to make a diagnosis. The doctors found an abscess caused by the parasitic infection toxoplasmosis—an opportunistic infection that preys on AIDS patients because of their weakened immunity. A positive HIV test before the brain surgery would have alerted Mr. Ashe's doctors to test him for toxoplasmosis and a dangerous surgery could have been avoided.

When patients who have had prior blood transfusions get AIDS-related symptoms, doctors may be appallingly remiss in testing them for HIV. It appears they are afraid to look for AIDS. If Mr. Ashe had been in his 70's like my parents were, his central nervous system dysfunction would have been shrugged off as an affliction of old age. There are only 40% of those who get infected with HIV from transfusions who survive their original illness but those who do can go through a lot of useless medical care before a diagnosis is made. And it isn't known how many of them die without *ever* being diagnosed as having AIDS-related conditions.

It is also imperative to know if you're HIV-positive so that members of your family can be protected. Persons who have been infected with AIDS through blood transfusions can unknowingly infect others in a number of ways. The greatest danger is to sexual partners. Strict precautions or abstinence is required. The CDC has documented a case in which a mother got AIDS from caring for her baby after it had been given an AIDS-tainted transfusion. Not knowing the child was infected, the mother did not use gloves to protect herself from the baby's bodily fluids which contained blood.

Unlike hospital care, when families care for ill members in the home, prevention of infectious disease is not emphasized. Unless a family knows someone in the home carries HIV, gloves will not be worn when handling bodily fluids and blood. There is also some danger of the spread of general organisms (germs) in a family setting. People whose immune systems are weakening from HIV may excrete high concentrations of many infectious diseases such as cytomegalorvirus, hepatitis B, herpes simplex virus, Epstein-Barr and tuberculosis. It is advisable to take precautions against the spread of these germs, especially around babies, pregnant women and the elderly. All things considered, it's better to know if you are infected.

Deaths from one contaminated blood donation can multiply at a frightening rate. When a young woman is transfused with AIDS blood she has a good chance of passing the infection to any babies she gives birth to. The unknowing mother can also pass the virus to her baby through breast feeding.

The family of actor and film director Paul Michael Glaser, former TV star of "Starsky and Hutch," is a tragic example of this type of infectious spread. Glaser's wife, Elizabeth, hemorrhaged after the birth of their daughter in 1981 and was transfused with AIDS-contaminated blood. Mrs. Glaser nursed the baby for eight months and the child became infected. Three years later the couple's son was born. He, too, was infected with the deadly virus.

The family did not realize Mrs. Glaser and the two children were HIV-positive until the little girl was diagnosed with AIDS when she was four years old. The child died at the age of seven. The same fate awaits the other two infected family members.

As any recipient of an AIDS-contaminated transfusion or blood product is capable of infecting others sexually, a significant percentage of the spouses of these recipients are now infected. A Marine became sexually infected with AIDS by his wife after she received a tainted transfusion at a government hospital during childbirth. Martin Gaffney and his wife later had a son who was born with HIV. An older daughter is the only member of the family who was not infected. After his wife and son died of AIDS, Gaffney sued the government to provide for her financially. Mr. Gaffney has since died.

Unfortunately, the tragedy of transfusion AIDS is heaped upon families already having health crises. According to Grace Powers Monaco, there are 48 children in the nation who were cured of cancer and later developed AIDS through blood transfusions given to treat their earlier illness. Ms. Monaco, a Washington, DC, attorney, is one of the founders of Candlelighters, a support group for families of children with cancer.

How Do You Get Tested for AIDS?

A test for HIV requires about one tablespoon of blood to be drawn from your arm for the ELISA test which detects antibodies to the virus. It can be done in your doctor's office or at your local health department. Test results are usually available within a few days to a week.

However, many doctors still don't realize the extent of the previous AIDS contamination of the blood supply and discourage people from getting tested. It's common for them to deny that *their* patients could get AIDS. Last year I went into my local emergency center with a severe nosebleed. It was messy. As the doctor started to pack my nose with his bare hands I asked, "Why aren't you wearing gloves?"

"You don't look like an AIDS patient," he answered.

"Neither did my parents who died of the disease."

The doctor rushed to the sink, washed his hands and gloved.

There is a mistaken belief that you can tell by a person's looks and lifestyle if he or she carries HIV. But when the virus is transmitted through transfusion, a nun could have it and her doctor would have difficulty considering her a valid candidate for a blood test. Remember that during the 1980s 78% of New York City doctors never ordered an AIDS test for a single patient.

If your doctor tries to discourage you from being tested for AIDS either insist on the test or go to your local health department for one. When she was 63 years old, Dorothy L. Polikoff testified before the Presidential Commission on AIDS. She told how she and her ailing husband, a prior transfusion recipient, had asked their doctors to test them for AIDS after reading a magazine article about HIV contamination in the blood supply. The doctors refused. "They told us there was no need to worry and that it was not necessary," she said. The next year, as their health continued to worsen, the Polikoffs went to the county health department on their own and got tested for AIDS. "We learned that we had both tested positive for the (AIDS) virus," Mrs. Polikoff said. "We brought the slips to our doctor and told him the results. We were both upset. I was almost hysterical and my husband was furious."

There are some advantages to being tested at a public site where the personnel are trained in protecting patient confidentiality. In 1988 doctors advised our entire family to get tested every six months. I went to the health department facility in Colorado Springs and was very impressed with the measures taken to ensure privacy. Records were kept in locked files and never left unattended. In Colorado, patients' medical records indicating HIV status are protected from any form of legal process, including search warrants, subpoenas and discovery in civil lawsuits. Nor can they be released to physicians, health care agencies, government institutions, employers or insurance companies. Although most states have similar laws, private doctors' offices not used to handling HIV test results may have employees untrained in confidentiality procedures.

My sister and her family had a disconcerting experience with testing done in their doctor's office. After she, her husband and their three children got an HIV test, the community knew the results before they did. At a social event several people told them how relieved they were to hear that their test for AIDS were negative. An office employee had leaked the information before the doctor had a chance to inform the family.

You may wish to consider keeping your HIV test off your health insurance records. An AIDS test can raise a red flag because companies may assume transfusion recipients are patients with continuing high risk lifestyles. Some insurance companies won't pay for an AIDS test. But an HIV test at the health department is often free although some states may charge up to $50 for one. While the majority of testing sites ask for names, often pseudonyms will be accepted and a few sites are totally anonymous. Call your health department to determine local policy and if there is a charge for the test.

I do not believe that a Swain-type concealment of a positive AIDS test is as likely today as it was in 1987. But it's still a possibility. There is far less chance of this occurring at a health department and no chance at all if you say you prefer not to discuss your exposure route until after you get the test results. At least at the health department if the test comes back positive you would not be working with a doctor who referred you for surgery and has close ties to the hospital where you had it. And doctors usually report a positive HIV test result of a prior transfusion recipient to the blood bank. It's best that that report is made *after* the patient has been given the positive test results.

How Reliable Are the Test Results?

If it has been a year or longer since your transfusion and your HIV test comes back negative you can accept that result with a very high degree of confidence. The test is almost 100% perfect for detecting infections after that length of time. However, other tests are often used to diagnose HIV infection in babies because they cannot always make antibodies to the virus. Any concerns you have after a negative ELISA test for HIV should be discussed with your doctor. Do not worry in silence.

False positive results are common with the ELISA test. That's why the lab will repeat the test at least once. If it still shows as positive, your blood sample will then be tested by another method, the Western Blot, which eliminates nearly all false positives. Sadly, a positive ELISA test confirmed by Western Blot is considered to be almost a certain guarantee of HIV infection.

I have tremendous empathy for the very small percentage of patients who test positive for the AIDS virus after getting transfusions. The emotional devastation suffered when a person learns they are HIV-positive is compounded when transmission was by transfusion because self-serving efforts are frequently made to discredit the victims. Bearers of bad news have never been well-received and HIV-positive blood recipients are a group the health establishment would prefer not to recognize. Support groups with those in a similar situation are usually nonexistent. This results in an incredible sense of isolation.

In 1989 a middle-aged couple in Texas were in a serious car accident and neither were expected to live. They did survive but the wife received large amounts of transfused blood which had been tested for AIDS. A year later both she and her husband tested HIV-positive. There is no doubt in this couple's minds that the woman got AIDS through the transfusions and passed the infection to her husband. She told the press, "I am 1,000% sure. There just couldn't have been any other source." Although the couple knows they had no other exposures, the tendency will be to doubt them. This is one of the reasons many choose to die in silence.

Those Who Have Had Transfusions During the Last 20 Years Should Be Tested for Hepatitis C

Those who received blood after 1977 should be tested for both AIDS and hepatitis C and those who received blood between 1970 and 1977 need to be tested for hepatitis C only.

Ross Eckert, who sits on the FDA's blood advisory committee, complained to the House Subcommittee that there appeared to have been a prior consensus by the blood banking industry and various health agencies, including the FDA and NIH, not to require a look back for hepatitis C after testing began in May 1990. When the matter came before the Blood and Blood Products Advisory Committee, Eckert had argued to no avail that those who had received prior donations from donors who would be testing positive for hepatitis C should be notified.

However, the public health service and blood industry, knowing that the numbers of hepatitis C infections given by transfusion were in the millions, simply passed the buck to the consumer. For the record, in May 1990 a joint statement was issued by the AABB, the American Red Cross and the Council of Community Blood Centers recommending that patients who had received blood transfusions within the last 20 years should ask their doctors for a hepatitis C test. On this issue consumers should take the advice of the Red Cross and blood industry trade associations.

It is important that prior transfusion recipients persuade their doctors to do the test because hepatitis C, a viral infection of the liver, usually goes undiagnosed. Initial symptoms of the disease are mild in most patients—just a general "run down" feeling. Only 10% have an obvious yellowing of the skin. Unfortunately, about 50% of the transfusion recipients who get hepatitis C will develop chronic active hepatitis and 10% will get cirrhosis of the liver. Others will develop liver cancer. Anyone who has been infected with hepatitis C by a contaminated transfusion is considered to have a low possibility of transmitting the infection to family members even though they may just be carriers of the virus and do not have symptoms.

The condition of a patient with hepatitis C needs to be monitored by a doctor and supportive care given in an effort to slow liver damage. There have been trial studies using interferon to relieve or even cure lingering hepatitis B and hepatitis C. Researchers expect that interferon can cure 10% of the chronic hepatitis cases and improve another 40% to 50%. An advisory committee of the FDA has recommended that interferon be marketed for hepatitis. If you test positive for hepatitis C and the virus is in the active state, ask your doctor about interferon.

As your doctor is very busy you should not rely on him or her to determine if you or other members of your family have had transfusions during the past two decades. If you are in the "had transfusion" category you must bring it to your doctor's attention. Because hepatitis C is not entangled in politics or social stigma like AIDS, getting tested for it should not present a problem. Seeing that any transfused members of your family are tested for AIDS and hepatitis C is as sensible as carrying health insurance.

Chapter 18

Take Responsibility for Safe Transfusion Therapy

Have you ever heard anyone say they were shopping around for some good used blood? That they were comparing what is available in transfusions—looking for something that would be trouble free for the next 12 years? Of course not.

People don't comparison shop for transfusions the way they do for important purchases like lawnmowers. Yet every family will eventually need one, and when they do the choice becomes a matter of life and death. But, historically, patients and their families have not had any input into the type of transfusion they buy. Until AIDS that choice was left entirely up to their doctors.

Most consumers are vaguely aware of what has been reported in the media on blood safety but that reporting is superficial and often inaccurate. Consequently, when they become patients they know nothing about how blood banks work or what precautions or procedures to ask for. They sense that medical staffs consider voiced concern over blood safety to be unwarranted and assume that the FDA is protecting consumers. But the FDA's blood committee doesn't hear from those who get the blood infused into their veins—it hears from the blood industry. Consumer non-involvement has perpetuated the ignorance that surrounds transfusion therapy and its options.

Patients can no longer afford to place blind faith in medical professionals and hospitals. Not all doctors are responsive to their patients' best interests or honest about failures and risks. Some of the medical care practiced in the United States during the past few decades has been hazardous. And the transfusion of large amounts of homologous blood grew into one of those unchecked hazards. Before AIDS many doctors ordered blood as casually as they told patients to take a couple of aspirin. I did not write this book, however, with a critical pencil that has no solutions. Many steps can now be taken to eliminate or greatly reduce the risks of homologous transfusion. But patients cannot remain passive. You must assume some of the responsibility for your own transfusion therapy and realize that the only patient rights you have are the ones you assert.

Surprisingly there is no medical controversy over autologous blood being the safest form of transfusion. It is endorsed by numerous medical organizations including the American Medical Association and the Public Health Service. The AABB has been on record for over 12 years recommending autologous blood as superior to regular banked blood. There is no question that, medically, the best transfusion patients can buy is the one they give themselves.

Then Why Must Patients Be Assertive to Get the Best Therapy?

It can take half a century for a new medical change to become accepted medical practice. Technology for intraoperative autologous transfusion (IAT) has been available since the early 1970s. But the procedures outdistanced their usage by more than a decade and are still used on a very limited basis.

The medical profession is resistant to change and doctors are conservative—hesitant to stray from the old standard treatment. Perhaps more importantly, autologous blood programs can be a pain in the neck to administer, requiring more patient-doctor interaction and extra work for blood banks. And there is no money incentive for hospitals and blood banks to reduce the amount of homologous blood sold.

If these obstacles are to be overcome, each hospital must have a dedicated doctor who will direct the move toward adequate blood replacement with the patients' own safe blood. Without a well-organized approach which integrates the various types of autologous blood programs, results will often be minimal. Consequently, though nearly all hospitals provide predonation for surgery patients and many also have some IAT equipment, programs are rarely used to full potential. A patient-directed push would hasten the transition to safer blood transfusion.

Doctors act as the purchasing agents for blood, placing orders for their patients through the hospital transfusion service or blood bank. Although the use of blood is controlled by physicians, there has been a failure in medical schools to educate students in when blood is necessary and in the risks of its use. In the past, young doctors learned when to give a patient blood by observing older doctors, resulting in an overuse of blood with little recognition of its dangers. Dr. Edgar Engleman, director of Stanford's blood center, told the House Subcommittee, "Many physicians and nurses are relatively poorly trained with respect to the indications for transfusion, and they are even less knowledgeable about the potential complications."

However, if doctors have been slow to pick up on the dangers of homologous blood, it was partially due to the downplaying of those dangers by blood bankers and health authorities. Health care professionals were unaware of how little blood banks did before 1985 to protect the blood supply. Few doctors read the CDC Surveillance Reports for hepatitis and AIDS which the agency will provide upon request. As longtime targets of safe-blood propaganda, physicians today are incorrectly told in the medical literature that there are just a handful of "confirmed" AIDS cases from blood given since testing began. And many doctors prefer to believe those few cases are the extent of the present HIV infection in banked blood.

Neither are all hospitals dedicated to providing the safest transfusion therapy. While hospitals that perform open heart surgery now have IAT capability, there is no guarantee that it will be used for *every* eligible heart operation. On a full surgery schedule, some surgeons still choose to do the procedure the old way and use homologous blood. Approximately 50% of the nation's hospitals do not have IAT capability and many of them do not utilize companies that bring machines and operators in as needed. Medical facilities have been slow to change old habits.

For instance, an emergency room may have a cell saver to salvage the blood of a hemorrhaging patient, but—though it takes just a couple of minutes to plug it in and secure tubing—it may be not be used on every patient whose condition merits it. Perhaps a trained operator is not available, or the staff on duty may not be committed to the patient benefits it offers. The California law requiring presurgery patients to be informed of transfusion risks and options got off to a rocky start. Although many hospitals and doctors used the information brochure, others did not have enough interest in safer transfusion to give the brochures to their patients. This is rather incredible considering the liability risks of that omission.

The Presidential Commission on AIDS was concerned with the lack of knowledge in medical facilities regarding transfusion therapy. In 1988 the commission stated, "Health care facilities should offer aggressive in-service training to their staff, particularly blood banking and transfusion services personnel, to bring them up-to-date on current autologous transfusion therapy techniques." Two years later, Dr. Engleman told the House Subcommittee panel that nurses and doctors still needed to be re-educated in transfusion medicine so "that consumers and professionals will be more cautious and knowledgeable in the future."

Is the Safest Transfusion the One Not Given?

The knowledge that a variety of major surgeries can often be safely performed without blood transfusion has been documented for over 25 years. During the 1960s it was found that it was unnecessary for patients to have a hemoglobin of over 10 to tolerate anesthesia or for their wounds to heal. This was evidenced by the number of Jehovah Witnesses who refused blood for surgeries which normally required transfusion support. Although surgical death rates for this group are higher, the majority of Witnesses survive their bloodless operations and have adequate recoveries. Moreover, Jehovah Witnesses are aware that their chance of death increases in direct proportion to the amount of unre-placed blood loss. For this reason they try to seek out the best surgeons whose skilled techniques keep bleeding to a minimum.

Such a surgeon is Dr. Ronald Lapin who founded the Institute of Bloodless Surgery and Medicine in 1983 and maintains there are very few operations that cannot be performed without homologous blood. The following techniques are employed by Dr. Lapin and his associates in the operating rooms at Coast Plaza Medical Center in Norwalk, California:

- Giving the patient medication to lower blood pressure so less blood will be lost

- Operating as quickly as possible to reduce bleeding time

- Trading scalpels for lasers and electric knives which seal off bleeding tissue

- Using cell savers to return red cells to the patient during and after surgery

- Collection of autologous blood before surgery

Dr. Lapin believes that homologous blood is the most dangerous substance used in medicine and should only be given in extreme cases to save a life. Since 1973 Dr. Lapin and his associates have performed over 15,000 surgeries without the use of homologous blood. The doctor says his patients have had an infection rate *after surgery* of less than 1% compared to the national post-surgical infection rate of 10%. "Our hospital stays are two days shorter than those of patients who have the same type of surgeries and get homologous blood," Lapin said. "Our cancer recurrence rates are lower, too. These patient benefits are a result of avoiding the adverse reactions and immune suppression caused by donor blood."

For nearly 15 years Dr. Lapin was severely criticized by the medical community for operating outside of the standard of care because he did not transfuse patients when hemoglobin dropped below 10. That guideline, which was used for decades to determine transfusion need, originated in the Mayo Clinic anesthesia department in 1941. Known as the 10/30 rule, transfusion was recommended for patients with a hemoglobin below 10 or a hematocrit below 30. For more than 40 years there was a generous use of blood without the guideline ever being challenged.

Not until after the arrival of AIDS, as patients contracted HIV from transfusions and started filing lawsuits, did the guideline for when to transfuse a patient come under scrutiny and move downward. In 1988 the National Institutes of Health concluded that homologous transfusions should be kept to a minimum. It is now the NIH position that patients with hemoglobin values of 10 or greater rarely require transfusion and those with values of less then 7 generally do. Thus, the transfusion trigger has dropped from 10 down to below 7. Consequently, today it is common practice to *not* transfuse patients who have an acute blood loss of 20% to 30% or more of their total blood volume. Instead, the loss is replaced by an IV solution of sterile salt water. There is no doubt the present conservative approach to transfusion reduces patient risks of adverse reactions and the spread of viral diseases.

But although there is medical agreement that before the mid 1980s doctors ordered too much blood, there is now a question of how far the pendulum can swing in the opposite direction without putting some patients at risk. Body tissues need a sufficient amount of oxygen which is supplied by the red blood cells. Even after just a moderate blood loss, the remaining red cells may be unable to supply adequate oxygen to meet the needs of some patients. The greater the oxygen deficit, the greater is the risk for multiple organ insufficiency or failure. Complications may include respiratory failure, kidney failure, liver failure and coma. In addition, the heart needs a minimum volume of blood to pump properly. Without it a patient may be at risk for heart attack or stroke. Older people having constricted blood vessels are the most vulnerable. And heart attacks and strokes are so common that if they do occur from undertransfusion, patients and their families never suspect the cause.

I have spoken with doctors who are concerned that an unknown number of patients are suffering damage and possible death because of a well-meaning reluctance to transfuse them with other people's blood. But due to lack of hospital monitoring, the frequency of the adverse effects of undertransfusion remain unstudied. Said one doctor, "No one is anxious to monitor complications that may lead to lawsuits."

It is obvious that the risks of homologous transfusion must be carefully weighed against the risks of giving too little blood. Consumers need to understand that the amount of blood that can be lost before a transfusion is necessary varies from patient to patient. There is a minimum hemoglobin level for *each* person below which severe illness and death occur. Unfortunately, a single measurement cannot be used to determine when a patient needs a transfusion. In addition to hematocrit and hemoglobin, doctors must consider a number of factors including the duration of the anemia, the type of operation, the probability of massive blood loss, the presence of coexisting disease conditions and intravascular volume.

The final, complex decision of whether to transfuse a patient is made by the surgeon and anesthesiologist. And neither of the two options they often have are without risk: giving homologous blood or leaving the patient undertransfused.

Fortunately for consumers, both these unacceptable options have the same solution—transfusion with the patient's own safe blood. While it is *not* always true that the safest transfusion is the one not given, it is true that the safest transfusion is the one you give yourself. But giving yourself a transfusion requires advance preparation and the cooperation of your surgeon. Very often the extent of that cooperation is influenced by patient involvement and knowledge.

A Safe Alternative

It happened less than a year ago when my uncle, Darreld Swain, had emergency heart surgery at the Humana Hospital in Aurora, near Denver. Darreld made it plain that he was more worried about being transfused with AIDS than dying a quick death from his heart condition.

"Having my grandson and my brother both get AIDS in blood transfusions is enough for one family," he said.

The surgeon's placatory look turned to astonishment. "What did you say?" he asked.

"My brother and grandson got AIDS from transfusions. I'm sure you've seen Jonathan on TV."

"Is that little boy your grandson?"

"He sure is. And my brother and his wife are already dead because of the AIDS blood he got during heart surgery."

It was then that the stunned surgeon made my uncle a promise. "We'll do everything possible to make sure you do not receive any blood except your own."

The doctors and hospital staff pulled out all the autologous stops. Immediately before Darreld's surgery, some of his platelet-rich plasma, which contains clotting factors to stop bleeding, was skimmed off by apheresis and saved for later reinfusion. Those factors can be lost by lengthy recycling of the patient's blood during surgery and often have to be replaced with packs of platelets from six to ten different donors. By donating his own plasma and platelets before surgery, Darreld avoided that exposure. Blood lost during his surgery was salvaged, washed and returned to him while the surgeon repaired five of his arteries. Darreld did not require any homologous blood or blood products even though there had not been time for him to donate his blood before the operation.

The cooperation of the doctors and hospital staff in providing the best possible transfusion support was outstanding. My uncle suffers from several other major diseases in addition to his heart condition and was 73 years of age, yet he made a remarkable recovery. "They finally did the blood thing right," he told me.

"Yes," I responded, "but your family's transfusion history was a powerful incentive. Your case proves what can be done."

Unfortunately, it is far more difficult for patients who are scheduled for surgeries that do not usually have much blood loss to get cooperation to participate in autologous blood programs. Blood banks and surgeons usually try to discourage such patients from donating their own blood before surgery. There is a likelihood that transfusion will not be needed and because predonation is burdensome to blood banks and hospitals, the institutions want to play the odds. But why should patients take the unnecessary risks of those odds?

Dr. Leora Traynor, an Ohio physician who has practiced medicine for nearly 30 years said, "A doctor cannot always anticipate a surgical event which will require blood replacement." Dr. Traynor shared a personal experience she had with her own family. In 1991 her 80-year-old mother was scheduled to have a vaginal hysterectomy—a surgery that is not supposed to require blood transfusion. The surgeon insisted that none of *his* patients lost blood with that procedure and said there was absolutely no reason to donate any blood before the operation.

But because Dr. Traynor did not wish to gamble on the probability of her mother not needing a transfusion, she herself wrote an order for the blood bank to collect and store three units of her mother's blood. She requested that the first two units be frozen so that donations could be spaced further apart to prevent anemia. When Dr. Traynor's mother was admitted for surgery, her hemoglobin was at 14 grams and there were three units of her autologous blood waiting at the hospital.

Unfortunately, a member of the hospital staff accidently punctured one of the bags of blood and it had to be discarded. However, at the end of her surgery, Dr. Traynor's mother was transfused with one autologous unit. And then, with a single unit of blood left, an unexpected postoperative emergency occurred. The elderly patient hemorrhaged in the recovery room. She was returned to the operating room and Dr. Traynor was *assured* that the final unit of autologous blood was being given to the patient. *But no blood was administered* and when her mother was later moved from the recovery room, Dr. Traynor found the autologous unit on the shelf under the gurney. The patient's hemoglobin was at 9—down 5 grams from the previous day. Nevertheless, she would not have received that last unit of her own blood if it had not been for her assertive daughter.

"The difficulties and roadblocks some patients meet when they try to prepare for a safe transfusion are incredible," said Dr. Traynor. "Even after receiving her two units of blood, my mother left the hospital with a hemoglobin of 10 grams. According to present medical guidelines, hemoglobin could have been allowed to drop to below 7 (or even 5 for healthy patients) before she would have been given homologous blood. But that conservative and, in some cases, harmful standard should not apply when autologous blood is available. Why shouldn't patients have full cooperation in *donating* and *receiving* their own safe blood?"

Hospitals may have policies against allowing patients to donate their blood before minor surgery. A medical study concluded that a blood program attempting to prevent all use of homologous "exposure for every elective surgical patient, will incur unacceptable costs." Unacceptable to whom? In the past, lives have been destroyed at horrendous medical cost by post-transfusion hepatitis and AIDS after patients received just one or two component units of someone else's blood. The Swain family has experienced medical costs in seven figures due to transfusion AIDS. To us the small cost of predonating a couple of pints of blood is infinitesimal.

My mother used to say, "The squeaky wheel will get the grease." In the 1990s, it will be the squeaky patients who have the better chance of receiving safe autologous transfusion. How to be a squeaking wheel is covered in a later chapter.

However, not all homologous blood can be avoided. Many accident victims must be given donor blood to save their lives. Newborn babies may need transfusions. And cancer and kidney patients and those who have certain blood disorders require homologous blood—some on a regular basis. Homologous blood is needed for some emergency surgeries and for a small number of elective surgeries.

Fortunately, in these situations it is possible to obtain homologous blood that is safer than the regular banked supply. For example, newborns can nearly always receive the blood of one or both parents. And knowledgeable selection of directed donors can provide safer blood products and greatly reduce the number of donors. If time permits and the HIV antigen test is commercially available, you could request that all units of regular banked blood be tested with it. Although the antigen test is not infallible, it is capable of detecting the virus itself soon after the donor is infected.

Doctors are wary about lay persons making therapeutic decisions regarding health care. This book does not suggest that patients should make final decisions for their transfusion therapy. It does suggest they should equip themselves with a knowledge of the alternatives to homologous transfusion and discuss them with their doctor to determine which procedures they may qualify for. Consumers should understand, however, that they do have the *right* to make decisions on their transfusion therapy or obtain second or third opinions from other doctors. But *refusing* a transfusion should be done with great caution because it could result in the patient's death. It is the author's opinion that the patient should retain the right to choose the safest type of transfusion and request autologous blood replacement to a known safe level.

After a discussion with your doctor, it may be necessary to reschedule surgery at a hospital having a more complete line of IAT equipment or to request that the first hospital bring in a mobile service to furnish machines and an operator. If you have a surgeon who appears disinterested in minimizing your exposure to donor blood, consider finding another who is willing to work with you. If you are told your surgery rarely requires blood transfusions, you may wish to find a surgeon who will let you prepare for blood replacement. It cannot be determined for sure before surgery that a transfusion will not be needed.

It's Up to the Consumer to Become Knowledgeable

I have emphasized infectious risk and neglected another very significant risk of homologous blood that would still prevail if all germs were forever removed from the blood supply. I was told by Dr. Ronald Lapin that "As bad as hepatitis and AIDS are, the complications that occur from incompatibility between donor and recipient blood are just as threatening. Consumers should think of homologous blood as a liquid transplant."

That is exactly what receiving someone else's blood is—a transplant. An essential part of another person's body is injected into a patient's veins and that patient's immune mechanisms may object to the intrusion like a chagrined host to an unwelcome house guest.

The host-body will do one of three things:

1. Accept the situation and live peacefully with the guest.

2. Be uncomfortable but not complain until days or months later when a confrontational illness occurs.

3. Upon transfusion, engage in a battle against the guest-blood with the outcome being either recovery, long term illness or death of the host.

Adverse transfusion reactions center around the antigen-antibody response of the recipient's immune system. The most serious blood incompatibility reactions are to A and B antigens in the ABO blood group and to D antigen in the Rh blood group. Antigen determinants on the outside of blood cells are programmed by genetic inheritance. If a donor's blood is Rh positive it will carry the D antigen and if it is Rh negative, the D antigen will be absent. But antibodies to some blood antigens occur naturally in the blood of those who do not have that antigen on their own blood cells. This is true of A and B antibodies. For example, a type A recipient without B antigen would almost always have antibodies to B and if type B blood were transfused into that person a life threatening reaction could occur—the transfused red cells would be attacked and destroyed by the recipient's immune system. Like some people with the same last name, antigens and antibodies with the same name do not get along.

In addition to ABO and D, there are 600 known blood types and subtypes. However, only those most likely to cause problems are crossmatched to the patient before transfusion. It's little wonder that the chance of getting an exact matching homologous transfusion is less than one in 100,000. Consequently, transfusions expose recipients to large numbers of foreign antigens whose effects on human health are not yet well understood. It is understood that homologous transfusion may result in the immunization of recipients against other people's blood types by exposing them to foreign blood antigens which cause the body's immune system to respond in the same way as a vaccination.

The immune transfusion reactions that can occur from homologous blood are as follows:

1. Immediate hemolytic reactions

2. Delayed hemolytic reactions

3. Chill-fever reactions

4. Allergic reactions

5. Post-transfusion purpura

6. Noncardiac pulmonary edema

7. Graft-versus-host disease

Immediate hemolytic reactions occur as patient antibodies break down and destroy incompatible red blood cells. These reactions are classified as catastrophic and are usually caused by ABO incompatibility resulting from human error made in the crossmatching and delivery of donor blood to the patient. Incorrect labeling of the patient's blood sample taken for testing is the most common error. Another significant error is transfusion of a unit of blood other than the one intended for the patient.

Immediate hemolytic reactions vary greatly in severity with symptoms including fever, chills, chest pain, nausea and shock. In the United States the chance of this type of transfusion reaction is one in 25,000 units of blood. About one in 20 acute hemolytic reactions are fatal.

Delayed hemolytic reactions are caused by antibody to blood groups other than ABO which was too weak to be detected in the patient's blood before transfusion. This is a result of the patient being previously immunized to antigen in the donor's blood by either a prior transfusion or a pregnancy. Exposure to antigen may occur between mother and infant during pregnancy or delivery and, as with initial transfusion exposure, fade after time. Upon a repeat transfusion exposure, the antibodies are too weak to cause a reaction until antibody levels rise 5 to 10 days later. The symptoms of delayed hemolytic reactions do not tend to be as serious as the acute reactions and rarely cause death. Transfusing females before menopause presents a potential for future problems. If Rh positive red blood cells are given to a Rh negative woman, a later pregnancy with a Rh positive fetus is very likely to cause severe hemolytic disease in the newborn.

Chill-fever reactions are a frequent complication, occurring in one out of 100 transfused patients. The symptoms appear during or within a few hours of transfusion and may start with severe chills followed by a fever of 104° or 105°. There may be vomiting and collapse although many cases are less severe. Chill-fever reactions are not usually life threatening—a fact difficult for the patient who is experiencing one to believe.

This reaction is more likely to be caused by recipient antibodies reacting to donor white cells rather than red cells. These antibodies develop in at least 20% of women during pregnancy and in 70% of people who have had prior multiple transfusions.

Allergic reactions occur when the transfused blood contains something to which the patient is allergic. Antibody to the offending substance triggers the immune response, causing hives, itching, asthma and in rare cases, anaphylactic shock. As many as 5 in 100 patients react with hives after transfusion but other allergic symptoms are not as common.

Post-transfusion purpura is a rare but serious condition which comes on 7 to 10 days after transfusion. The patient's own platelets are destroyed, causing bleeding to occur under the skin and internally. Previous immunization by transfusion or pregnancy sets the stage for antibody in the patient's blood to react to infused platelets from nearly all blood donors. Post-transfusion purpura can be fatal but most patients recover spontaneously.

Noncardiac pulmonary edema causes acute breathing difficulty without heart failure. This transfusion reaction is rare and usually due to antibodies in the donor's blood reacting with the recipient's white blood cells.

Graft-versus-host disease is now increasingly recognized as a complication of transfusion in small babies or immunosuppressed patients and can cause death soon after transfusion—or years later. Symptoms of this disease are inflammation of the skin, stomach problems and liver dysfunction. The illness can be prevented by irradiating blood products before transfusion, but this treatment is not routinely done.

Immune Suppression

In addition to the above reactions, homologous blood confuses the immune system and can result in depressed patient immunity for some time after transfusion. For over a decade, studies have shown that infusing a person with another's blood exposes the recipient to foreign cellular or soluble antigens which stimulate T lymphocytes and suppress immunity.

Physicians have found that patients having homologous transfusion at the time of cancer surgery have a much higher recurrence of cancer than those not transfused. One study compared survival rates of patients with colon cancer and found that, after five years, 74% of those who did not get transfusions were still alive compared to only 48% of those who had transfusions. Another study of 100 patients found the recurrence rate for all cancers of the larynx was 14% for those who did not have blood transfused, while 65% of the transfused patients had their cancer return. For cancer of the mouth, pharynx and nose, the recurrence rate was 31% without transfusion and 71% with transfusion.

These studies have confirmed there is a significant adverse effect on the survival of cancer patients who receive homologous blood. Other studies found an increased frequency of postoperative bacterial infections in patients receiving donor blood. These infections require antibiotic treatment and prolong hospital stays an average of three days.

Because transfusion often complicates the recovery of surgical patients, it is as important to protect the immune system from donor blood as to guard against the risk of viral transmission. Those who are able to avoid homologous transfusion have less chance of getting bacterial infections after operations because their immune response is stronger. And homologous blood can also activate viruses that are dormant in the patient's own body. Cytomegalovirus may produce a latent infection that can be activated by multidonor transfusion.

The Advantages of Giving Yourself a Transfusion

1. The risk of getting infectious diseases is eliminated.

2. You can't have incompatibility reactions to your own blood.

3. Allergic reactions are avoided.

4. Immune suppression is avoided.

These are all powerful incentives for consumers to insist on using autologous blood options—rather than receiving homologous blood—whenever possible.

Chapter 19

Your Own Blood Is Better

The practice of blood transfusion grew rapidly in the United States during the two decades preceding 1980. There was a slight drop after the advent of AIDS but a study published in the *New England Journal of Medicine* reported that by 1987 the cost of transfusing some 20 million units of blood and components to patients reached approximately $3.2 billion per year.

In recent years, the use of autologous blood has increased while homologous blood usage has started to decline. Out of the approximately 20 million units of blood transfused in 1987, 3% were autologous. According to information provided by the AABB, during the next four years autologous blood donations continued to grow and in early 1992 accounted for 5% of the total donations being made. In 1987, 49,000 operations utilized IAT to salvage patients' blood during surgery—a small fraction of the estimated 2.4 million operations per year that have significant blood loss. Although the use of various autologous blood programs is increasing, they are still underutilized because of inadequate education of both the medical establishment and the public.

Today however, all blood banks and nearly all hospitals will allow patients to donate their blood before surgeries having high blood loss. Capability for IAT has increased. Half of the nation's hospitals now have at least limited equipment for recycling a patient's own blood. There are also 24-hour mobile services that will provide machines and technicians to those hospitals lacking their own capability. As the public becomes more aware that the transfer of a part of one human being's body to another person is a high risk procedure, autologous blood programs will become the wave of the future. The day will arrive when both elective and emergency surgical patients will provide much of their own blood. This will be an exciting medical advance because blood transfusion is often vital to health care, especially for complex surgeries that last several hours.

Today a number of medical tools are available which enable blood replacement without the risky infusion of someone else's blood. These tools or procedures are divided into five different modalities. When patients learn of these options, their response and cooperation is favorable. Nearly everyone is enthusiastic about getting his or her own blood.

Donating Your Blood Before Surgery

The safest transfusion is the one which uses your own predonated blood. Blood donated before surgery has an advantage over blood salvaged by IAT because it does not contain debris, drugs or contamination from the surgical site. Donating your own blood is the autologous option to consider first.

The medical exclusions for volunteer blood donors do not apply to people donating blood for their own use. There are no age limits and even those in their seventies and eighties can usually predonate at least part of their own blood replacement needs. According to the AABB it is possible for babies to donate small amounts of blood if a small needle is used along with a pump to maintain blood flow. However, the theory appears to exceed the practice because I haven't spoken with a single blood bank that collects blood from babies. I found many blood banks don't collect from children unless they are in their early teens and that usually the blood needs of children are handled by regular banked blood or by directed donation. Nevertheless, when a survey was conducted of 180 children between 8 and 18 who were allowed to donate their blood before surgery, only four experienced a mild reaction and 88% of them supplied all their own blood requirements.

Generally, doctors believe that if patients are in good enough condition to undergo elective surgery they can donate blood, but certain heart conditions and a few other illnesses will exclude some people. A hemoglobin test measures the amount of iron-containing red material in red blood cells and is an indicator of anemia. Because you must have a hemoglobin of 11 or greater before each donation, oral iron supplements are prescribed one week before the first donation and until hospital admission. Older or underweight patient donors may be given an IV as their blood is being drawn to prevent a reaction due to loss of blood volume.

You may have read that you can donate up to six pints of blood during the six weeks before surgery. For most patients that's an unrealistic goal. The majority of people are only able to donate one to three pints of blood about a week apart and not be anemic when they go into surgery. While younger people can regenerate a pint of blood in a week or two, it takes older people about three weeks. Predonation requires a common sense approach for each individual.

From the consumer viewpoint, the most frustrating aspect of pre-donation is the unknown factor of how much blood, if any, will be needed during or after surgery. A good percentage of surgeries do not require blood but there is no way to know with total certainty which ones won't. However, it is well-known which operations rarely need blood. An expected blood loss can be fairly accurately predicted by your surgeon from clinical evaluation and his or her personal experience in that procedure. It is recommended that whenever possible, patients donate their total estimated blood need, but many fall short of that goal. Those donating blood before surgery should keep in mind that even one or two pints stored as whole blood or as component units of red cells and plasma may provide the safe margin that protects them from homologous blood or the complications of undertransfusion.

In modern transfusion therapy a patient will usually just be given red cells during a surgery that requires blood replacement. Plasma and platelets will not be transfused unless tests indicate that they are needed to help blood to clot. For surgeries having a moderate blood loss of three or four pints, red cells from two predonated units of blood would probably be sufficient. However, patients donating their own blood may want the extra protection of having both red cells and plasma stored for their possible use. Units collected within 10 days of surgery can be stored as whole blood and will provide the benefits of both red cells and plasma. Even in surgeries having massive blood loss, two donations can reduce exposure from 16 donors to 5 donors providing you insist on single-donor platelets or have a directed platelet monodonor. And when predonation is combined with IAT and preoperative plateletpheresis, you will likely avoid all donor exposure. These issues are covered in more depth later in the book.

The donation of blood during pregnancy, for possible use at the time of delivery or Caesarean section, is a new medical concept that gained popularity during the last decade. It appears to be a safe procedure for most women, and doctors say up to four pints can be donated after the

34th week of pregnancy, or much sooner if the component units are frozen.

The majority of women have their babies without receiving transfusions but many lose a fourth to a third of their blood which leaves them weak and fatigued for many weeks. Some doctors believe all pregnant women should store their blood and, if it is needed after delivery, it should be transfused up to full replacement levels. The following conditions increase the likelihood of excessive blood loss during delivery: a history of multiple miscarriages, a history of previous blood transfusions, placenta previa, eclampsia and C section. If the donated blood is not transfused to the mother, it can be kept for possible use by the baby. Children will almost always have blood that is compatible with at least one of their parents.

Preparation and Use of Predonated Blood

Component	Maximum Storage Time	Reason Transfused
Whole blood	35 days	For oxygen delivery and to expand blood volume
Red blood cells	35 or 42 days*	For oxygen delivery and to expand blood volume
Fresh frozen plasma	1 year	For clotting and to expand blood volume
Platelet concentrate	5 days	To stop excessive bleeding
Frozen red blood cells	10 years	For oxygen delivery

* Depends on the preparation

How much mileage you get out of the donations you make depends on how your surgeon orders them to be prepared. Usually the plasma is separated and only the red cells are kept for the patient donor. If your blood tests negative for infectious diseases, the plasma which accounts for 55% of the total volume of your donation is sold to another patient. You will notice in the above table that in addition to providing clotting factors, autologous plasma can also be used as a volume expander. At a time when your body is facing the stress of surgery, why should it be asked to replace donated blood when less than half of that donated will be available for reinfusion? This is one of the issues listed in the next chapter for discussion with your surgeon.

If your total donation is stored for your needs it can either be prepared as whole blood or as component units of red cells and frozen plasma. Whole blood is cheaper, but after storage of one day or less, the clotting factors begin to decrease in effectiveness. Fresh frozen plasma is of higher quality and, when teamed with red cells, provides more options in covering plasma and red cell replacement needs.

When your blood is stored as packed red cells, you have six weeks in which to donate. If your surgery isn't pressing, the donation period can be extended beyond six weeks and the first unit or two of red cells can be frozen. Any prepared plasma will always be fresh frozen and is good for one year. If your hemoglobin doesn't drop below 11 you are allowed to make donations three *days* apart and up to 72 hours before surgery, but this is an unrealistic schedule for most patients.

In perspective, a healthy volunteer donor is only allowed to donate blood six times a year and no more frequently than once every eight weeks. Patients might question their doctors about the wisdom of donating more than three pints of blood in a six week period. Your goal is to reach the surgery room in the best physical condition possible and have an uncomplicated recovery. However, blood bankers maintain that when daily iron pills are taken to ensure that bone marrow produces replacement blood cells, patients can often donate up to 10% of their total blood volume per week.

A new drug, erythropoietin, is now available which helps the body recover faster from blood loss. Some doctors have found that erythropoietin therapy enables patients to donate twice as much blood before surgery. If a patient-donor becomes slightly anemic, half units of blood may be collected at one week intervals and pooled to make a unit. And there can be a health benefit from predonating your blood because bone marrow will already be stimulated to replace blood lost during and after surgery. The amount of blood that can be donated safely before surgery varies greatly between patients and requires close monitoring by doctors.

Initially, most blood banks were less than ecstatic about preoperative donation. It's cumbersome. Each donor's health must be evaluated, collection times scheduled, people gotten to the right place and donations meticulously labeled and segregated for storage. Later all the blood units drawn have to be sent to the right surgery room at the proper time. And presurgery patients are not typical, healthy donors. They are often apprehensive and require more attention from blood bank personnel. It is not surprising that during the 1980s some blood banks performed autologous donation services grudgingly and limited collection hours to discourage patients from donating. However, today you can generally expect a cooperative attitude. This is important because an effective donation of blood before surgery depends on cooperation between you, your doctor, the blood bank and the hospital.

Your doctor acts as the purchasing agent for all transfused blood whether it is someone else's or your own. You cannot donate before surgery unless your surgeon initiates the order by contacting the blood bank and making a written request. The request will indicate the kind and number of blood components needed and the type of surgery, date and location. Your health problems will also be communicated to the blood bank. An appointment is made for you with the blood bank to ascertain if you are able to give blood and if the requested units can be collected in time for surgery.

The blood units donated before surgery are usually labeled "autologous only" or "autologous-homologous." If labeled "autologous only" it means the blood cannot be used for anyone else and if you do not need it for surgery you will likely be charged for it anyway at full or reduced rates. When you are billed for leftover units, it's doubtful your insurance will cover the cost which is why some blood banks require you to pay in advance for predonation. If you and your blood pass the screening criteria and testing used for regular donors and your units are marked "autologous-homologous" they can be sold to other patients if you don't need them. In this case you shouldn't be charged a full price.

All blood donations are required to have ABO and Rh typing prior to labeling and autologous donations are also tested for hepatitis B and AIDS. Should either hepatitis B or AIDS infection be found in the blood, most facilities will not process and transfuse it to the patient-donor because of risk to blood bank and hospital personnel. Of course, the blood poses no additional risk of infectious diseases to the patient who donated it because he or she already has those infections.

Your units of predonated blood are marked with special identifying tags with your signature which you will sign again before surgery. The signature helps prevent mixups and reassures patients that they are getting their own blood. One woman signed hers with a bright marker so it could be seen from her bed and she would know it was her correct unit. After all your donations are collected, the blood bank should inform you, your surgeon and the hospital of the number and kinds of components prepared and where they are stored. The hospital will record this information on the front of your hospital chart and if the blood is being held at a blood bank outside the hospital, arrangements are made for its transfer. Your doctor's admission order should also alert hospital personnel to confirm that your blood is in the proper place.

The risk of anemia for patients who donate their own blood has already been discussed. It is also possible to have a brief reaction of dizziness, nausea and low blood pressure when the blood is drawn. This reaction is experienced by 2% to 5% of all blood donors including healthy volunteers. Other problems associated with autologous donations are due to blood bank or hospital errors and include:

1. Losing the blood and not being able to find it in time for surgery

2. Transfusing it to the wrong patient

3. Breakage of a stored unit

4. Not getting the blood to the surgery room

Suggestions for reducing the chance of these errors are found in the next chapter.

The exact cost to the patient for predonating blood cannot be determined before surgery. It will depend on numerous variables. Were all units transfused to the patient? Were leftover units labeled "autologous-homologous"? Were crossmatching fees avoided? Other factors are: the blood bank's policy, hospital markup, testing and transfusion fees and the patient's insurance coverage. However, consumers are usually charged more for their own blood than for someone else's blood. But if IAT is used during an operation the total costs of it and predonation can be *cheaper* than buying large amounts of homologous blood.

During the summer of 1991, I compared the autologous and homologous prices charged for whole blood and red cells at a number of blood centers and hospitals around the nation. Generally, after hospital charges are added, a unit of autologous red cells or whole blood will cost over $200 and if transfused will be covered by insurance. Usually included in the price is an extra handling, drawing or storage fee of $20 to $30 which makes your predonated autologous blood slightly more costly than banked homologous blood.

The nonprofit side of the blood industry has always gotten its product free—previously from volunteer donors and presently from volunteers and a growing number of donor-patients. Although it takes blood banks more time to collect autologous units, the cost of recruiting volunteer donors is eliminated for those units. In a book on autologous blood programs published by the AABB, the cost of providing autologous and homologous blood was judged to be "about equal." Blood banking costs have been driven up by the additional tests now being done, but consumers can be confident that the industry is finding ways to compensate. However, few knowledgeable patients would object to paying a little more to get their own blood. When costs of the myriad problems caused by homologous blood transfusions are considered, autologous blood becomes a bargain at any price. It is heartening that most of the patients who donate blood before surgery avoid homologous exposure. In a study done at the Mayo Clinic doctors found that 90% of those predonating did not require blood from anyone else.

The other methods of autologous transfusion do not require the patient involvement or inconvenience that preoperative donation does. They are performed in the surgery or recovery room while the patient is usually under the effects of anesthesia. However, it is important for health consumers to understand these procedures because it may be necessary to combine one or more of them with predonation if the goal is to avoid all homologous blood. And when patients are unable to donate any blood before surgery, it's possible that a combination of autotransfusion techniques will cover their blood requirements.

Intraoperative Autologous Transfusion

IAT is the collection, processing and reinfusion of a patient's blood when it is lost because of injury or surgery. A machine called a cell saver can recycle much of the blood in your body over and over again. Although not all blood lost during surgery can be salvaged, between 50% and 70% may be collected and reinfused to the patient.

Unlike patient donation before surgery, IAT eliminates any chance of getting the wrong blood due to a mixup in the labeling and handling of donated units. Salvaged blood comes from your body and returns to it without chance of clerical error. The quality of the blood is excellent and contains more oxygen than predonated red cells which lose oxygen during storage. It is compatible with your body, available and free of the infectious risk of homologous blood. As it is salvaged the blood passes through disposable plastic tubes and containers. In addition to red cells, salvaged blood may contain platelets, white cells and clotting factors depending on the device used for collection and if it is washed or unwashed. However, when blood is recycled *during* surgery it is almost always washed and just the red cells are returned to the patient.

IAT is used more frequently than any other autologous blood practice except preoperative donation. As salvaged blood can be collected, washed, filtered and returned to the patient from a bag under pressure within ten minutes after it is lost, valuable time is saved when treating emergency bleeding due to injury. Surgery will not be delayed while homologous blood is being obtained and crossmatched for the patient.

IAT can be used for all surgical specialties but is most often utilized in cardiac and vascular surgery, orthopedic surgery, liver transplants and repair of traumatic injuries. Use of IAT is also expanding into neurosurgery, urology, plastic surgery and some OB/GYN procedures. It is not used for open bowel surgery or when blood would be suctioned from a site of infection or malignancy because of concern that germs or cancer cells could be spread throughout the patient's body. Although many adolescents can benefit from the use of IAT, the volume of blood that can be salvaged from younger children is small. Machines capable of efficient blood recovery during the surgeries of small children have not yet been developed.

There are two methods of IAT. In the simpler one, blood is mixed with a drug that prevents clotting as it is vacuumed into a portable canister. When the plastic liner inside the canister is full, the contents are either filtered and transfused as whole blood or washed, filtered and returned to the patient as red cells. Canister devices are inexpensive and easy to use but may be too slow to keep up with heavy blood loss.

The second method of IAT was developed with the help of doctors at the Mayo Clinic and resulted in the Haemonetics Cell Saver which was introduced in 1974. It took nearly 20 years and the AIDS scare for cell savers to become common surgery room equipment. Today these machines are sophisticated cell washing devices which cost $18,000 or more.

Cell savers suction lost blood into a rotating centrifuge bowl where plasma and other components are separated from the red blood cells by spinning. The red cells are washed with a normal saline solution, pumped into a reinfusion bag and returned to the patient. The fast return makes the more expensive machines ideal for surgeries having a rapid, high volume blood loss because most all blood recycled during an operation will have to be washed. The filtering and washing process is effective in removing anti-clotting agents, bone chips and other debris, byproducts from the breakdown of red cells and most bacteria.

The development of safer and more efficient equipment has dramatically decreased the complications of IAT since the 1970s. An earlier machine with a history for causing air embolism is no longer manufactured. There have not been any major risks reported with the new machines hospitals use today because they filter out air and have a warning signal if it should get into the system.

The chance of IAT spreading malignant cells during cancer operations is avoided because it is rarely ever used for those surgeries. However, a new machine is being developed to remove cancer cells from a patient's blood and filters are being improved to eliminate bacteria. Although sepsis (infection of the bloodstream) is a potential risk of all blood salvage procedures it is extremely rare if blood is suctioned from an uninfected site. And the risk of delayed clotting and mild non-immune hemolytic complications are significantly reduced by filtering and washing the blood. Doctors who have had over a decade of experience with IAT consider it a very safe procedure which eliminates the medical problems associated with homologous blood.

Postoperative Autologous Transfusion

Some patients lose as much or more blood after surgery as during it. Consequently, a hospital with a complete autologous blood program will also provide postoperative blood salvage. Blood lost from the surgical wound can be collected, processed and returned to the patient in the same way it was during surgery. For the first four to 12 hours after an operation, blood draining from the wound is collected and run through a cell saver or immediate return device.

Occasionally postoperative blood salvage is not done in some hospitals because after patients leave the operating room there isn't anyone assigned to take over the duty in the recovery room. IAT operators are usually specially trained nurses or hospital transfusion service personnel who work under the supervision of surgeons and anesthesiologists in the operating room. Nurses in the recovery room are often hesitant to assume the responsibility.

In recovery rooms, it has been more convenient for hospitals to use less expensive equipment which does not require the constant attention of a dedicated operator to run. As there is not as much debris in blood lost after surgery, transfusing unwashed post-operative blood became accepted practice in many hospitals because it could be easily accomplished with canister or immediate return devices. There is no question that unwashed blood salvage is more convenient for hospital personnel but there is medical controversy over its safety. And studies supporting both sides of the argument further confuse the issue.

Unwashed salvaged blood contains large amounts of damaged red cells, free hemoglobin and clumps of fibrin which can prolong bleeding time and cause mild hemolytic reactions. Although the clinical significance of the byproducts left in unwashed blood is still controversial, there is no disagreement that washed red cells lessen the risk of complications. Some surgeons will not infuse their patients with unwashed blood and many hospitals use smaller cell savers to wash blood in recovery rooms or send the blood to the lab for washing. This may be another issue to discuss with your doctor when surgery is scheduled.

In past years some insurance companies did not fully cover IAT procedures, but today they are routinely paid for by insurance carriers, including Medicare and Medicaid, if they are billed in the proper format. It appears that the cost of IAT and other autologous surgical modalities are being absorbed as part of a surgery's total cost—insurance companies have ceiling payments for specific surgeries and hospitals keep their charges within that guideline. You could check with the billing or accounting department of the hospital where surgery is scheduled to make sure IAT is being covered. Hospital cost of providing IAT is much less than transfusing a heavy-blood-loss patient with homologous blood. The break-even point between banked homologous blood and IAT is around a two-unit blood replacement. Patient cost for IAT is the same regardless of how many units of blood are recycled.

For surgeries having low blood loss which usually do not require transfusion, a less sophisticated standby collection canister can be used at a cost to the hospital of around $100. This device suctions blood lost during surgery into a sterile canister and, if a unit is collected, it can be taken to the hospital blood bank or lab and washed with a cell washer before transfusion. Or a cell saver can be wheeled into the surgery room to complete the procedure. There is a new machine by Haemonetics designed specifically for low blood-loss procedures. However, it may be awhile before many hospitals purchase the new machines because in 1992 just 2% to 5% of surgeries having low blood loss utilize red cell salvage. In the meantime, canister collection provides an option. The purpose of collection during low blood-loss procedures is to reserve lost blood in the event that it *is* needed. With this precaution the patient is not asked to take the unnecessary risk of getting a homologous transfusion he or she wasn't supposed to need. The small cost of the standby device is absorbed in the total surgery charge.

Preoperative Apheresis

Recently a new application of plasmapheresis has been utilized in some surgeries having an expected high blood loss. Immediately before surgery a machine draws off plasma from the patient's blood which contains clotting proteins and platelets. This platelet-rich plasma is saved for later reinfusion and solves the problem caused by the loss of vital clotting factors which result from lengthy recycling of cells by IAT. Although the vast majority of transfused patients don't require plasma or platelets, those who do are often given platelets from six to ten donors. For those cases, preoperative apheresis can be the deciding factor in a patient being able to avoid all donor blood.

Platelet-rich plasma is not needed during an operation because doctors do not want blood to clot while they do surgery. But at the end of the operation as many as 200 billion platelets are given back to the patient to control postoperative bleeding. The fresh, undamaged clotting substances can reduce the amount of blood lost after surgery and enable the patient to heal faster.

Some patients will have medical problems such as very low blood pressure, certain heart conditions and anemia which prevent the use of preoperative apheresis. And in *extreme* emergency operations there isn't time to do the procedure. However, for those who are eligible for apheresis there is no risk to the patient if the plasma is collected by sterile methods and stored and transfused properly. Preoperative apheresis is the most recent advance in autologous transfusion and does not have universal acceptance in the surgical community. However, some surgical teams use the procedure routinely and when combined with the salvage of red blood cells it may offer a total autologous program for those having heavy blood loss surgeries.

Hemodilution

If this autologous procedure is used, it will be done immediately before surgery as the patient is undergoing anesthesia. Blood is withdrawn by the anesthesiologist and saved for later reinfusion. The patient is given an IV solution of saline and albumin to maintain volume for adequate circulation.

A hematocrit test shows the percentage of red blood cells in a patient's blood. If a patient goes into surgery with a hematocrit of 40 and is hemodiluted to a hematocrit of 20 he or she will lose 50% fewer red cells. Although the patient will lose the same amount of blood the actual loss of red cells will be less. The whole blood which was drawn off before surgery is infused back to the patient when it is needed.

Hemodilution is the least performed type of autologous blood practice. Although it is an old procedure, the National Institutes of Health takes the position that more studies are needed to determine the safe lower limits of hematocrit after hemodilution. Doctors who use hemodilution usually only draw off one or two units. The amount of blood that can be withdrawn depends on the size of the patient, the hematocrit and the expected surgical blood loss. Consumers should be aware that the blood withdrawn by hemodilution may occasionally not be returned to the patient. A doctor has suggested that if you or a family member has hemodilution you should get the surgeon to guarantee the withdrawn blood will be reinfused.

Hemodilution is mostly used in cardiac bypass surgery in combination with IAT. It is also considered an option for surgeries that have a low blood loss and for a number of children's operations, including cardiac surgery. When hemodilution is used in a pediatric surgery, fresh red cells, platelets and clotting factors can be returned to small children who have few autologous blood options. However, this procedure cannot be used for patients who have anemia, serious heart disease or kidney disease.

The autologous options discussed here can be used alone or in any combinations to eliminate or reduce exposure to someone else's blood. Any increased costs in providing patients with their own blood pale into insignificance when the costs of virus-laced homologous blood are considered. Because of the infectious diseases my parents contracted from my father's 18-donor transfusion, the last three and a half years of their lives were a descent into hell. Their conditions required the following services: Home Health Care for two years, 105 days in convalescent homes and 201 days in hospitals. In addition, one or two family members were needed to provide care 24 hours a day which resulted in two lost incomes. When medical costs of the health problems caused by the use of homologous blood are considered, arguments over autologous blood not being cost effective, or depleting blood bank and hospital resources, become absurd.

Chapter 20

How to Work With Your Doctor

If you or a member of your family has an elective surgery scheduled, or a medical condition that may eventually require surgery, advance planning to use the patient's own blood is essential. This chapter helps consumers work with blood banks, hospitals and doctors to obtain the safest transfusion therapy available.

Paul Gann Blood Safety Act

In 1978 I was living in California with my husband and children when Howard Jarvis and Paul Gann co-authored Proposition 13 and ignited a nationwide taxpayer revolt. The state's voters overwhelmingly approved the initiative and California's soaring property taxes were rolled back. Although Paul Gann was never elected to public office, he went on to sponsor a total of six ballot measures and is credited with directing more far-reaching legal and state constitutional changes than any other Californian.

Unfortunately, in 1982 Gann had open heart surgery. He was transfused with 43 units of blood and blood products from 43 different donors. Five years later the 75-year-old Gann held a press conference at the state capitol and acknowledged that he was facing an AIDS death. He tearfully told reporters that the blood he had been transfused with had been contaminated with HIV. "When my doctor told me I had AIDS I felt more anger and frustration than ever before in my life."

Gann vowed to make AIDS his last campaign and shortly before his death in 1989 the California Legislature passed the Paul Gann Blood Safety Act. The act requires physicians and surgeons in California to advise patients of the risks and alternatives to homologous blood whenever the reasonable possibility of a transfusion exists because of surgery or procedures such as hemodialysis or chemotherapy. The Gann Act mandates that there be written documentation of notification in the patient's medical file. When there is no life-threatening emergency and the patient's condition permits, doctors are required to allow enough time before surgery so that patients wishing to predonate their blood may do so.

The public could assume that the Paul Gann Blood Safety Act would have had the support of medical and consumer groups charged with the responsibility of assuring quality health care. This was not the case. On reviewing the bill, I was shocked to learn that four very powerful organizations were listed as opposing it. They were: the California Medical Association, the Board of Medical Quality Assurance, the Department of Consumer Affairs and the Department of Health Services.

Opposition to the Gann Act partially stemmed from the resistance medical groups have to legislators telling them how to provide medical care. In addition, the bill did not provide funding, and doctors and surgeons would be charged for the information brochure they were required to give patients. The California Medical Association took the position that the state should pay the cost. The Department of Consumer Affairs and the Board of Medical Quality Assurance were being asked to make the brochures available to the public at no cost. The Department of Health Services, which was required to prepare the brochure, argued that it was unnecessary and that patients were already being informed of transfusion options.

The opposition to the Gann Act is an example of how consumer needs can be ignored in a complex medical bureaucracy. While it is doubtful that there was any group deliberately trying to keep health consumers uninformed, there was the usual resistance to change and a reluctance to shoulder increased responsibility. And it should also be noted that health authorities prefer to avoid situations that may cause public concern over blood safety.

The Paul Gann Blood Safety Act was sponsored by State Senator John Doolittle with the active support of Dr. Theresa Crenshaw and the dying Paul Gann. A number of individual doctors went on record supporting the act and the State Legislative Committee of American Association of Retired Persons gave it a support position. The California Legislature, deeply touched by Gann's tragedy, ignored the opposition and passed the bill. New Jersey is the only other state to enact similar legislation. However, two state legislatures are presently considering blood safety bills: one in Pennsylvania sponsored by State Representative Michael Sturla, and another in New York sponsored by State Senator Guy Velella.

The following brochure was prepared by the California Department of Health Services in response to the Paul Gann Blood Safety Act. It is not copyrighted. I suggest that you make copies and put them in the glove compartments of your cars. Also keep one with your family health information. Make the brochure readily available so that you can have a copy for discussing transfusion options with doctors in case a family emergency requiring blood should arise. In emergency situations where blood becomes trapped inside the chest or abdomen, it can often be suctioned out and infused back into the patient. Remember that IAT can be used during and after most emergency surgeries.

Preparing for Elective Surgery

In most cases, there will be adequate time before elective surgery to plan for transfusion needs. If approached in a well-informed and cooperative manner, a surgeon should not be offended if you explain that you want to do everything possible to avoid getting other people's blood. Although surgeons will not actively object to that concept, some may discourage you and many will play down the risks of homologous blood. The best of intentions can get lost in hospital logistics. For these reasons the consumer cannot afford to remain uninvolved.

A good autologous blood program does not just happen in a hospital. It takes directed organization and the cooperation of several departments. For example, if the blood bank and surgery department do not work together, a patient can donate blood and then have the goal of avoiding homologous exposure undermined by being given a six-pack of donor platelets.

From the patient viewpoint a hospital offering excellent transfusion therapy would have:

- An approved written protocol integrating all autologous blood options

- A separate policy or guideline allowing autologous blood to be transfused at higher hemoglobin and/or hematocrit levels than the conservative levels now used for homologous blood

- A transfusion committee with representatives from administration, blood banking, various surgery departments, pathology, anesthesiology and recovery room staff

The Safest Blood is Your Own.
Use It Whenever Possible.

Many surgeries do not require blood transfusions. However, if you need blood, you have several options. Although you have the right to refuse a blood transfusion, this decision may hold life-threatening consequences. Please carefully review this brochure and decide with your doctor which option(s) you prefer.

The methods of using your own blood can be used independently or together to eliminate or minimize the need for donor blood, as well as virtually eliminate transfusion risks of infection and allergic reaction.

Option	Explanation	Advantages	Disadvantages
PRE-OPERATIVE DONATION Donating Your Own Blood Before Surgery	The blood bank draws your blood and stores it until you need it, during or after surgery. For elective surgery only.	✓ Eliminates or minimizes the need for someone else's blood during and after surgery.	• Requires advance planning. • May delay surgery. • Medical conditions may prevent pre-operative donation.
INTRA-OPERATIVE AUTOLOGOUS TRANSFUSION Recycling Your Blood During Surgery	Instead of being discarded, blood lost during surgery is filtered, and put back into your body during surgery. For elective and emergency surgery.	✓ Eliminates or minimizes need for someone else's blood during surgery. Large amounts of blood can be recycled.	• Not for use if cancer or infection present.
POST-OPERATIVE AUTOLOGOUS TRANSFUSION Recycling Your Blood After Surgery	Blood lost after surgery is collected, filtered and returned. For elective and emergency surgery.	✓ Eliminates or minimizes the need for someone else's blood after surgery.	• Not for use if cancer or infection present.
HEMODILUTION Donating Your Own Blood During Surgery	Immediately before surgery, some of your blood is taken and replaced with I.V. fluids. After surgery, your blood is filtered and returned to you. For elective surgery.	✓ Eliminates or minimizes the need for someone else's blood during and after surgery. Dilutes your blood so you lose less concentrated blood during surgery.	• Limited number of units can be drawn. • Medical conditions may prevent hemodilution.
APHERESIS Donating Your Own Platelets and Plasma	Before surgery, your platelets and plasma, which help stop bleeding, are withdrawn, filtered, and returned to you when you need it. For elective surgery.	✓ May eliminate the need for donor platelets and plasma, especially in high blood-loss procedures.	• Medical conditions may prevent apheresis. • Procedure has limited application.

This brochure was developed by the California Department of Health Services, NOT copyrighted

- An objective to eliminate the use of homologous blood whenever possible by transfusing patients with their own blood to known safe levels

- A knowledge that failure to make autologous blood programs available can lead to legal jeopardy as more cases go to court with patients claiming they got hepatitis or AIDS because they were not offered transfusion alternatives

- A dedicated doctor to head the committee and assume responsibility for the program

- A flexible predonation policy for patients who wish to donate for those procedures which usually have a low blood loss

- A standard policy to collect the blood lost during surgeries not expected to need transfusion

- Adequate IAT equipment for all surgical departments

- Trained personnel in recovery rooms to take over the salvage of red cells after the patient leaves the operating room

However, because the vast majority of hospitals do not have a transfusion service department, lack of leadership has often resulted in underutilization of the advances in transfusion medicine. But when the hospital blood bank or transfusion service also assumes the responsibility of autotransfusion, autologous programs run smoothly. The Mayo Clinic's Blood Bank and Transfusion Services has administered all aspects of autotransfusion since 1983. Blood bank personnel operate IAT equipment in operating rooms and take untransfused salvaged red blood cells to the blood bank for storage in case the patient should need them in the days following surgery. This is an example of one of many small details that can get overlooked if efforts are not organized. In the surgery room, IAT operators generally work under the supervision of the surgeon and anesthesiologist who come to a joint decision on the transfusion needs of the patient.

Although a growing number of hospitals have well-coordinated autologous programs, there are still many surgeons who are either disinterested or do not take the extra time to order them for their patients. The Mayo Clinic implemented an automatic referral system which had secretaries instead of surgeons write the order for patients to be evaluated for probable donation of their blood before surgery and IAT during surgery. Under this program, 86% of patients avoided all homologous exposure. When surgeons had to initiate the request for collection of the patient's own blood, only 26% did not get homologous blood.

This study suggests that many surgeons are apathetic about helping patients give themselves a transfusion. Though options for autologous transfusion are available, patients cannot depend on doctors to routinely arrange for them. Some patients have found it helpful to enlist the aid of the surgeon's office staff in obtaining an evaluation for autologous blood procedures. They explain to secretaries and nurses their desire to avoid homologous blood and ask for their assistance.

The vast majority of hospitals and blood banks have policies indicating it is "inappropriate" to request predonation for patients having surgery that rarely requires blood—surgeries like tonsillectomies, gall bladder operations and vaginal hysterectomies. The blood banking position is that units donated for low blood loss procedures are merely "psychological insurance" for the patient. They maintain that if one unit is stored for a surgery in which blood is seldom needed and something goes wrong, one unit will probably not be enough. Consequently, most, but not all, blood banks will try to talk the patient out of donating or have surgeons discourage it and never make the request.

But the "appropriateness" of a patient predonating blood that will likely not be needed is a decision that should be made by the person being asked to take the unnecessary risk. In the spring of 1990, a woman I know had a D & C—a procedure which almost never requires blood transfusion. The woman asked her gynecologist about predonation and he adamantly assured her that she would "definitely not need any blood." As a result, when the woman signed the hospital treatment form she refused to give permission for a blood transfusion. Immediately before her D & C the patient was asked to sign a form releasing the hospital from liability in the event that she did need a transfusion after all and they couldn't give it. The assumption of risk which was "appropriate" when the patient was asked to assume it had become totally "inappropriate" when placed on the hospital. Fortunately, she did not need blood.

But a 17-year-old girl in Ventura, California, was not so lucky. After her D & C, the teenager was given two units of blood from which she contracted AIDS. According to a study published in the *New England Journal of Medicine* in June 1990, "Units of whole blood and red cells are given in small numbers to large numbers of people." Many of those units go to people having surgeries that were not expected to require blood. Few knowledgeable consumers would volunteer to take that risk when there are a number of options.

Those scheduled for low blood loss surgeries can either insist on donating one or two units of blood or they can request that all blood lost during surgery be suctioned into a canister device and saved. Then, if it is needed, cell washing capability can be added and the blood can be infused at a small cost to the hospital.

Or the two options may be combined. You can donate a single unit of blood and ask your surgeon to have the blood bank prepare from it a component unit of red cells and a component unit of fresh frozen plasma. In addition, your lost blood can be suctioned during surgery and saved. This combination provides good insurance at low cost in case something should go wrong and considerable blood is lost.

There is no reason that patients who do not want to take the risk of getting homologous blood in marginal blood loss surgeries should be asked to do so. Nor is there any reason for surgeons to be placed in the difficult position of having a patient unexpectedly require blood after the patient had been assured he or she would not need it. In this situation, surgeons can be so hesitant to give homologous blood that the patient is left at risk from complications of undertransfusion.

People having surgeries with significant or heavy blood loss have an edge—their concerns about homologous transfusion are viewed as valid and they are allowed to donate their own blood without a hassle. However, these cases will not automatically have access to the latest advances in autologous blood technology. And few patients who could benefit from preoperative apheresis will be offered the procedure. All the equipment manufacturers I've talked with have made the same observation. "Doctors who have had experience with IAT and preoperative apheresis are very enthusiastic about patient benefits. Those unfamiliar with the procedures tend to be skeptical." Because there is a lag between technology and actual practice, patients continue to be unnecessarily exposed to the blood of other people. Most hospitals lacking equipment and trained personnel believe they can't afford it.

However, hospitals lacking IAT equipment can request machines and operators from Red Cross blood centers or private companies as they are needed. Not all Red Cross blood centers currently provide this service but in the recent organizational overhaul more monies were pledged to supplying IAT equipment. Companies that were once completely outside of transfusion medicine are competing with the Red Cross. PSICOR, Inc. of San Diego, California, offers a nationwide service providing IAT machines and highly trained personnel to hospitals on a 24-hour notice. The company's charges are covered by all medical insurers but surgeons or hospitals must request the service. The patient cannot arrange for it.

There are now private, for-profit blood banks that draw and store autologous blood either at the request of surgeons for a scheduled surgery or at the patient's request for long-term storage. Red blood cells can be frozen and kept for at least 10 years and plasma for one to five years depending on the preparation.

Nonprofit blood banks maintain that in case of an emergency, the blood cannot be thawed and gotten to the patient in time. However, current thawing methods can reconstitute a unit of blood in less than an hour which is adequate time for all elective surgeries and many emergency situations. Today, transfusions are rarely given within the first six hours after an emergency hospitalization. A private blood bank that collects, freezes and stores blood for a client's future use can air-express that blood to hospitals nationwide in approximately six hours. And blood that is stored in a patient's own city can be thawed and transported to local hospitals in approximately one and a half hours. However, frozen blood must be used within 24 hours after thawing.

The Pentagon is presently collecting and freezing blood in an effort to stockpile a quarter of a million units for use in combat or a national disaster. That blood will be used for homologous transfusions but it would be ideal if individuals could have three units of red cells and perhaps plasma on permanent storage for their own use. Cost would be a major disadvantage but some extended families store blood and share the expense. As blood types are inherited, there is a good chance of several family members sharing a common blood type and in an emergency, type O red cells can be given to people having other blood types. All premature babies can receive type O blood, especially O negative.

People who have a health condition that may eventually require transfusion should consider long-term storage of their own frozen blood. You may check with the AABB at their new location in Bethesda, Maryland—301-907-6977—to determine an autologous blood bank's accreditation and certification. Most of these banks ship blood across state lines which requires them to have an FDA license and regular FDA inspections. Autologous blood banks are run by doctors and trained medical personnel.

A person wanting to always have three units of red blood cells stored at Idant Laboratories, the nation's oldest and most established autologous blood bank, would pay $705 for collection, testing and storage for one year and $450 per year for storage thereafter. During the seven years Idant has been storing autologous blood, the company has never had a client who has been transfused with the blood of another person. Their clients' own blood has not only been thawed and flown long distances to reach hospitals on time, but the amount stored has been adequate for patient need.

Another autologous blood bank that just offers service in the state of California will collect and store three units of red cells for *10 years* for a total, upfront charge of $1,704—a bargain if you could be confident that a company will be in business for 10 years. (Do not confuse the high cost of lengthy storage with the small cost of predonating your blood before a scheduled surgery.)

In the past, some hospitals and nonprofit blood banks stored frozen, unused, autologous units that were not needed for surgery at a cost of $40 to $100 a year per unit. However, now most of those facilities will not provide long-term storage unless the patient has a rare blood type, another planned surgery or blood containing antibodies which make it incompatible with most donor blood. If you have leftover units and any of the above conditions, ask the hospital about storage.

It's a good idea for anyone who is having to pay for unused blood units to ask the hospital about long-term storage. There is a small chance that a few might still store blood at a minimal price. Patients who can afford it and are interested in long-term storage should have any unused units they donated for surgery transferred to a private autologous blood bank. This avoids collection and testing fees plus the inconvenience of donating again. However, if there is not an autologous blood bank in your area (look in the Yellow Pages under "blood") it will be necessary to call a national bank such as Idant Laboratories—212-935-1430. It would be much simpler if we could store our blood in our home freezers but we can't. Frozen blood requires close monitoring at exact temperatures.

A Confusing Marketplace

I made random phone calls to hospitals around the nation to determine the transfusion therapy being offered in the marketplace. It was a revealing eye-opener. I am convinced that top transfusion programs are a rare find and that their implementation in smaller hospitals will be a long time in coming. The rural hospitals I talked with did well to collect a few autologous units a year but those hospitals were not performing heart surgeries or many other high blood loss operations. However, many hospitals in larger cities lack high-quality, centralized blood programs. In one area serving over 500,000 people not one hospital had an integrated autologous blood program or adequate IAT capability. Two of the hospitals in the city perform a large number of heart and orthopedic surgeries.

In many hospitals there are inconsistencies in the availability of IAT equipment between surgical specialties. If one department purchases equipment it probably is not available for other departments to use. Attitude also can vary between specialties. Orthopedic surgeons tend to be more dedicated in assisting their patients in the avoidance of homologous exposure. The autologous interest is often more erratic in other specialties and many hospitals have far too little IAT equipment and operators to cover their surgical needs. Consumers cannot assume they will get adequate autologous transfusion therapy without effort on their part. They have to determine for themselves which hospitals and surgeons offer the best care.

But it is difficult for people to view transfusion as a consumer item because for over 40 years blood banks have conditioned the public to think of blood as a gift. According to blood banks they never sell blood—they "provide blood," they "make it available to patients," they "give blood to save lives," they "offer the gift of life" and so on. In their public relations releases to the press they never mention that blood costs a patient anything.

Recently I asked a large, regional blood center what it charged for various blood products. The spokesperson, who knew I was writing a book on autologous blood programs, lectured me.

"It's important for you to understand that we never charge anything for blood," she said. "If you write that we do charge for blood that will be incorrect and discredit your book."

"Well, what do you charge for?"

"We charge for the cost of collecting, testing and providing the blood but we never charge for the blood itself. You can't write that we do."

"Oh, I see," I replied. "It's like when I buy a 7-Up. The contents are free and I'm just paying for the can." My simile was met with silence.

Undoubtedly, the effort to preserve the concept that blood is a service or gift is rooted in the statutes requiring it to be a service. But perhaps the major cause of the discomfort is that if blood were classified as a product, blood banks could be held to strict liability for transmitting hepatitis and AIDS.

As previously discussed, nonprofit blood banks have charged enough for blood to earn higher profit margins than the majority of Fortune 500 companies. But they call their earnings "excesses" rather than profits. Because it is necessary for patients to view a transfusion as just another purchase, I have used the verb "sell" when referring to the exchange of blood.

It should be remembered that the amount patients pay for blood includes hospital costs and profits which may be more than double what the blood bank charged. There are as many differences in quality of services and pricing between hospitals as between blood banks. And many larger hospitals have their own in-house blood bank which provides at least part of the blood the hospital uses.

What to Do

I wish I could tell you that it's easy to buy a safe transfusion but the task can make purchasing a used car look like child's play. There are numerous variables to consider. All hospitals will tell you they have excellent transfusion programs. Most are sincere—they don't realize they are behind in a rapidly changing technology or that the autologous methods they use are not integrated to provide maximum patient benefits. However, if you are willing to spend a couple of hours making phone calls you can determine which hospitals in your area offer the best transfusion therapy.

When you are told you or a member of your family needs elective surgery, approach it as if you were shopping for a roofer to make improvements on your house. If your roof needed replacing, you would be involved in the selection of the materials you want—tar, shingles or tile. You would not leave the decision entirely up to the contractor. Together you would agree on the best roof for the condition of your house and then the roofer would purchase the materials and do the job.

View an elective surgery in the same way. The surgeon you decide to use for your operation will be ordering any blood transfusion you may need. But you should be involved to make sure he or she brings the best available materials and equipment to the operating table. And the surgeon's options may be limited by hospital policy or lack of equipment. Before you commit to elective surgery you should have already surveyed the autologous blood programs offered by the hospital or hospitals the surgeon is associated with.

If you are referred to a specialist and you know there is a possibility of surgery, call the specialist's office before your appointment and ask which hospitals he or she operates at. Be brief. It isn't necessary to identify yourself or explain.

Now you're ready to call each of the hospitals where the doctor practices to see which one has the most progressive transfusion program. If the surgeon only operates at one hospital, call at least one other, preferably the largest hospital in your area or one associated with a medical school. Surgeons can be granted "temporary privileges" at almost any hospital. Don't hesitate to ask the surgeon to change hospitals if you feel that another has superior transfusion therapy. Or you may request a second opinion from another specialist and discuss both the advisability of surgery and transfusion options with the consulting doctor. A discussion on getting a second opinion follows shortly.

Both Dr. Theresa Crenshaw, who worked on the issue of blood safety while a member of the Presidential Commission on AIDS, and Dr. Ronald Lapin of the Institute of Bloodless Surgery and Medicine, believe that those having surgeries with a low expected blood loss should plan in advance for autologous replacement in the event that it *is* needed. However, if your surgery falls into that category, you may choose, after doing the survey and talking with the surgeon, to "play the odds" and hope you won't need transfusing. Whatever you decide, you will have made an informed decision, understanding the risk you take and what would be required to avoid it. But the Swains found that after two members of our family got AIDS from two contaminated transfusions the oft-quoted statistical risks mean zip.

Call each of the hospitals you are checking out. If you are not sure that the surgery you're considering usually requires blood transfusion, speak with the surgery department and ask if it does. After you have that information ask to talk with the hospital blood bank, the transfusion service or the lab—in that order. Some hospitals do not have an in-house blood bank or a transfusion service department. Often the main hospital lab assumes all responsibility for transfusion functions. When you locate the proper department, ask the questions in one of the following lists, depending on whether your surgery usually requires transfusion.

List Number One—For Those Whose Surgery Does *Not* Usually Require Blood

1. Ask if patients having surgeries that are not expected to need transfusion are discouraged from donating their own blood.

2. If the answer is "yes," ask what happens if the patient absolutely insists on donating. Will the blood bank which supplies the hospital's blood draw and prepare all units your surgeon orders? This is important because the "refusal buck" can get passed between the blood bank and surgeon. If the bank will draw what is ordered you can tell your surgeon that the bank has agreed to collect whatever blood he or she requests.

   But if the blood bank will not draw autologous blood for surgeries which seldom need transfusion, you should be aware that there is a liability issue. If necessary, you can call the administrator of the hospital and explain that you have been refused the opportunity to donate your blood because it is believed you likely will not need it. Ask if the hospital will assume full responsibility for any adverse reactions or infectious diseases you may get from homologous blood in the event a transfusion is needed. Will they sign a statement indicating that intent? I'm confident you will be allowed to donate. If not, consider taking your business to another hospital.

3. Ask how much the patient is charged for an unused unit of autologous blood. The cost varies widely. A hospital blood bank in my area only charges $28 even if the blood isn't sold to another patient. Check with your insurance company for their reimbursement policy on leftover units. Very often companies just pay for what is transfused to you.

4. Ask the blood bank if during a low blood-loss procedure the lost blood can be salvaged either by a cell saver machine or a simple canister collection device. If no one at the blood bank can answer this question you may assume the hospital does not have a well-integrated autologous blood program. Call the surgery department and ask the same question. You may have to talk with a surgical nurse. You want to find out if, in those surgeries that normally do not need transfusion, blood is ever salvaged.

After you've talked with each hospital on your list you'll know what autologous programs, if any, are being used for surgeries not expected to need blood. Since the AIDS epidemic, the move toward safer transfusion has been influenced by patient concern. The risk patients are asked to take when they have low blood loss surgeries can be eliminated with a consumer nudge. Those not willing to take the chance of a possible emergency requiring blood can request that their surgeons provide predonation and/or a collection device during surgery.

List Number Two—For Those Whose Surgery Usually Requires Blood

Patients having heavy blood loss operations face a different set of obstacles. They will get full cooperation in predonating their blood but the challenge to this group is in obtaining a combination of IAT, apheresis or hemodilution modalities according to individual need.

1. Call each of the hospitals where your prospective surgeon operates. Speak with the blood bank or lab and ask if IAT is under their supervision. If it isn't you will probably be referred to the surgery department or, if the hospital is progressive, to a transfusion service.

2. When you locate where the function is administered, ask if both cell savers and plasma savers are used in the operating rooms at the facility.

3. Is hemodilution done at the hospital? If it is, ask what percentage of the units are returned to the patient. If units are not returned, hemodilution becomes an additional blood loss instead of a protective measure.

4. Is lost blood salvaged in recovery rooms? (If the answers to questions 2, 3 and 4 are yes, the hospital is using all the presently available autologous modalities.)

5. But if the hospital lacks IAT capability, ask if it has outside providers bring in equipment and operators. This service is available in most areas but some hospitals and surgeons aren't aware that it is. Find out what is available so you can ask your surgeon to make the request if necessary. Call your local Red Cross or PSICOR at 1-800-521-9757.

After talking with the hospitals where your surgeon practices, it will be fairly obvious which one has the most up-to-date autologous transfusion program. Does the hospital's right hand know what the left hand is doing? If you were not impressed with what you heard, call the largest medical center in your area and compare services. Remember, you can get a new surgeon at another hospital or request yours to get temporary privileges at another facility if machines and operators can't be brought in to one lacking them. It is not necessary to settle for inferior care.

Although you will now have some knowledge of the autologous therapies practiced in your area, you do not know which ones are the better choices for your medical condition. Your surgeon will evaluate your options at the time of your appointment. You may wish to give him or her a copy of the California Department of Health Service brochure and ask which methods would work best for you. Your medical condition could rule out some of them and if you predonate blood, sufficient time before surgery must be allowed.

What to Ask Your Surgeon if Your Surgery Does Not Usually Require Blood

1. May I predonate some blood even if I won't likely need it? Is there a local autologous blood bank?

2. If not prepared as whole blood, could both red cells and plasma be reserved for my possible use?

3. During surgery, could I have all the blood I lose collected with a canister device just in case I do need transfusion?

4. At what level would you transfuse me with my own blood? At the very least the old 10/30 rule should apply for autologous blood because it does not carry a risk of viral infection.

5. If the hospital where you plan to schedule my surgery is not willing to allow me to prepare for blood replacement with my own safe blood, could you do my surgery at another hospital?

Remember you have the right to insist on predonation; the blood bank will likely back down and cooperate. Or the surgeon can ask an autologous bank to draw your blood if the hospital will accept blood from that bank. If you should change hospitals, call the administration office of the first facility and let them know you were unhappy with their transfusion program. A few calls of this type will bring changes in hospital policy.

What to Ask Your Surgeon if Your Surgery Usually Requires Blood

1. Are there any new advances in transfusion medicine that are not listed on this California Health Service brochure?

2. Can I donate my own blood before surgery?

3. If not prepared as whole blood, could both red cells and plasma be reserved for my use?

4. Am I eligible for IAT?

5. Will the blood I lose in the recovery room be salvaged and returned to me? Will it be washed?

6. Does the hospital where you operate have adequate salvage equipment for both surgery and recovery rooms? Can you guarantee machines will be available? If the answer is "No," can a machine and operator be provided by the Red Cross or a private company?

7. Could I benefit from hemodilution or preoperative apheresis?

8. Will any autologous blood that is not transfused to me be kept for a few days after my surgery?

9. Does the transfusion guideline you use for giving the patient's own blood differ from the conservative one used for regular banked blood?

10. If I lose more than one pint of blood will you transfuse me with my own blood?

If the surgeon is impatient, patronizing or uncooperative, refrain from reacting negatively. Stall and say you will call the office in a couple of days with your decision on whether to proceed with the operation. Be secure in the knowledge that you have every right to interview the provider of a service that you and your insurance company will pay for. You are the one with the medical condition and how it is managed will affect your health for the remainder of your life. It is essential for you to have a surgeon you thoroughly trust. If you're unhappy with this choice, call your referring doctor, explain your concerns and ask for another surgeon who practices at a hospital having an adequate autologous transfusion program or arrange for a second opinion.

However, if you are impressed with the surgeon and he or she meets your other criteria, surgery can be scheduled. Be aware that arranging for autologous blood transfusion requires considerable interaction and logistical support within the hospital. Busy doctors and hospital staffs may not always follow through on their intent to utilize autologous methods. And getting the blood transfused back to the patient presents another challenge.

The Mayo Clinic study referred to earlier stated that doctors "used essentially the same amount of autologous blood as was usually ordered for homologous transfusions for equivalent cases." Remember that the new 1988 guidelines for transfusion allow over 30% of a patient's blood to be lost without replacement. Even newer guidelines in 1992 allow the hemoglobin of healthy patients to drop to five grams before a transfusion is started—over a 50% blood loss! If a hospital uses the lower transfusion guideline and patients don't get their own safe blood back, they could be at a disadvantage. Having just recently donated blood, they may be at more risk for complications of anemia than those who did not donate before surgery. The reluctance to risk transfusing homologous blood is understandable. However, treating patients who have their own blood available by the same conservative standard as those who do not, is questionable. It is reasonable to suggest that the old 10/30 rule that was accepted by the medical establishment for nearly half a century to determine when to transfuse blood should be the *minimum* guide for patients who have autologous blood available. (The normal hemoglobin range for women is between 12 and 15; men are between 14 and 18. Normal hematocrit readings range from 40% to 50% for men and slightly lower for women.)

Dr. Joseph Feldschuh, a cardiologist and assistant professor at Cornell Medical School, believes patients should be transfused with autologous blood to a normal level. In his book, *Safe Blood*, Dr. Feldschuh writes, "No patient missing any amount of blood after surgery should be denied a transfusion with his own safe blood when it is available on the grounds that he does not really need it. No hospital should give an anemic patient's blood to another patient without written consent. Patients should insist that they get their own blood back and be transfused to a full normal level."

Because of the complexity of turning an intended autologous transfusion into reality and the tendency of some surgical staffs to use autologous blood as sparingly as homologous blood, you may want to write your surgeon a letter immediately after your surgery is scheduled. In it, reaffirm your dedication to lessening transfusion risks. If you don't want to write your own letter, you have permission to copy the one on the next page.

Study the listed transfusion options A through G in the letter. By the time surgery is scheduled you will have discussed the various options with your surgeon and know if you'll be donating your blood in the weeks before your operation (option A). And you will have made a decision on whether to arrange for directed donors (option G). Unless there is cancer or infection at the surgical site, almost all patients are eligible to have blood salvage (options B, C, *or* F). Options D and E are seldom used, but your surgeon may have indicated an intent to utilize one of them. Make a check in the square next to each option you and the doctor decided to use. You will probably have more than one item checked. Sign the letter, make a photocopy for your records, then mail the original to your surgeon's office.

It would also be helpful to take a copy of this letter to the hospital when you check in for surgery. I recommend that the patient or a family member give the letter to the surgeon *before* surgery. Explain that it is a copy of the letter that was sent to his or her office and ask if the surgeon has seen it. Suggest that it be placed in the patient's hospital file.

Although it is an unwise health decision, you do have the right to refuse homologous blood. But many surgeons will not operate under that restriction and refuse to guarantee that you will not receive the blood of someone else. Dr. Ronald Lapin and his staff at Coast Plaza Medical Center in Norwalk, California, will make such a guarantee. They have a 24-hour hotline, 1-800-NO-BLOOD. People whose religious beliefs prevent them from accepting transfusions should keep this number by their phone. Of course, no facility can guarantee any patient that they will survive surgery, with or without the use of homologous blood. In medicine there is no such thing as zero risk.

Patients should not put off having an essential surgery because of concern over contaminated transfusions. While it is true that blood from the regular banked supply carries an infectious risk, the options in transfusion medicine make procrastination foolish.

Date _____
Dear Dr. _____:

Thank you for your cooperation in helping me avoid or reduce exposure to homologous blood. During our recent discussion we agreed that, unless my condition changes, the following checked options will be used for my surgery:

A. ☐ predonation before surgery
B. ☐ intraoperative autologous transfusion (IAT)
C. ☐ postoperative autologous transfusion
D. ☐ preoperative apheresis
E. ☐ hemodilution
F. ☐ salvage with a simple collection device for minor surgery
G. ☐ directed donation

I trust that advance arrangements will be made to ensure that the proper equipment is scheduled for options B and C, or F. Also, that any autologous or directed donor blood collected for me will be: waiting in the proper place on the day of surgery, transfused to me *before* blood from the regular supply, and if not used, properly stored and kept for a few days after surgery in case I need it later.

Knowing that adequate blood replacement is important to an uncomplicated recovery I wish, at the very least, to be transfused with my own blood in accordance with the previous 10/30 rule. Should I lose more than one pint of blood and have autologous whole blood or red cells available, I prefer to be transfused even though my hemoglobin and hematocrit are above 10/30. I would like a minimum of two postoperative tests to determine hemoglobin or hematocrit—one test when I arrive in the recovery room and another the day after surgery.

If homologous blood must be given, I assume that every effort will be made to keep the number of donors to a minimum. Should platelets be required, I request that they be provided by plateletpheresis from a single donor.

I realize that providing ultrasafe transfusions requires more time and coordination for doctors, hospitals and blood banks. Your effort to ensure these extra patient benefits is greatly appreciated.

Sincerely yours,

_____
    (signature)

Tips for Predonating Your Own Blood

1. Do not delay in making your first donation and try to keep on schedule. Donations that are properly spaced will lessen the chance of anemia.

2. Do not insist on delaying surgery for a longer donation period than your surgeon recommends. In certain cardiovascular surgeries, delay can be critical and in many cases blood needs can be covered by preoperative apheresis and IAT.

3. Faithfully take the iron supplements and any other pills prescribed by your doctor.

4. Pay attention to your diet. Eat healthy, well-balanced meals with an emphasis on iron-containing foods: liver, chicken, pork, beef, whole wheat, oats, raisins, etc.

5. If your hemoglobin drops too low during the time you're donating, ask your surgeon about erythropoietin therapy. The drug often allows more blood to be donated and prevents an anemia which could weaken your immune system and complicate post-surgical recovery. It makes no sense to predonate if the donated blood has to be reinfused later to treat anemia caused by the donation. That is why a hemoglobin of at least 11 is required before each donation. Don't be afraid to ask questions or call your surgeon if you are concerned about how your donations are progressing.

6. Let your surgeon know you want to be transfused with your own blood to a near normal level. If the hospital does not have a separate transfusion guideline for when to transfuse homologous and autologous blood, you may have to discuss this with the hospital administrator.

7. Should your surgery be postponed, donated units can be frozen and stored for you at the blood bank where they were drawn. Cost for freezing and thawing varies widely between facilities but you can expect to pay about double for each frozen unit. However, it is often only necessary to freeze the first unit or two that you donated.

8. Mixups or loss of your predonated blood are always a possibility in a busy blood bank whose main business is supplying homologous blood. But private autologous facilities have predonation down to a routine because preparing and storing autologous

blood is their only business. If one is in your area you may choose to make your donation there. However, you must first ascertain that the hospital where you're having surgery will accept blood from that autologous bank. If your surgeon orders your blood to be drawn at a private blood bank, insurance coverage is the same as for service at a nonprofit blood bank or center.

If you plan to have any units that might be left over after surgery stored for future use, private banks can handle the details. They will pick up the units from the hospital, freeze the red cells and store them for up to 10 years if you desire. Your fresh frozen plasma can be stored for one year. You must be prompt in making the arrangements before the units expire, get destroyed or are given to someone else. If there is no private blood bank in your area, accredited Idant Laboratories will pick up your unused units and store them. The company provides service across the nation. Call 1-212-935-1430.

9. When you make the final donation before your surgery, ask the blood bank if they will be informing you, your surgeon and the hospital in writing of the number, the kind of components prepared and where they are stored.

10. If the site of your operation should be changed to a different hospital than was planned, call the newly scheduled hospital's blood bank or lab a day or two before surgery and make sure arrangements have been made for the transfer of your blood.

11. When you check into the hospital for surgery (even if the site was not changed), have a family member go into the hospital's bank or lab and tell them you are in the hospital and when your surgery is scheduled. Ask if your blood is in the proper place. This is especially important if the blood was drawn at a blood bank outside of the hospital.

An unhappy post-surgery patient told me, "I donated four pints of blood and they got left in a refrigerator at a blood center a few blocks away. They gave me a transfusion with the blood of three people." Lessen the chance of mistakes by assuming some of the responsibility.

Chapter 21

Directed Donation and Other Options

There will always be patients who have no choice but to accept blood from other people. There are few autologous blood options for young children except for hemodilution, in some surgical cases, or an occasional blood bank that will cooperate in collecting blood from them before an operation. However, only a small amount of blood can be drawn from children at one time and they do not make enthusiastic donors. In certain types of cancer conditions there is no alternative to transfusing both adults and children with homologous blood. The same is true of other illnesses which require transfusion on a regular basis in addition to some accident victims and surgery patients.

Directed Donation

One of the steps that can be taken to reduce the risk of homologous blood is directed donation which has gained popular appeal during the AIDS epidemic. Directed donation is not an autologous blood option—it is choosing your own blood donors. Although receiving blood from blood relatives can reduce the risk of transfusion reactions, any blood from another person carries a risk of transmissible disease. In fact, you will probably be told that the blood of directed donors is no safer than regular banked blood and that studies have shown that it carries the same risk.

But if you have the knowledge to make good donor choices and know how to reduce the number of donors used, you will get a safer transfusion than if you accepted "potluck" blood.

In choosing donors, much depends on how objectively you can look at friends and relatives and factor in all the clues you have to their past health and lifestyles. Do not naively assume that just because you have known someone for a long time that person could not be in a high risk group for AIDS.

Dr. Julian Schorr who has been with the Red Cross Blood Services throughout the AIDS epidemic asks a question that deserves thoughtful consideration. "Will your cousin admit that he is gay or will your nephew admit he shared a needle at a party a few weeks ago?" Dr. Schorr recommends selecting middle aged females who are not likely to be involved with drugs or bisexuals. "Your brother's 20-year-old son is not any safer than the average Red Cross donor," he said.

However, Dr. Dennis Goldfinger, director of the blood bank at Cedar-Sinai Medical Center in Los Angeles, is an advocate of directed donations. Writing in the *Hastings Center Report*, Dr. Goldfinger's favorable opinion was based on studies of directed donors at his blood bank. "Directed donors are likely to be more truthful, because they know the patient for whom this blood is intended and would not want to transmit disease to a close friend or relative. Furthermore, we believe that in many cases the patient actually is capable of selecting a safer donor than that randomly provided by the blood bank."

I cannot forget that in 1983 the doctor and hospital refused to allow Jonathan's family to donate blood for him. That refusal sentenced a newborn child to a lifetime of AIDS. After nine years none of the family-selected-and-refused donors have AIDS—something that cannot be said for one of the blood bank's selections.

But today the chance of being refused directed donation is slight and nearly all blood banks and hospitals will provide the service upon request. Yet directed donation was discouraged or refused at a time when just one hepatitis test and no AIDS test was being done. Why is it offered now? The blood banks responded to public demand! Consumers have more power than they realize in shaping transfusion therapy. And the availability of directed donation has another major safety advantage.

Reduce the Number of Donors

Directed donation does more than allow you to choose donors you believe are safer than random volunteers. It provides an opportunity to reduce the number of blood donors you will be exposed to. Keep in mind that the risk of both transfusion reactions and infection transmission multiplies with each additional donor you have. One donation is usually processed into three units of blood products—red cells, plasma and platelets. A patient having a surgery with massive blood loss may be given all three products but blood banks do not keep the components processed from a single donation together so they can be transfused as a set. Neither are hospital inventories of banked blood segregated by donors. Consequently, patients often get blood from three donors when they could get the same products from just one donor.

Currently a patient who has the same kind of heart surgery my father had could receive five component units of red cells, four component units of plasma and 10 packs of platelets all from separate people. In this case the patient would be exposed to the blood of 19 donors. However, it is possible by using a procedure called plateletpheresis to skim off all the needed platelets from a single donor.

You can arrange for a single platelet donor to have his or her platelets drawn off by a machine that returns the rest of the blood to the donor. Large amounts of platelets are harvested in this way without causing harm to the donor, whose body can replace the lost platelets in less than five days. This collection from a single directed donor can cut platelet exposure from a possible 10 donors down to one. Just as important as avoiding viral infections from nine unnecessary donors is the patient's avoidance of developing antibodies to their platelets. When recipients are infused with platelets from multiple donors, the host's immune system can form antibodies to them within a few days which causes a transfusion reaction if more platelets are given to the patient. This creates a serious problem for people having illnesses such as leukemia which require repeated platelet transfusion.

Inasmuch as platelets have a life span of around five days they must be donated shortly before transfusing. However, as long as a month before transfusion you can choose someone to donate platelets and that person can be tested and accepted as your platelet donor. Plateletpheresis can then be done a day or two before surgery and it will not be necessary to run tests on the platelets themselves.

The heart surgery mentioned before could require the blood of 19 or more donors. By using a single directed platelet donor and four other directed donors from whom the patient receives both red cells and plasma, total donor exposure is cut from 19 donors to five or six. Total donor exposure would be lessened even further if one or two of the donors made more than one donation or if IAT was used during surgery. How can blood banks continue to maintain that directed donation is not an effective method for reducing transfusion-associated health problems from homologous blood?

Patients should understand that one directed donor may be allowed to make several donations. FDA regulation 640.3-F states that directed donors do not have to wait eight weeks between donations. A few days after making one donation, a directed donor may be examined by a doctor at the blood bank and, if found in good health, be allowed to make another donation. It's possible for one donor to be examined several times and donate several pints of blood which greatly reduces the number of donors the patient is exposed to.

Donor exposure can also be significantly reduced when newborn babies require transfusion. Infants are given tiny amounts of blood prepared in quadpacks which contain only a fourth or a fifth as much as an adult unit of red cells. Blood banks send the quadpacks from a single donor out together but it is common for hospitals to transfuse the small packs to different babies. They don't bother to keep the quadpacks from one donor segregated and reserved for one infant. As a result, a newborn needing a series of small transfusions can be exposed to 20 donors instead of four or five. Directed donation for infants will prevent much of this exposure. Fathers often act as donors for newborns and if the mother predonated her blood before delivery it will probably already be available.

Parents should never allow their babies to be transfused with blood carrying a four or fivefold risk just because providing packs from the same donor causes more bookkeeping for the hospital. If there isn't time to collect and process compatible directed donor blood, request that the hospital guarantee in writing that they will use quadpacks from a single donor until directed donor blood can be prepared. If the hospital inventory has been mixed, ask for a new supply of packs from the blood bank.

Contrary to public belief, even in emergency blood loss situations patients are rarely transfused immediately after hospitalization. A recent medical study found that only 2% of the transfusion recipients at Cedars Sinai Hospital in Los Angeles received blood during the four hours after their admission. If transfusion is delayed for 24 hours or longer, blood banks have time to test directed donations for infectious diseases. Therefore, directed donation should not be ruled out for all emergency cases.

Although there is a law requiring that blood be tested for AIDS, the FDA does not interfere in the practice of medicine. If blood is urgently needed, a patient's doctor can waive testing for all infections. It is my personal opinion that a patient should not take this risk. It is generally better to accept tested blood from the regular blood supply than untested blood from donors you have selected.

If you can't predonate your own blood and are having a surgery that is not expected to need a transfusion, consider directed donation. You could ask a couple of family members who you know have your same blood type to each donate a unit of blood for you during the week before your operation. Tell your surgeon you would prefer that each unit be prepared as red cells, plasma and platelets and all be reserved for you. Platelets, which can only be stored for five to seven days, are typically separated from a single donation of blood which yields a small number. In surgeries usually having moderate blood loss it is unlikely that the large number of platelets skimmed by apheresis would be necessary.

The component units prepared from the blood of your two selected donors can be used along with a canister collection device during surgery to cover any "unexpected" blood loss. If you don't need the donated units, they will be sold to other patients and you should not be charged for them. However, you could check with hospital billing to determine if there are any charges to the patient for unused directed units. There is a possibility that you could be charged a handling fee even though the blood is used by other patients.

Actually, the blood bank makes good money on directed donations. When it collects the blood of two directed donors, it gets two pints of raw product from which it can process six to eight units of blood products. Without spending any money for recruitment costs it also gets two new, healthy donors who may later be persuaded to become regular volunteer donors. Nevertheless, most of the blood facilities I called had higher handling fees for directed donation than for autologous predonation. However, the designated patient's insurance will pay for the units that are transfused to him or her.

Directed donation is an important blood option. It can supply all of a patient's transfusion requirements or be used in combination with one or more autologous options. For example, with massive blood loss surgery you might donate one unit of blood yourself, have a couple of directed donors for red cells and plasma plus a platelet monodonor, and also have your own red cells salvaged during and after surgery.

How to Proceed if You Want Directed Donation

- If your surgery will have heavy blood loss, discuss your transfusion needs with the surgeon during your first appointment. If you are ineligible to predonate your own blood and can't have preoperative apheresis:

  1. Request directed donation.

2. Make sure when the surgeon orders directed donation for you he or she asks that both red cells and plasma will be prepared for your use.

3. Request plateletpheresis from a single donor which you will recruit.

4. Request that IAT be used in the operating and recovery room.

- If your surgery has a low expected blood loss but you do not want to risk getting a transfusion you weren't supposed to need, discuss it with your surgeon. If you are ineligible to donate blood for yourself:

1. Request directed donation.

2. Inform the surgeon that in the week before your operation you want to have one or two directed donations prepared as red cells, plasma and platelets.

3. Request a canister collection device to save blood lost during surgery.

- If you have an infant who needs transfusion:

1. Insist that as the child's parents you or other blood relatives be allowed to donate for all the blood products the baby needs.

2. Obtain assurance from your pediatrician and hospital that all quadpacks prepared will be carefully tagged and reserved for your child.

3. If surgery is planned for children, ask if hemodilution, IAT or autologous donation could reduce or eliminate the need for directed donation. Those modalities can be used for older children and sometimes for younger ones.

- Take total responsibility for the recruitment of your donors. Some blood banks require a seven-day advance notice to provide directed donation and it usually takes 12 to 48 hours to test and process each unit.

- Before sending donors to the blood bank make sure the bank has your doctor's orders. Determine the hours and location where donations can be made and inform your donors.

- Ask them to make more than one donation for you which will reduce the number of donors needed.

- When recruiting donors for surgeries with heavy blood loss, give high priority to getting a platelet monodonor. This one selection can eliminate up to nine donors, but the process of plateletpheresis requires some donor time and inconvenience.

- When asking friends or family members to give blood for you try to avoid a sense of urgency or pressure. There is concern in blood banking circles that directed donors may consent to donate blood—and then are too embarrassed to give an honest medical history.

- Don't recruit those who are casual acquaintances or the friends of your friends. Know your donors well and don't have a "blind spot" to something in their lifestyle that may put them at risk for blood-borne disease.

- Don't avoid asking women to donate for you. A medical study found that female donors have less transmissible infections than men. Middle-aged women are considered to be the safest.

- Avoid recruiting health care workers as donors, especially surgeons, dentists, emergency room personnel and others who are in contact with the blood of many people.

- Do not recruit donors who have had blood transfusions during the past 20 years, especially between 1977 and 1986.

- If you are a woman of childbearing age, don't send your husband or sexual partner to the blood bank to donate for you. Being transfused with their blood could cause health problems in future unborn children.

- Regular donors whose blood has been repeatedly tested for years and found to be safe are excellent choices, providing they also meet the above criteria. If you are fortunate enough to know any regular donors don't hesitate to ask for their help.

- If you are informed that the blood of a directed donor is unsuitable for you but you know that donor has your same blood group and type, do not ask prying questions. Respect the donor's privacy in case he or she was disqualified by a positive test for a transmittable disease. Except for incompatibility, the blood bank cannot tell you why a donor's blood is unsuitable, due to strict confidentiality laws.

- If surgery is a few hours away and there is not enough processed directed donor blood available to cover estimated need, don't delay a pressing surgery. Some surgeons, under patient and family pressure, will request the blood bank to release donations that have not been tested for infectious disease. Not all blood banks will comply with this request but some do. It is advisable to inform your surgeon that you do not want any untested directed donor blood except platelets from a donor who has been tested within the past 30 days.

Remember that the donors you select will receive the same screening by the blood bank that regular donors get. However, if the above suggestions are followed your donors will have passed two exclusions the blood bank does not use. Your donors will not be health care workers or prior transfusion recipients and you will have some personal knowledge of their past health and lifestyles. More importantly, you will not receive blood from as many donors.

The Worst Case Scenario

The worst case scenario for obtaining safer transfusion therapy occurs when a patient must have blood within a few hours of an emergency hospital admission and the patient's condition rules out the major autologous blood options. In this situation there would not be enough time to get directed donations processed. The only way regular banked blood could be avoided altogether is if the patient already had a stored supply of his or her own frozen blood. Because very few people today have such a supply, patients have no option to accepting regular donor blood. However, there are still steps that can be taken to reduce the risk.

Reduce Donors When Receiving Regular Banked Blood

In current blood banking practice, very little effort is made to limit exposure to multiple donors. As we've discussed, a donation of whole blood is separated into a unit each of red cells, plasma and platelets and transfused into three patients. Inventorying blood by donors so that components from one donor could be given in sets of three would require blood banks and hospitals to do more recordkeeping. In addition, blood banks generally supply platelets pooled from up to 10 blood donations instead of from a single plateletpheresis donor because they don't want the platelets that are left over after red cell and plasma are prepared to be "wasted." Wasted platelets translate into less revenues. On this issue, blood banking and consumer interests collide—consumers prefer not to watch "wasted" family members die from hepatitis and AIDS.

If a member of your family is in a worst case scenario you may choose to become very assertive. Be aware that it's possible for hospitals to provide both single donor plasma and single donor platelets collected by apheresis. Demand them. Or at the very least demand that single component units of red cells, plasma and platelets from the same donor be provided in sets. They can use blood that has been recently processed, before it gets mixed into the general inventory. But medical facilities don't like to transfuse recently dated red cells—they use older blood first so it doesn't outdate and "waste." Again, consumer interests are in conflict with the interests of medical facilities.

Ask the hospital administrator to guarantee in writing that the number of donors will be kept to a minimum and if a large number of platelets are transfused that they will come from a single donor. If the hospital does not have such platelets available, the staff should make an effort to obtain them from other blood banks or hospitals in the area. Only after all efforts to get single donor platelets have failed should a family relent and accept a potpourri platelet concentrate prepared from random-donor collections.

The consumer should be aware of another factor. Experts believe that although plasma contains numerous proteins with myriad functions, the transfusion of *homologous* plasma should be limited to replacement of clinically significant clotting factors that can't be replaced by safer alternatives. Ask questions to determine the kinds and numbers of blood components the doctor is ordering and how many donors gave them. If plasma is ordered, ask the doctor to explain why its use is necessary. According to the AABB, homologous plasma should only be given if the patient has documented clotting factor deficiencies.

Additional Tests For Homologous Blood

HIV Antigen Test

As previously discussed there is an antigen test for AIDS which detects the virus itself rather than antibodies to it. Unlike the ELISA this test does not have a window period during which an infected person will test negative. Very few blood banks use the HIV antigen test on blood donations and in mid-1992 it is not commercially available. However, if a member of your family needs homologous blood and time permits, you may ask your doctor if the antigen test is available for testing the units that will be transfused.

CMV Test

One of the most frequent infections transmitted by transfusion is cytomegalovirus (CMV). CMV is a herpes virus which can have devastating consequences for infants, pregnant women, the elderly and others with impaired immunity. While it is capable of causing death in weakened patients, healthy immune systems can keep it under control. Over 50% of the population carries the virus. A simple blood test to detect CMV has been available since 1980 but the test, which costs just $2, is not usually used by blood banks.

However, some doctors advocate testing all patients for CMV before they are given a transfusion. If the patient does not have the virus then each unit of donor blood can be tested for CMV and only those units which do *not* carry it should be transfused to the patient. If patients are already infected with CMV it's not necessary to test transfused units for the virus.

At the present time only newborn babies are routinely tested for CMV before transfusion. But inasmuch as the test is both available and inexpensive, patients who want extra protection may request their doctors to test them for CMV and, if they are negative, the blood for their transfusion can be tested for the virus.

Tips for Reducing Transfusion Need

1. Choose the surgeon carefully. A highly skilled surgeon using the latest techniques can considerably reduce the amount of blood lost during surgery. Make sure a resident will *not* be allowed to perform the surgery.

2. Patients require a number of blood tests before surgery. Ask the doctor to order small "pediatric" amounts of blood to be drawn for laboratory testing. Even for adults, smaller amounts than are normally collected are adequate for testing purposes.

3. Inquire if hypotensive anesthesia will be used for the surgery. It lowers blood pressure so less blood is lost.

4. Ask the surgeon about medication that you might take after surgery to help your body regenerate red blood cells faster.

Is That Elective Surgery Really Necessary?

There is another obvious way to avoid the risk of a blood transfusion—avoid having elective surgical procedures that have only marginal benefits. Contrary to public belief and media hype, high technology medicine is not always good medicine. Sometimes less is better. Writing in the *Journal of the American Medical Association*, Dr. Marcia Angell, the respected deputy editor of the *New England Journal of Medicine*, penned a sharp criticism of the medical system. "Far from being beneficial much of the medical care in this country is unnecessary—by which I mean that it is of no demonstrated value to those who receive it and some of it is harmful." At the top of Dr. Angell's list of surgeries that are often unnecessarily performed was coronary artery bypass surgery, an operation that has historically required a lot of blood for transfusion and given a large number of AIDS infections.

New medical tests, devices and drugs are evaluated by the FDA before they are released for public use. However, the FDA does not provide regulatory oversight for surgical procedures and a surgery can gain widespread medical acceptance before studies are conducted to judge its benefits and risks. Coronary bypass gained popularity long before its effectiveness was assessed. In some executive circles being a member of a "bypass zipper club" actually became a status symbol.

First performed in the late 1960s, coronary bypass is a surgery in which a blood vessel from another part of the body is fashioned into a graft to make a detour around a blocked coronary artery. But it wasn't until 1983, when the results of a 10-year study were published, that it became evident that only patients with severe blockage of the left main coronary artery were living longer as a result of bypass surgery. And less than 5% of patients with coronary artery disease have a diseased left main artery! Study findings indicated that for patients without left main disease, the single possible advantage of bypass is a reduction of angina (chest pain) which can improve the quality of life. However, some patients will still suffer varying degrees of angina pain after bypass. Moreover, many times patients can be effectively treated with drugs and avoid surgery altogether. Today the newer procedures of balloon angioplasty, laser angioplasty and atherectomy offer additional alternatives to bypass surgery.

In his book *Medical Mayhem*, noted cardiologist Dr. David Nash concludes that two categories of patients should have coronary bypass—those with serious left main artery disease and those whose pain symptoms cannot be controlled with drugs and other medical procedures and management. Patients should make sure they have copies of the results of any heart studies done. If an arteriography indicates a 70% stenosis of the left main artery it is considered a serious blockage. Heart patients should understand that arteries that are grafted or cleaned out will very often clog up again after a few years.

A study published in 1987 from the Harvard School of Public Health compared patients who had refused to have bypass surgery with those who did. The results were startling. A full 70% of the patients who did *not* have surgery and were treated with drugs were fully employed two years later. However, two years after surgery only 45% of the patients who had bypass were well enough to work. The hazards of coronary bypass range from death to long-term depression, but patients considering the surgery must also factor in the risks of receiving massive blood transfusion. Bypass surgery is a major reason that people over 50 receive the majority of the transfusions given in the United States.

After studies were published showing that bypass rarely prolongs survival, consumers would expect that the number of surgeries would have dropped. This did not occur. Estimates of unnecessary bypass surgeries range from 25% to at least 33%. Yet between 1984 and 1988 the number of people over 65 having the operation *doubled*. In 1988 the national cost of coronary bypass surgery was $7 billion.

In addition to bypass there are a number of other surgeries with a reputation for overuse. These include hysterectomies, tonsillectomies and gall bladder operations. In the hands of an over-zealous surgeon, any type of surgery can be over-performed. Yet effective measures are not taken to identify and eliminate unnecessary or ill-advised surgeries. Despite growing concern over soaring health care costs, which in 1990 rose to $672 billion and 12.2% of the gross national product, little is done to protect either the national budget or the consumer from unnecessary health procedures.

Get a Second Opinion

Regardless of the type of surgery being considered you have the right to request that your condition be reviewed by another specialist for a second opinion. You're entitled to understand the full range of choices open to you. Each year approximately 23 million surgeries are performed in the United States. Not all of them are necessary; some are even unwarranted. Many operations could either be deferred or the patient's condition could have been treated just as effectively without surgery.

It has been shown that second opinions significantly reduce the number of operations performed. One medical study concluded that getting a second opinion reduced bypass surgery "by as much as 50%" and afforded a safe option for patients. Hysterectomies and gall bladder operations are commonly done—yet if a second opinion is sought, a patient has a good chance of having them judged unnecessary or ill-advised.

Medical indications for certain surgeries are often murky and require a judgment call but a decision to operate is weighted on the side of the surgeon. According to Dr. David Nash "Surgeons benefit from performing surgery because it permits them to practice and improve their skills, as well as rewarding them financially." However, some patients have unnecessary surgeries because they *want* them and a few even shop around until they get them.

Medicare, as well as many private insurance companies, encourage and pay for second opinions. Some insurers require them. You can either arrange for one yourself or ask your doctor to arrange one for you. You needn't worry about offending the surgeon—second opinions are routine medical practice. Always ask for your records to be sent to the second doctor so that tests will not have to be repeated. If you are the rare but wise patient who always asks for copies of all your test results, you will have your own medical file and won't need to involve the doctor.

Getting an independent second opinion can be a challenge. You want an opinion from an uninvolved doctor who will not feel pressure to rubber-stamp the surgery recommendation. For this reason you may prefer to choose the second physician yourself. Ask your primary care physician for additional referrals. Try to locate a board-certified specialist who does not practice in the same office or hospital as the first surgeon. Call your county medical society for the names of several doctors who specialize in the field in which your illness falls. You can call Medicare's toll-free number (800-638-6833) to find out how to locate a doctor in your area or call your local Social Security office. You may also get names of specialists from medical schools or large hospitals.

Questions to Ask the Second Physician

1. What are the likely benefits of this surgery?

2. Will surgery result in a permanent correction of my condition?

3. If I have this surgery, what are the complications or risks?

4. What is the failure rate of this procedure?

5. How long is the recovery period? Will full function return?

6. What are the emotional problems associated with this procedure?

7. If I don't have the surgery, what do I risk?

8. What do I risk if surgery is delayed?

9. Are there alternative treatments that should be tried first?

10. Would you please send a copy of your written opinion to me?

★   ★   ★

- Keep asking questions until you understand the position of the consulting doctor. You can always go to a public or medical library and research your medical condition. Ask reference personnel for help.

- If the second opinion conflicts with the original recommendation, you can obtain a third opinion or make the decision yourself based on the information received and your own research.

- In addition to surgical risks, consider the hazards associated with general anesthesia and homologous blood transfusion.

- Before any surgery, determine that the operation will be performed by the surgeon himself or a senior member of the hospital surgical staff and not a resident who is still in training.

Protect the Elderly Members of Your Family

The elderly need family intervention and support to avoid questionable surgeries and risky transfusion therapies. When confronted with complex, high-tech medical care, older patients are vulnerable and may be easily frightened into ill-advised surgeries without understanding the risks. Many, like my father, have a total trust in doctors and are medically uninformed. The September 1992 issue of AARP Bulletin commented on the needless exposure of patients to health risks due to unnecessary surgeries. "This is especially true of older Americans who receive the bulk of the 23 million operations performed each year."

Every year more and more major surgeries are being performed on people in their 70's and 80's—surgeries like bypass and hip and knee replacements requiring a lot of blood. I'm not suggesting that the majority of these surgeries shouldn't be done but I know from firsthand experience they have pitfalls that need to be more fully understood by patients and their families. Generally, the older a patient is the less likely he or she is to question the present claim that "virtually every unit of AIDS infected blood is removed by the HIV test."

I am deeply concerned by my conviction that a significant number of older people suffer the consequences of transfusion-associated hepatitis and AIDS without their true illnesses ever being diagnosed. To my knowledge no medical studies have been conducted to determine how fast AIDS advances in people over 70. Persons of advanced age can already have weakened immune systems and decreased mental function. It could be assumed that the AIDS virus would break them down faster. It would be expedient for relatives to ask the doctors of prior transfusion recipients to run hepatitis and HIV tests to make sure the symptoms of "senility" are not actually the symptoms of viral disease. AIDS can be found within any age group—it doesn't just affect the young. The November 1991 issue of *Modern Maturity* stated, "Complicating matters, some HIV symptoms manifested in older patients are often misdiagnosed and attributed to other diseases." What the three-paragraph writing left unsaid was that when people over 60 get AIDS it is almost always a result of blood transfusion.

I have not found any studies of the risk that women over 70 have of contracting AIDS sexually. I've been told by epidemiologists that because older women produce little estrogen there is an increased chance of vaginal abrasions through which the virus can enter. My mother's infection from only three exposures is not an isolated case. A number of elderly women have gotten AIDS after minimum sexual contact with infected partners.

When older people acquire AIDS, it is nearly always through tainted blood transfusions or sex with an infected transfusion recipient—yet very few realize the danger or what may be done to avoid it. In a letter written to California State Senator John Doolittle, Dr. Walter Bortz, a past president of the American Geriatrics Society, said, "We are seeing increased numbers of older people with AIDS. Although I'm not aware of any study dealing with this topic, I would hazard an informed guess that virtually all of these cases are secondary to transfusion of contaminated blood." This is not surprising because 70% of all the red cell transfusions given in America go to people over age 50.

Nine of the first 15 confirmed transfusion AIDS cases from HIV-tested blood were patients over age 59. We will never know how many are dying without being diagnosed and reported. Even today, transfusion-caused AIDS is not insignificant—it still happens and the consequences are enormous. And a patient's only protection is to change risky behavior, the risky behavior of trusting the safety of the blood supply.

How Effective Is Consumer Involvement?

The improvements made in blood banking since early 1985 occurred after public outcry. Blood bankers were content to use just one test for hepatitis until AIDS focused attention on the blood supply. They now use four. Consumers forced blood banks into allowing directed donation and the Hemophilia Foundation pressured plasma manufacturers until safe clotting factors were provided.

But AIDS and hepatitis contamination has not been eliminated from the present blood supply and consumer pressure cannot be relaxed. There are still safety measures that could, and should, be implemented. They include: using a second or more effective test for HIV-1, improving management and computer systems to reduce blood bank errors, reducing the number of donors per transfusion, excluding more high-risk donors and provision of frozen blood storage to allow more time to donate blood before surgery and for long-term storage. More honesty in the public statements made by the blood industry and public health officials would also be a huge step toward safer transfusion therapy.

At the present time hospital policy is an additional bottleneck in obtaining safe therapy because autologous blood options are underutilized in many facilities. This is where informed consumers can wield significant influence. If people requested ultrasafe transfusions as a condition of surgery, it wouldn't be long before sweeping policy changes occurred. Today hospitals compete for patients—let them offer the safest possible transfusion therapy as an enticement.

Since the AIDS epidemic, blood bankers have done a lot of grousing about the public's "unrealistic demand" for blood safety and how "hysteria has won out over science." They often use lofty, idealistic arguments maintaining that a consumer push for safer transfusions would result in a two-tier blood system in which the well-informed, more aggressive and affluent patients get safer therapy than poor, shy, unknowledgeable patients. While the last statement could prove to be temporarily true, very soon consumer demand would result in universal changes that would be available to all patients just as directed donation now is. The more informed and involved patients become, the faster improvements will be made.

Righting the Wrongs

Paris, France

During the summer of 1992, four senior officials of the French national health care system were on trial. They were being prosecuted by the French government for fraud leading to the AIDS deaths of clotting factor and transfusion recipients. The trial focused on hemophiliacs because the four accused doctors delayed for six months the use of a decontamination process which cleanses HIV from clotting factors.

There was also a six-month delay in testing blood donations for AIDS. The French officials did not use the American HIV test while they waited for the Pasteur Institute to develop one. These delays in protecting French blood recipients occurred in 1985 during a time when the doctors admit they knew the blood supply was contaminated with AIDS but issued no warnings of the danger.

Approximately 50% of the 4,000 hemophiliacs in France are now infected with AIDS. However, about 50% of America's 20,000 hemophiliacs are also infected. By 1985 it was too late to save most hemophiliacs who took clotting factors because adequate steps to protect blood supplies weren't taken in 1983. But had France used the process in early 1985, some *new* hemophilia infections could have been avoided. Moreover, testing blood donations for HIV would have saved a good number of transfusion recipients.

As the trial continues in Paris, police outside the courtroom have to hold demonstrators at bay. For weeks AIDS activists and families of the dying victims have marched with pickets and chanted, "Murderers!" France's Finance Ministry has said it will move quickly to compensate recipients who became infected with AIDS from transfusions and clotting factors between 1980 and 1985.

Denver, Colorado

The Colorado Supreme Court recently ruled that juries of lay people may decide if the entire U.S. blood industry was negligent in protecting the blood supply during the years before the HIV test was available. In the summer of 1992, the trial of Susie Quintana against the nation's second largest blood collector, United Blood Services, was the first case heard under that ruling. Mrs. Quintana contracted AIDS in 1983 from a transfusion.

At the trial, Dr. Don Francis, an international epidemics expert recently retired from the CDC, presented testimony. Dr. Francis stated that tens of thousands of Americans could have been saved from AIDS infections if the blood industry had followed the steps the CDC recommended in late 1982 and 1983. Those steps were direct questioning of donors to determine sexual preference and using one or more of the five blood tests the CDC doctors advocated. Dr. Francis explained how the CDC had interviewed hundreds of men with AIDS and evaluated their blood before recommending tests that could weed out most infected donors.

A major witness for the defense was Dr. Harvey Klein, chief of transfusion medicine at the National Institutes of Health. He testified that testing blood would have *endangered* the blood supply because homosexuals, bisexuals and drug abusers would have flooded the banks to give blood to determine if they were infected. Dr. Klein said there was no evidence that the CDC-recommended tests would have saved lives. Another witness, social scientist Jane Piliavin, testified it would have been "unthinkable" in 1983 to ask blood donors their sexual preference.

After deliberating five hours, the jury found both United Blood Services and the blood industry negligent. Jurors blasted the industry, saying its standards in 1983 were unreasonably deficient in safeguarding the lives of blood recipients. Unfortunately, Susie Quintana never heard the verdict. She died as her attorney was delivering the closing argument.

Iowa City, Iowa

In the late spring of 1992 a precedent-setting lawsuit was filed in Iowa charging a conspiracy by the American Red Cross, the American Association of Blood Banks, the Community Council of Blood Centers and several 1983 blood leaders. The defendants are accused of disseminating false and misleading information about the AIDS crisis and the risk of contracting AIDS through the nation's blood supply. The suit alleges blood leaders conspired to hide the facts from the public while they delayed direct questioning of donors and refused to test blood for indicators of AIDS. The lawsuit continues as we go to press.

Bureaucratic Inaction

As previously discussed in Chapter 13, the House Energy and Commerce Committee recently initiated an investigation into possible endangerment of the U.S. blood supply in 1986. There is evidence that the FDA allowed the Abbott HIV blood test to be used for 10 months after it was known to be flawed. When the Dupont and French tests came out in early '86, independent laboratory comparisons found them to be twice as efficient in weeding out AIDS infected donations as the Abbott test. But the government did not require blood banks to use one of the other tests while Abbott improved its test. Consequently, there was a 10-month period when twice as many AIDS-infected units could have been unnecessarily transfused to patients.

The FDA also failed to take prompt action when the AIDS test was released in 1985. The agency did not require testing of the blood inventories already waiting to be delivered to hospitals. Some blood facilities tested the units in stock; others did not. There are documented cases where patients got AIDS because of that failure. Even more disturbing is that the FDA did not mandate use of the test when it was first released! For a short time some blood banks delayed testing donations for HIV. There are more known AIDS cases from that omission. It was not until January 1988—nearly three years later—that the FDA finally mandated testing blood donations for AIDS!

The *Wall Street Journal* commented on the failure of bureaucracies to act in the public good. Writing on the French blood trial, the editor stated the defendants had operated a system of great power and authority under which no individual was responsible—"the system was assigned responsibility. And now they claim they were not at fault." The *Journal* called the deaths of the French blood victims "murder by bureaucracy."

In the United States, blood leaders are quick to blame the bureaucracy. Dr. Jay Menitove, one of the leaders being sued for conspiracy, insists it was not the blood industry's duty to inform the public about the possibility of AIDS being transmitted through blood transfusions. Dr. Menitove claims that was the duty of the nation's health agencies. But judging from the agencies' safe-blood assurances in response to a possible new AIDS virus, the bureaucracy is unaware of its responsibility. Perhaps, consumers should explain responsibility to both the blood industry and the bureaucracy.

My father, the tough old greasewood, taught me that while being passive and not speaking out about impending danger may be the easy thing to do, it is not the honorable one. And so it is that I have written the unvarnished events that swept away my parents' lives. May other families use the knowledge found within these pages to make informed choices for the protection of their own health and longevity.

Notes

Chapter 1: Betrayal
No notes

Chapter 2: A Harsh Life
No notes

Chapter 3: An Ill-Fated Surgery
P.34 CDC studies indicate that only about 40% of the persons infected with AIDS through transfusion will survive the condition for which they were hospitalized and given transfusion. Ward et al., "Transmission of HIV by Blood Transfusion Screened as Negative for HIV Antibody," *New England Journal of Medicine*. February 1988;318:473.

Also see Peterman et al., "Estimating the Risks of Transfusion-Associated AIDS and HIV Infection," *Transfusion*. September 1987;27:371.

Chapter 4: Unsuspecting Victims
P.42 Information on the acute infection which may occur within three weeks of exposure to HIV and the few patients who have ongoing AIDS-related symptoms was taken from the *Report of the Presidential Commission on the HIV Epidemic*, No. 02 14-701, U.S. Government Printing Office, Washington, DC. 1988, p. 7-11.

Chapter 5: Unmasking the AIDS Coverup

P.56 Research finding injury of neurons in the brain and central nervous system due to HIV was reported in the *San Francisco Chronicle* on the following days: February 4, 1991 and February 19, 1991.

P.61 The protective attire used by doctors and surgical staffs at San Francisco General Hospital to prevent exposure to HIV is detailed in an article by Carol Pogash, "Bad Blood," *Image*, January 1989.

Chapter 6: Total Disillusionment

P.78 Jonathan's medical costs were itemized in an article by Robin Micheli, "When AIDS Hits Home," *Money*, November 1987.

Chapter 7: Blood, Thunder and Confrontation

P.90-91 The drugs used to treat pneumocystis carinii pneumonia (PCP) are discussed by Bruce Nussbaum in his book *Good Intentions*, Atlantic Monthly Press, New York, NY. 1990, p. 231.

P.94 Information on Dr. Kristen Ries was taken from an article by Judy Rollins, "Treating Patients with Humanistic Sensitivity," *Salt Lake Tribune*, March 20, 1988.

Chapter 8: Homecoming

No notes

Chapter 9: Death in the Slow Lane

P.109 The quote of Albert Camus is found in his book *The Plague*, Vintage Books, New York, NY. 1972, p. 287.

P.109 The newspaper account of Sweden's AIDS Alcatraz was taken from an article by Ron Laytner, "Sweden is Building an AIDS Alcatraz," *Deseret News*, January 20, 1988.

P.111 The suicide of Doug Folsom was reported by the *San Francisco Examiner* on July 29, 1990.

Chapter 10: A Boy Named Jonathan

P.122 Decorating the Christmas tree with Jonathan and his puppy was from a writing by Renate Robey, "Christmas an Extra Special Holiday for Jonathan," *Denver Post*, December 25, 1988.

P.122 Jonathan's seventh birthday party was described by Michelle Fulcher, "Jonathan's 7—and Family of AIDS Child Glad to Celebrate," *Denver Post*, March 19, 1990.

P.122-23 The book which educates children about AIDS was written by Sharon Schilling with Jonathan's help. *My Name is Jonathan (and I Have AIDS)*, Prickly Pear Press, Denver, CO. 1990.

P.123   Doctor Franklyn Judson's quote is from the front pages of the book cited above.

Chapter 11:   All Swain Family AIDS Infections Were Avoidable

P.128   The study concluding that blood banks feared directed donation programs would erode public confidence in the regular blood supply was presented at the NIH Development Conference, *Program and Abstracts.* July 1986, pp. 83-87.

P.128   In interrogatory answers dated March 9, 1992, Civil No. C-88-5095, Third Judicial District Court of Salt Lake County, State of Utah, Dr. Myron Laub stated one of Orville Swain's donors tested HIV-positive in June 1985. This was later confirmed by the donor during deposition.

P.129   The explanation of the tests used to detect present and prior hepatitis B infection is recorded in a book edited by R. Madhok, C. D. Forbes, and B. L. Evatt, *Blood, Blood Products and AIDS*, John Hopkins University Press, Baltimore, MD. 1987, p. 126.

Chapter 12:   Safe Blood Crock-Talk

P.131-32   Dr. Joseph Bove's statistical risks for acquiring AIDS in a transfusion are recorded by Randy Shilts, *And the Band Played On*, St. Martin's Press, New York, NY. 1987, pp. 361, 433.

P.132   Statistics on the number of transfusions per year and average component units used for each are from Cumming et al., *Annual Blood Facts*, American Red Cross Documents No. BSL87-82, Washington, DC. 1987.

P.132   The CDC statistical estimate of HIV infections (29,000) given via transfusions before testing began in spring 1985 was by Peterman et al., "Estimating the Risks of Transfusion-Associated AIDS and HIV Infection," *Transfusion.* September 1987;27:371.

P.132   The study finding up to a 1 in 100 risk of acquiring HIV infection in a blood transfusion in some areas before testing began was by Pepkowitz et al., "High Incidence of Transfusion-Associated HIV Infection in Patients Transfused from 1979-1985 As Determined by AIDS Look-Back Studies," *Transfusion.* 1987;27:541.

P.133   A CDC study stated that about 60% of those who receive transfusions die from their underlying condition. Ward et al., "Transfusion of HIV by Blood Screened as Negative for HIV Antibody," *New England Journal of Medicine.* 1988;318:473.

P.133   A later study acknowledged that the majority of recipients of HIV-positive transfusions die from their original disease before AIDS appears. Donegan et al., "Infection with HIV-1 Among Recipients of Antibody-Positive Blood Donations," *Annals of Internal Medicine.* 1990;113:733.

P.133   Dr. Elizabeth Donegan's quote was reported by Associated Press, November 15, 1990.

P.133   Secretary of Health Margaret Heckler's assertion that the blood was 100% safe is reported by Randy Shilts, *And the Band Played On*, St. Martin's Press, New York, NY. 1987, p. 345.

P.133   Brian McDonough's statement stressing the dangers of homologous blood was made during an appearance on ABC-TV's "20/20", "When Blood Kills," No. 645, December 11, 1986.

P.133-34   Many of the infectious agents that can be transmitted by blood transfusion are listed in the book edited by R. Madhok, C.D. Forbes, and B.L. Evatt, *Blood, Blood Products and AIDS*, John Hopkins University Press, Baltimore, Md. 1987, Table 2.1.

P.134   Margaret Heckler's quote is a continuation of the one cited previously. Randy Shilts, *And the Band Played On*, St. Martin's Press, New York, NY. 1987, p. 345.

P.134   The tragic fate of the nation's hemophiliacs was lamented by Dr. Theresa Crenshaw in her article, "Challenging the Traditional Transfusion," *Saturday Evening Post*, April 1989.

P.134   Statistics on the number of hemophilia and transfusion AIDS cases were taken from the monthly report, *HIV/AIDS Surveillance*, Center for Disease Control, Atlanta, GA. July 1992.

P.135-36   I am indebted to Randy Shilts for the account of the meeting called by the CDC in Atlanta on January 4, 1983. *And the Band Played On*, St. Martin's Press, New York, NY. 1987, pp. 220, 222, 223.

P.136   The quote of Dr. Don Francis is from testimony presented at a trial in Denver in which United Blood Services was sued for negligence by Susie Quintana. Howard Pankratz, "Doc: AIDS Toll Avoidable," *Denver Post*, July 18, 1992.

P.136   The memo written by Dr. Joseph Bove was presented at the *Hearing of the House Subcommittee on Blood Supply Safety*, Serial No. 101-169, U.S. Government Printing Office, Washington, DC. July 1990, pp. 73, 74, Exhibit C.

P.137   Andera Rock asserts that taking steps to make the blood supply safer does not feed blood industry revenues in her article, "Inside the Billion-Dollar Business of Blood," *Money*, March 1986.

P.137   Ross D. Eckert's quote was reported by Jan Pekkansen in an article, "How Safe Is the Nation's Blood Supply?" *Readers' Digest*, July 1988.

P.138   The study estimating that up to 460 transfusion recipients a year could be infected with AIDS by blood that tested negative for HIV is by Ward et al., "Transmission of HIV by Blood Transfusions Screened as Negative for HIV Antibody," *New England Journal of Medicine*. February 1988;318:473.

P.139 The statement that human error causes the release of infected blood donations more often than inadequate blood tests do is from the book edited by R. Madhok, C. D. Forbes and B. L. Evatt, *Blood, Blood Products, and AIDS*, John Hopkins University Press, Baltimore, MD. 1987, p. 176.

P.139 Statistics on FDA recalls of blood components and plasma medicines were gathered by Gilbert Gaul for a series of articles on the blood industry. "Errors Increase as Blood Business Grows," *Philadelphia Inquirer*, September 24, 1989.

P.139-40 Safety problems at Belle Bonfils Blood Center in Denver were reported by the following: *Associated Press, Deseret News*, and the *Denver Post*, April 28 and 29, 1990.

P.140 The press was instructed on its responsibility to not alarm the public about the blood supply during the first session of the *House Subcommittee Hearings on Blood Supply Safety*, Serial No. 101-169, U.S. Government Printing Office, Washington, DC. July 1990, pp. 4, 6.

P.140 The blood banker quoted in the San Francisco newspaper on the availability of blood was Dr. Herbert Perkins, medical director of Irwin Memorial Blood Bank, *San Francisco Chronicle*, April 6, 1989.

P.141 The medical study concluding there was a safe excess of blood in the U.S. during the 1980's was by Surgenor et al., "Collection and Transfusion of Blood in the United States," *New England Journal of Medicine.* June 1990;322:23.

P.141 Dr. Dennis Donohue's statement that during the early 1980's doctors were ordering too much blood was made on ABC-TV's "20/20", "When Blood Kills," No. 645. December 11, 1986.

P.141 The estimate that half of all surgical procedures could be performed by using only autologous blood was from the writing of Dr. Ronald Gilcher in the book *Autologous and Directed Blood Programs*, American Association of Blood Banks, Arlington, VA. 1987, p. 4.

P.141 The Watkins Commission concluded that some blood banks were slow to promote blood conservation because revenues depended on the sale of blood. *Report of the Presidential Commission on the HIV Epidemic*, No. 0-214-701, U.S. Government Printing Office, Washington, DC. p. 78.

P.142 The reaction of blood bankers to Dr. Edgar Engleman's use of a surrogate test for AIDS is recorded by Randy Shilts, *And the Band Played On*, St. Martin's Press, New York, NY. 1987, p. 307.

P.142-43 The pleas of doctors urging protection of the blood supply went unheeded as blood leaders increased efforts to assure the public that the chance of getting AIDS in a transfusion was less than one in a million. Reported by Randy Shilts in the source cited above, pp. 332-33.

P.143 Surgeon General C. Everett Koop was interviewed from London on ABC-TV's "Good Morning America," on March 9, 1988. The statements he made were reported by Associated Press, March 10, 1988.

P.143-44 The syndicated response of Thomas Sowell to the criticism of the book *Crisis* was printed in the *Gazette Telegraph*, March 22, 1988.

Chapter 13: Scientific Intrigue, Politics and the AIDS Blood Test

P.145 Reduction in the number of FDA inspectors between 1977 and 1984 was reported in an article by Gilbert Gaul, "FDA Fails to Police Blood Industry," *Philadelphia Inquirer*, September 25, 1989.

P.145 Reductions in funding for public health agencies and the drop in CDC personnel are discussed by Sandra Panem in her book *The AIDS Bureaucracy*, Harvard University Press, Cambridge, MA. 1988, p. 87.

P.145-46 Rivalries within the public health service were described by Randy Shilts, *And the Band Played On*, St. Martin's Press. New York, NY. 1987, pp. 386, 387, 434.

P.146-49 The account of the scientific controversy surrounding the discovery of the AIDS virus and development of the HIV blood test is taken from a consortium of sources, the primary one being the Shilts tome cited above. pp. 386-88, 409, 419-20, 429-30, 435, 447, 515, 521, 528-30, 539.

Additional sources are:

1. "The Chronology of AIDS Research," *Nature*. April 1987;326:435.

2. Sandra Panem, *The AIDS Bureaucracy*, Harvard University Press, Cambridge, MA. 1988, pp. 25-30.

3. Tim Beardsley, "The Heat Is on Gallo—Again," *Scientific American*, May 1990.

4. John Crewdson, "AIDS Doctor Probe A Study in Scrutiny," *Chicago Tribune*, October 7, 1990.

The comment of Sandra Panem is from her book cited above, p. 99.

P.150 Information on the investigation of the Gallo lab by the NIH Office of Scientific Integrity was taken from a writing by John Crewdson, "Lies, Errors Cited in AIDS Article," *Chicago Tribune*, September 15, 1991.

P.150-51 The inadequacy of the first Abott HIV blood test was reported by John Crewdson, "Flaws in 1st AIDS Blood Test Probed," *Chicago Tribune*, January 26, 1992.

P.151 The following sources provide information on the criminal charges France filed against three (later four) health officials in that country: *New York Times*, October 20, 1991, *Associated Press*, October 23, 1991 and the *San Francisco Chronicle*, October 23 and 31, 1991.

P.151 Also, see the article by John Crewdson, "Ex-Gallo Aide Charged with Embezzlement," *Chicago Tribune*, January 31, 1992 which reveals additional problems in the Gallo lab:

1. Dr. Prem Sarin, a former long-term deputy of Gallo was charged with embezzling $25,000 which was paid the U.S. government by a German pharmaceutical company for research in the Gallo lab.

2. The previous year another Gallo aide, Syed Salahuddin, pleaded guilty to accepting illegal payments from a company that supplied the lab with materials and services.

3. Another Gallo assistant was, in early 1992, still under investigation for his ties to that same company.

P.151 Also, see John Crewdson, "U.S. Agency Faulted in AIDS Vaccine Study," *Chicago Tribune*, July 16, 1991. A ten-month investigation of Gallo's association with French researcher Daniel Zagury and their efforts to develop an AIDS vaccine concluded that the two researchers had failed to protect the human subjects who received the vaccine.

Chapter 14: The Multibillion Dollar Business of Blood

P.153 Nonprofit blood revenues are approximately twice the $780 million 1991 revenues of the Red Cross reported by Pamela Sebastian, "Red Cross Is Strained by Disasters Even as It Revamps Its Programs," *Wall Street Journal*, September 15, 1992.

P.153 Revenues for the plasma business are adjusted from the 1988 $2 billion figure of Gilbert Gaul, "America the OPEC of the Global Plasma Industry," *Philadelphia Inquirer*, September 28, 1989.

The 1988 base figures were adjusted according to national health expenditure increases through 1991 as shown in the following sources:

1. *Statistical Abstract of the U.S.*, U.S. Department of Commerce, Washington, DC. 1991, p. 92.

2. *World Almanac Book of Facts*, Tharos Books, New York, NY. 1992, p. 948.

P.155 Information on the brokering of blood and the quote of Dr. Aaron Kellner was reported by Gilbert Gaul, "How Blood Became a Billion-Dollar Business," *Philadelphia Inquirer*, September 24, 1989.

P.155 An additional source on blood brokering was the *House Subcommittee Hearing on Blood Supply and Safety*, Serial No. 102-7, U.S. Government Printing Office, Washington, DC. May 15, 1991, pp.171-173.

P.155-56 Information on the Gulf Coast Regional Blood Center is from testimony given at the House Hearing cited above, pp. 164-176.

P.156 Former FDA Commissioner Frank E. Young is quoted by Gilbert Gaul in "How Blood Became a Billion-Dollar Business," *Philadelphia Inquirer*, September 24, 1989.

P.157 The compensation of the president of Gulf Coast blood center was reviewed at the *House Subcommittee Hearing on Blood Supply Safety*, Serial No. 102-7, U.S. Government Printing Office, Washington, DC. May 15, 1991, pp. 272, 273.

P.157 The disparity in blood prices was surveyed by Gilbert Gaul and reported in "How Blood Became a Billion-Dollar Business," *Philadelphia Inquirer*, September 24, 1989.

P.158-59 Profitability of nonprofit blood banks is discussed by Gilbert Gaul in the article "Red Cross: From Disaster Relief to Blood," *Philadelphia Inquirer*, September 27, 1989.

P.158 Sidney Shainwald was quoted by Andera Rock, "Inside the Billion-Dollar Business of Blood," *Money*, March 1986.

P.159 The government-industry agreement which granted blood centers the right to certain geographical areas is detailed by Ross Eckert in the book *Securing a Safe Blood Supply*, American Enterprise Institute for Public Policy Research, Washington, DC. 1985, pp. 3, 4, 41-3, 80,81.

P.159-60 Red Cross expenditures are from the Gilbert Gaul article, "Red Cross: From Disaster Relief to Blood," *Philadelphia Inquirer*, September 27, 1989.

P.160-61 Information on Red Cross blood safety problems is from the following three sources:

1. Gilbert Gaul, *Philadelphia Inquirer*, September 25 and 27, 1989.

2. *House Subcommittee Blood Supply Safety Hearing*, Serial No. 101-169, 1990.

3. *House Subcommittee Blood Supply Safety Hearing*, Serial No. 102-7, 1991, U.S. Government Printing Office. Washington, DC.

P.161 Safety problems at Belle Bonfils Blood Bank in Denver were reported by the following: *Associated Press, Deseret News*, and the *Denver Post*, April 28 and 29, 1990.

P.162 Statistics on the plasma business are from the reporting of Gilbert Gaul, "America: The OPEC of the Global Plasma Industry," *Philadelphia Inquirer*, September 28, 1989.

P.163 Information on the overbleeding of plasma donors is taken from a writing by Lynn Telford, "Blood Money," *Utah Holiday*, November 1986.

P.163 Placentas as a source of plasma was discussed by Gilbert Gaul, "America: The OPEC of the Global Plasma Industry," *Philadelphia Inquirer*, September 28, 1989.

P.163 The study finding inappropriate infection control practices for plasma collection in some foreign countries was by Avila et al., "The Epidemiology of HIV Transmission Among Paid Plasma Donors," *AIDS*. 1989;3:631.

P.164 A study finding that 25% of the IV drug users in the U.S. still sell their plasma was researched by Nelson et al., "Blood and Plasma Donations Among A Cohort of Intravenous Drug Users," *Journal of the American Medical Association*. April 1990;263:2194.

P.164   The safety margin of plasma products is discussed by the CDC in the *Morbidity and Mortality Weekly Report.* April 1986;35:231.

P.165   The prevalence of hepatitis in the recipients of hemophilia clotting factors was reported by May et al., "Progressive Liver Disease in Hemophilia: An Understated Problem," *Lancet.* June 29, 1985. p. 1495.

P.165-66   The account of the commercialization of gay sex, the spread of STDs and the cooperation of gay men in the development of the hepatitis B vaccine are reported by Randy Shilts, *And the Band Played On*, St. Martin's Press, New York, NY. 1987. pp 18, 19, 67.

P.166   Statistics on HIV infection within the hemophilia community were provided by the National Hemophilia Foundation.

P.166   Dr. Gordon Muir asked the obvious question: "Why weren't gay men deferred from donating blood before the AIDS scare?" in the article "Gay Times and Disease," (Bachanan and Muir), *The American Spectator*, August 1984.

P.166-67   Gene Antonio makes his assertion that the contamination of the nation's blood supply with AIDS could have been avoided by tighter donor screening in his book, *The AIDS Coverup*, Ignatius Press, San Francisco, CA. 1986, p. 80.

P.167   Sandra Panem notes that a large percentage of the nation's blood supply was donated by single men between age 25 and 45 in her book *The AIDS Bureaucracy*, Harvard University Press, Cambridge, MA. 1988, p. 22.

P.167-68   Information on the loss of gay blood donations in San Francisco, the concern of a backlash against gays and costs of the hepatitis B core test are detailed in Randy Shilt's book, *And the Band Played On*, St. Martin's Press, New York, NY. 1987, pp. 223, 231, 308.

P.168-69   Dr. Don Francis' assertion that the FDA's biased attitude in 1983 resulted in a consensus against public health is reported by Howard Pankratz, "FDA Biased Toward Blood Banks in '83, Doctor Says," *Denver Post*, July 21, 1992.

P.169   A review by the *Philadelphia Inquirer* indicating that the FDA Blood Products Advisory Committee rarely has its recommendations rejected by the FDA was reported by Gilbert Gaul, "FDA Fails to Police Blood Industry," *Philadelphia Inquirer*, September 25, 1989.

P.169   Information on the American Blood Commission is from two sources:

1. Sandra Panem, *The AIDS Bureaucracy*, Harvard University Press, Cambridge, MA. 1988, pp. 21, 22.
2. Gilbert Gaul, "How Blood Became a Billion-Dollar Business," *Philadelphia Inquirer*, September 24, 1989.

P.169-70 Facts on hemophilia and the quote of Alan Brownstein, Executive Director of the National Hemophilia Foundation were taken from an interview with him on May 30, 1990.

P.170 The statement that the transmission of AIDS via transfusion is preventable is found in the *Report of the Presidential Commission on the HIV Epidemic*, No. 0-214-701, U.S. Government Printing Office, Washington, DC. p. 149.

Chapter 15: A Self-Serving Blood Monopoly

P.173-74 The interview with Dr. Myron Laub, "Utah Blood Recipients Have Little Chance of Getting AIDS," was published in the *Deseret News*, July 3, 1988.

P.173-74 Safety deficiencies found during an FDA inspection of the LDS Blood Bank, July 31, 1985 and August 1, 2, 1985 were written on FDA Form 483 by FDA inspector Edward M. Maticka and were obtained under the Freedom of Information Act.

P.174 Statistics on Utah AIDS cases and HIV infections acquired via transfusions were reported in *Total AIDS Cases—Utah and U.S. and Reported HIV Infections for Utah*, Utah Department of Health, Salt Lake City, UT. March 6, 1992.

P.175 Information on Intermountain Health Care (IHC) is from three sources:

1. *Intermountain Health Care 1991 Annual Report*, Salt Lake City, UT. 1991.

2. Twila Van Leer, "May 30 is Last Day S.L. Red Cross Will Collect, Distribute Blood," *Deseret News*, February 22, 1986.

3. Leanard Arrington, Davis Bitton, *The Mormon Experience: A History of the Latter-Day-Saints*, Alfred Knopf, New York, NY. 1979, pp. 271, 272.

P.176 The medical paper asserting it is unethical to withhold information of HIV infection from a patient was by Welsby et al., "A Personal View," *British Medical Journal*. 1986;292:954.

P.176 The quotation of Dr. Norwood Hill is from testimony he presented to the *House Subcommittee Hearing on Blood Supply Safety*, Serial No. 102-7, U.S. Government Printing Office, Washington, DC. May 1991, p. 160.

P.176-77 The account of Francis Borchelt's ordeal from transfusion-acquired AIDS is reported by Randy Shilts, *And the Band Played On*, St. Martin's Press, New York, NY. 1987, p. 501. Also see 'Borchelt' in index.

P.177 Mr. Shilts relates how Mary Johnstone's doctors kept her HIV infection concealed on page 432 of the book cited above.

P.177 The testimony of Dorothy L. Polikoff before the Presidential Commission on the HIV Epidemic was included in an article by Dr. Theresa Crenshaw, "It's a Bloody Shame," *Humanist,* May 1989.

P.177-79 Information on FDA inspections of the LDS Blood Bank, obtained under the Freedom of Information Act, are taken from the following documents:

1. FDA inspection of January 2, 4, 7, 1980 conducted by Russell W. Gripp and Edman E. Sturgeon.

2. FDA inspection of August 27, 1981 conducted by Charles M. Breen.

3. FDA inspection of June 6, 7, 1983 conducted by Charles M. Breen.

4. FDA inspection of August 31 and September 1, 2, 1985 conducted by Edward M. Maticka.

5. FDA inspection of December 21, 1985 conducted by Peter T. Regan.

P.179 Dr. Myron Laub told the press that in November 1989 the LDS Blood Bank began interviewing donors to determine if they were at high risk for AIDS. Jess Gomez, "Strong Dosage of Guidelines Help Safeguard Blood Against AIDS," *Salt Lake Tribune,* July 20, 1990.

P.179 The first 15 confirmed AIDS cases acquired from tested blood were detailed in a Letter to the Editor by Conley et al., "Transmission of AIDS from Blood Screened Negative for Antibody to HIV," *New England Journal of Medicine.* May 1992;326:1499.

P.180 A study concluding that the risk of getting AIDS in a transfusion depends more on local knowledge of the disease than the prevalence of AIDS within the community was by Kleinman et al., "Risk of HIV Transmission by Anti-HIV Negative Blood," *Transfusion.* 1988;28:499.

Chapter 16: Blood Safety in the 1990s

P.181 The CDC reported that 11% of all women with AIDS had acquired HIV infection via blood transfusion. *Morbidity and Mortality Weekly Report.* April 1989;38:14.

P.181 The statistic that 27% of the HIV-positive women in California were infected by blood transfusion was reported by the *San Francisco Examiner,* March 3, 1991.

P.182 Statistics on the potential for getting AIDS in a transfusion if testing and screening had not been done were presented by Dr. Gerald Quinnan to the *House Subcommittee Hearing on Blood Supply Safety,* Serial No. 102-7, U.S. Government Printing Office, Washington, DC. 1991. p. 34, Table 1, footnote.

P.182 The results of the General Accounting Office study on CDC AIDS surveillance was reported by Associated Press, June 26, 1989.

P.183 The CDC hierarchy of exposure categories is explained toward the back of each monthly *HIV/AIDS Surveillance Report,* Centers for Disease Control, Atlanta, GA.

P.183   CDC studies indicate that only about 40% of the persons infected with AIDS through transfusions will survive the condition for which they were hospitalized and given transfusion. Ward et al., "Transmission of HIV by Blood Transfusion Screened As Negative for HIV Antibody," *New England Journal of Medicine.* February 1988;318:473.

Also see Peterman et al., "Estimating the Risks of Transfusion-Associated AIDS and HIV Infection," *Transfusion.* September 1987;27:371.

P.184   To determine the number (by April 1992 4,741) of prior transfusion recipients whose AIDS cases have been reported to the CDC but are not listed in the transfusion exposure category see *HIV-AIDS Surveillance Report,* Centers for Disease Control, Atlanta, GA. April 1992, p. 15.

P.184   The small percentage of New York City dentists and doctors who ordered an AIDS test during the 1980s was taken from the *Annual Report to the President And Congress of the National Commission on AIDS,* U.S. Government Printing Office, Washington, DC. August 1990, p. 164.

P.184-85   A CDC study stated, "We estimate that 29,000 recipients of all ages from these years (1978-1984) received a unit of blood infected by HIV and that approximately 12,000 are still alive." Peterman et al., "Estimating the Risks of Transfusion-Associated AIDS and HIV Infection," *Transfusion.* September 1987;27:371.

P.185   Dr. William Roper's letter which stated that confirmed AIDS cases contracted from tested blood must have a positive donor identified is printed in the *House Subcommittee Hearing on Blood Supply Safety,* Serial No. 101-167, U.S. Government Printing Office, Washington, DC. July 1990, pp. 3, 4.

P.186   The Letter to the Editor revealing that 158 transfusion AIDS cases were reported from tested blood between 1985 and 1990 was by Conley et al., "Transmission of AIDS from Blood Screened Negative for Antibody to HIV," *New England Journal of Medicine.* May 1992;326:1499.

P.186   The 145 transfusion AIDS cases reported to the CDC before April 1985 from untested blood are from the *Morbidity and Mortality Weekly Report,* the Centers for Disease Control, Atlanta, GA. May 1985;34:245.

P.186-87   The Letter to the Editor detailing the CDC protocol for confirming an AIDS case from tested transfused blood was by Conley et al., "Transmission of AIDS from Blood Screened Negative for Antibody to HIV," *New England Journal of Medicine.* May 1992;326:1499.

P.187-89   Mary Carden testified at the *House Subcommittee Hearing on Blood Supply Safety,* Serial No. 101-169, U.S. Government Printing Office, Washington, DC. July 1990, p. 125.

Ms. Carden's written response to the Subcommittee includes her quotes on the following: the unwillingness of blood banks to share information on transfusion AIDS cases with federal agencies, p. 152 (source cited above), the difficulty of conducting donor investigations because of lack of records, p. 153, her assertion that transfusion AIDS acquired from tested blood is underreported, p. 152, and her observation that the FDA found 228 transfusion AIDS cases had been reported to only one Red Cross region, p. 153.

P.188   The 4,500 missing donor records at the Red Cross Washington, DC, Blood Region were cited in an FDA inspection of the American Red Cross National Headquarters FDA form 483, item 25, inspectors Carden and Morrison, June 24 to July 1991.

P.188   The FDA eventually determined that, out of 235 transfusion AIDS cases reported to the Washington, DC, region, there were some that had never been investigated after four years. This information is taken from an FDA communication sent to American Red Cross Headquarters on August 10, 1990 which was obtained under the Freedom of Information Act.

P.190   The editorial which downplayed transfusion AIDS was printed in the *Gazette Telegraph*, May 22, 1991.

P.190   The 4,023 transfusion AIDS cases reported between the time HIV testing began and the May 1991 editorial are the cases reported to the CDC by that date minus the 145 cases that had been reported by April 1985 when testing was initiated. See the *HIV/AIDS Surveillance Report*, Centers for Disease Control, Atlanta, GA. May 1991 and the *Morbidity and Mortality Weekly Report*, Centers for Disease Control, Atlanta, GA. May 1985;34:245.

P.190   The paragraph on blood supply safety, "Blood Supply Getting Safer All the Time," is from the insert of *AIDS Alert*, Volume 7, Number 5, American Health Consultants, Atlanta, GA. Summer 1992.

P.191-93   Information on FDA efforts to improve safety in the nation's Red Cross blood centers, the 1988 agreement with the American Red Cross and the organization's response was gathered from two sources:

1. *House Subcommittee Hearings on Blood Supply Safety*, Serial No. 101-169, July 1990.

2. *House Subcommittee Hearings on Blood Safety*, Serial No. 102-7, April and May 1991, U.S. Government Printing Office, Washington, DC.

P.192   Red Cross intent for safety improvements was detailed in a statement by Senior Vice President, Dr. Jefferey McCullough at the 1991 Hearing cited above, pp. 10-16.

P.193   The 51 FDA citations of the Pacific Northwest Regional Blood Center are listed in the *House Subcommittee Hearings on Blood Safety*, Serial No. 102-7, U.S. Government Printing Office, Washington, DC, April and May 1991, pp. 109-120.

P.193   The probation of the center's director and the requirement that samples of the blood collected at the center be sent to Minnesota for testing was detailed in an article by Angela Wilson, "Tapping the Vein," *Willamette Weekly*, April 15, 1992.

P.193   Dr. Marcus Simpson was quoted by *Associated Press*, May 21, 1991.

P.193   Comparison of safety violations by Red Cross and non-Red Cross blood establishments are taken from a statement by Dr. Gerald Quinnan, Acting Director of the FDA Center for Biologics, presented at the *House Subcommittee Hearings on Blood Supply Safety*, Serial No. 102-7, U.S. Government Printing Office, Washington, DC. April 1991, Table 5, p. 81.

P.193-94   Poor labeling of blood units at the New York Blood Center was cited during an FDA inspection of the center between April 3 and June 21, 1991, FDA Form 483, items 7-11, obtained by Freedom of Information Act.

P.194   Dr. Gerald Quinnan's statement on continuing transmission of infectious disease via transfusion is from the *House Subcommittee Hearings on Blood Supply Safety*, Serial No. 102-7, U.S. Government Printing Office, Washington, DC. April 1991, p. 46.

P.194   The increase in FDA recalls of suspect blood is from material presented by Dr. Quinnan, p. 80 of the source cited above.

P.195   Former FDA Commissioner Charles Edwards was quoted by the *Wall Street Journal*, May 16, 1991.

P.195   Statistics on the large number of post-transfusion hepatitis infections given before testing and donor screening were presented by Dr. Gerald Quinnan, *House Subcommittee Hearings on Blood Supply Safety*, Serial No. 102-7, U.S. Government Printing Office, Washington, DC. April 1991, p. 78, Table 1.

P.196   Statistics on hepatitis were presented by Dr. Edgar Engleman at the *House Subcommittee Hearings on Blood Supply Safety*, Serial No. 101-169, U.S. Government Printing Office, Washington, DC. July 1990, p. 36.

P.196   The Eckert quote and his estimate of hepatitis infections from transfusions were presented at the hearing cited above, p. 20.

P.196   The FDA estimated 54,000 hepatitis C infections a year were transmitted after blood banks implemented the hepatitis C test. Presented by Dr. Gerald Quinnan to the *House Subcommittee Hearings on Blood Supply Safety*, Serial No. 102-7, U.S. Government Printing Office, Washington, DC. April 1991, p. 78, Table 1.

P.196   Dr. Edgar Engleman's comments on the usefulness of the hepatitis B core test are recorded in *House Subcommittee Hearings on Blood Supply Safety*, Serial No. 101-169, U.S. Government Printing Office, Washington, DC. July 1990, p.91.

P.197   The ELISA test for HIV is considered 99% effective in excluding AIDS-infected donors. Dr. Carol Bell, *Conn's Current Therapy*, W.B. Sanders Company, Philadelphia, PA. 1990, p. 417.

P.197 Silent HIV infections in which antibodies cannot be detected by the ELISA and Western Blot tests are discussed in an Editorial by William A. Haseltine, "Silent HIV Infections," *New England Journal of Medicine.* June 1989;320:1487.

P.197 The study concluding that as many as 460 Americans a year could be infected with HIV by transfusions due to the ELISA test's inadequacy was by Ward et al., "Transmission of HIV by Blood Transfusions Screened As Negatives for HIV Antibody," *New England Journal of Medicine.* February 1988;318:473.

P.197 The two studies placing the risk of acquiring AIDS from tested blood at about 1 in 60,000 per unit are:

    1. Nelson, et al., "Transmission of Retroviruses from Seronegative Donors by Transfusion During Cardiac Surgery," *Annals of Internal Medicine.* Oct 1992;117:554.

    2. Busch et al., "Evaluation of Screened Blood Donations for HIV by Culture and DNA Amplification of Pooled Cells," *New England Journal of Medicine.* July 1991;325:1.

P.198 Studies indicating the AIDS virus can be contracted in the absence of broken skin were presented at the 1991 AIDS conference and reported by Laurie Garrett, "AIDS Virus Enters Body Through Membranes," *Newsday*, June 20, 1991.

P.198 Ross Eckert's concern about past transfusion recipients donating blood is recorded in the *House Subcommittee Hearings on Blood Supply Safety*, Serial No. 101-169, U.S. Government Printing Office. Washington, DC. July 1990, pp. 23, 103.

P.198-99 The study finding prior transfusion recipients to be the second highest group of HIV-positive blood donors was by Perkins et al., "How Well Has Self-Exclusion Worked?" *Transfusion.* 1988;28:601.

P.199 Dr. Marcus Conant expressed concern over blood donors who are health care workers in contact with the blood of numerous patients. *House Subcommittee Hearings on Blood Supply Safety*, Serial No. 101-169, U.S. Government Printing Office, Washington, DC. July 1990, p. 104.

P.199 A study finding a high percentage of residents and interns stick themselves with needles contaminated with HIV was by Klein et al., "Universal Precautions for Preventing Occupational Exposure to HIV," *American Journal of Medicine.* February 1991;90:141.

P.199 An editorial describing surgeries which require blind probing was written by Dr. Frank S. Rhame, "The HIV Infected Surgeon," *Journal of the American Medical Association.* July 1990;264:507.

P.200 Dr. Joseph Feldschuh writes of his concern for transfusion safety and makes his case for a national frozen autologous blood supply in his book, *Safe Blood*, The Free Press, New York, NY. 1990, pp. 118, 119, 164, 165.

P.200-01   Information on the AIDS-like mystery illness is taken from a consortium of sources:

1. Geoffrey Cowley, "Is a New AIDS Virus Emerging?" *Newsweek*, July 27, 1992.

2. Lawrence Altman, "AIDS Without a Trace of HIV," *New York Times*, July 22, 1992.

3. Marilyn Chase, "AIDS Meeting is Dominated by Reports of Disease in HIV-Negative Patients," *Wall Street Journal*, July 24, 1992.

P.202   Statistics on HTLV in the donor population are recorded by Dr. Carol Bell, *Conn's Current Therapy*, W.B. Saunders Company, Philadelphia, PA. 1990. p. 417.

P.202   The concern of Dr. Edgar Engleman that continued blood safety improvement won't last if public interest lags was stated at the *House Subcommittee Hearings on Blood Supply Safety*, Serial No. 101-169, U.S. Government Printing Office, Washington, DC. July 1990, p. 33.

P.204   Reassuring statements of past blood safety were made by Red Cross officials and spokespeople and reported by Associated Press during the week beginning May 20, 1991.

P.204   The reaction of Mary Carden to the reporting of Red Cross blood woes is taken from the *House Subcommittee Hearings on Blood Supply Safety*, Serial No. 101-169, U.S. Government Printing Office, Washington, DC. July 1990, p. 153.

P.204   Dr. James Allen was quoted by David Perlman, "Mysterious AIDS Cases Raise Concerns," *San Francisco Chronicle*, July 22, 1992.

Chapter 17:   Testing of Prior Transfusion Recipients

P.207-08   The recommendation that prior transfusion recipients should be alerted to their possible exposure to HIV and be tested is recorded in the *Report of the Presidential Commission on the HIV Epidemic*, No. 0-214-701, U.S. Government Printing Office, Washington, DC. 1988, pp. 75, 76.

P.207-08   The CDC also recommended that doctors test transfusion recipients for HIV in the *Morbidity and Mortality Weekly Report*, Centers for Disease Control, Atlanta, GA. March 27, 1987;36:137.

P.209   The study finding 634 donations had been made at Irwin Memorial Blood Bank by people known to have developed AIDS was by Perkins et al., "How Well Has Self-Exclusion Worked?," *Transfusion.* 1988;28:601.

P.210   The finding that up to 1 in 100 transfusion recipients were infected with HIV at Cedar-Sinai in Los Angeles is from a study by Pepkowitz et al., "High Incidence of Transfusion-Associated HIV Infection in Patients Transfused From 1979-1985 As Determined by Look-Back Studies," *Transfusion.* 1987;27:541.

P.210 A University of California study that looked back at recipients of blood between 1978 and 1985 found 1 in 56 was infected with the AIDS virus. Donegan et al., Letter to the Editor, "Mass Notification of Transfusion Recipients at Risk for HIV Infection," *Journal of the American Medical Association.* August 1988;260:922.

P.210-11 Information on Arthur Ashe's illness and HIV infection is taken from an article by Lawrence Altman, "Timing of Ashe's Surgery Put Him at Risk for AIDS," *New York Times*, April 9, 1992 and from *Associated Press*, April 9, 1992.

P.211 The case of a mother getting infected with HIV from her baby was reported in the *Morbidity and Mortality Weekly Report*, Centers for Disease Control, Atlanta, GA. February 7, 1986;35:76.

P.211-12 The tragic HIV infection of three members of actor Paul Glaser's family because of an AIDS-contaminated transfusion was reported in the *Los Angeles Times*, August 25, 1989.

P.212 Martin Gaffney and his son were infected with HIV by his wife after she received an AIDS-tainted transfusion. *New York Times*, June 22, 1988.

P.212 The number of children who were cured of cancer but contracted AIDS through the transfusions used to treat their disease was provided by Candlelighters and reported in the *Gazette Telegraph*, October 19, 1990.

P.213 The testimony of Dorothy L. Polikoff before the *Presidential Commission on the HIV Epidemic* was included in an article by Dr. Theresa Crenshaw, "It's A Bloody Shame," *Humanist*, May 1989.

P.214-15 The account of the couple who are HIV-positive after the wife's transfusion with large amounts of blood in 1989 was reported by the *Dallas Morning News*, August 5, 1991.

P.215 Ross Eckert's concern over the blood industry's refusal to do hepatitis C look-backs is recorded in the *House Subcommittee Hearings on Blood Supply Safety*, Serial No. 101-169. U.S. Government Printing Office, Washington, DC. July 1990, p. 101.

Chapter 18: Take Responsibility for Safe Transfusion Therapy
P.220 The inadequate training of hospital staffs in autologous blood techniques was addressed in the *Report of the Presidential Commission on the HIV Epidemic*, No. 0-214-701, U.S. Government Printing Office, Washington, DC. 1988, p. xix in front pages.

P.220 Dr. Edgar Engleman believes doctors and nurses need to be re-educated in transfusion medicine, *House Subcommittee Hearings on Blood Supply Safety*, Serial No. 101-169, U.S. Government Printing Office, Washington, DC. 1990, p. 36.

P.220-21 Information on the work of Dr. Ronald Lapin was provided by the Institute of Bloodless Surgery and in an interview with him, July 1991.

P.221 The 1988 NIH guideline for when a patient may require a transfusion is from "Perioperative Red Cell Transfusion," *National Institutes of Health Consensus Development Conference Statement.* June 27-29, 1988.

P.221 The risks of organ failure in patients having oxygen deficiency due to surgical blood loss were documented in a study by Shoemaker et al., "Tissue Oxygen Debt as a Determinant of Postoperative Organ Failure," *Critical Care Medicine.* November 1988;16:1117.

P.222 A recent study concludes that anemia may play a role in postoperative myocardial ischemia (insufficient blood supply to the heart muscle) and cardiac morbidity. Nelson et al., "The Relationship between Postoperative Anemia and Cardiac Morbidity in High Risk Vascular Patients in the ICU," *Critical Care Medicine.* 1992;20:571.

P.223-24 The account of the surgery of Dr. Leora Traynor's mother was told to me by Dr. Traynor and is used with permission.

P.224 The study that suggests it's too costly to try to prevent all homologous blood exposure for all patients concedes that the "undercollection of autologous blood places patients at unnecessary risk." Axelrod et al., "Establishment of a Schedule of Optimal Preoperative Collection of Autologous Blood," *Transfusion.* 1988;29:677.

P.226-28 Information on immune transfusion reactions was taken from the following three sources:

1. Dr. Herbert Perkins, "Blood Transfusion," *Cecil Textbook of Medicine*, B.W. Saunders and Company, Philadelphia, PA. 1988, Volume 1, 18th edition, pp. 947-50.

2. Dr. Carol Bell, "Adverse Reactions to Blood Transfusion," *Conn's Current Therapy*, W.B. Sanders and Company, Philadelphia, PA. 1990, pp. 411-16.

3. Dr. Ira Shulman, "Adverse Reactions to Blood Transfusion," University of Southern California, Los Angeles, CA. November 1989.

P.228 Immune suppression in post-transfusion recipients was reported by R. Madhok, C.D. Forbes, and B.L. Evatt in the book *Blood, Blood Products and AIDS*, John Hopkins University Press, Baltimore, MD. 1987, p. 105.

P.229 The study of breast and colon cancer patients was by Voogt et al., "Perioperative Blood Transfusion and Cancer Prognosis," *Cancer.* February 1987;59:836.

P.229 A study of the recurrence rates for cancer of the larynx, mouth and nose was by Jackson et al., "Blood Transfusion and Recurrence in Head and Neck Cancer," *Annals of Otology, Rhinology and Laryngology.* March 1989;93:171.

Chapter 19: Your Own Blood Is Better

P.231 Statistics on blood usage between 1982 and 1988 was taken from a study by Surgenor et al., "The Collection and Transfusion of Blood in the U.S. - 1982-1988," *New England Journal of Medicine.* June 1990;322:1646.

P.231 The statistic that in 1992 only 5% of the blood collected at blood banks was autologous was provided by the American Association of Blood Banks, May 1992.

P.232 The study finding that children who donated their blood before surgery usually avoided homologous blood exposure was by Silvergleid et al., "Safety and Effectiveness of Predeposit Autologous Transfusion in Preteen and Adolescent Children," *Journal of the American Medical Association.* 1987;257:3403.

P.233 Reduction of donor exposure is discussed by Dr. Joseph Feldschuh in his book, *Safe Blood*, The Free Press, New York, NY. 1990, pp. 168-172.

P.234-36 The majority of the facts on autologous donation and information for the chart on the preparation and use of blood are from the writing of Dr. Ronald Gilcher in the book *Autologous Blood Programs*, Editors Garner and Silvergleid, American Association of Blood Banks, Arlington, VA. 1987, pp. 15-29.

P.237 Comparison of the cost of providing homologous and autologous blood is from p. 9 of the book cited above.

P.238 A study at the Mayo Clinic found that 86% of the patients who donated blood before surgery did not require homologous blood. Moore et al., "Simplified Enrollment for Autologous Transfusion: Automatic Referral of Presurgical Patients for Assessment for Autologous Blood Collection," *Mayo Clinic Proceedings.* 1992;67:323.

P.238-43 Information on intraoperative and postoperative autologous transfusion, preoperative apheresis and hemodilution was taken from the following sources:

1. Sandler, Naiman, Fletcher, "Alternative Approaches to Transfusions: Autologous Blood and Directed Blood Donations," *Progress in Hematology*, Volume XV, Grune and Stratton, Philadelphia, PA. 1987, pp. 183-219.

2. Dr. Howard Zauder, *Intraoperative and Postoperative Blood Salvage Devices*, (booklet) University of New Mexico School of Medicine, Albuquerque, NM. pp. 25-36.

3. *Transfusion Alert: Use of Autologous Blood*, Publication No. 91-3038, National Institutes of Health, Bethesda, MD. 1991, pp. 1-13.

4. Garner, Silvergleid, Editors, *Autologous and Directed blood Programs*, American Association of Blood Banks, Arlington, VA. 1987, pp. 47-63.

5. Susan Butler, "Current Trends in Autologous Transfusion," *RN*, November 1989.

Chapter 20: How to Work With Your Doctor

P.245-46 The Paul Gann quote and background information is provided by Robert Gunnison, "Gann talks of Facing an AIDS Death," *San Francisco Chronicle*, June 10, 1987.

P.246 Gann's accomplishments and death were reported by Robert Gunnison and Mark Barabak, "Prop 13's Gann Dies of AIDS," *San Francisco Chronicle*, September 12, 1989.

P.246 The objections of groups in opposition to the Gann Blood Safety Act are recorded in the State of California *Ways and Means Committee Analysis*, Bill No. SB-37. August 23, 1989, p. 3.

P.247-48 The consumer brochure mandated by the Gann Blood Safety Act was prepared by the California Department of Health Services, Dr. Kenneth Kizer, Director, Sacramento, CA.

P.249 A Mayo Clinic study found that if secretaries referred patients to be evaluated for autologous blood programs the percentage who avoided all homologous blood went up 60%. Moore et al., "Simplified Enrollment for Autologous Transfusion: Automatic Referral of Presurgical Patients for Assessment for Autologous Blood Collection," *Mayo Clinic Proceedings*. 1992;67:323.

P.250 A Harvard study observes that a good many transfusion recipients only receive a unit or two of red cells. Surgenor et al., "Collection and Transfusion of Blood in the U.S. 1982-1988," *New England Journal of Medicine*. June 1990;322:1649.

P.260 The statement from the Mayo Clinic study is by authors Moore et al., "Simplified Enrollment for Autologous Transfusion: Automatic Referral of Presurgical Patients for Assessment for Autologous Blood Collection," *Mayo Clinic Proceedings*. 1992;67:323.

P.260 Guidelines issued in February 1992 by the American College of Physicians allowing the hemoglobin level to drop to five grams before transfusing healthy patients were reported by Jane Brody, "Know the Options for Safer Blood Transfusions," *New York Times*, September 9, 1992.

P.260 Concern over the uncertainty about when transfusion is necessary is discussed in a paper by Dr. P.C. Malone, "Might the Aphorism 'There is no Indication In Medicine for a Pint of Blood' Lie Behind Some of the Residual Morbidity and Mortality of Surgery?," *Medical Hypotheses*. February 1991;10:55.

P.260-61 Dr. Joseph Feldschuh states that patients should insist on getting their own blood back and be transfused to a normal level in his book, *Safe Blood*, The Free Press, New York, NY. 1990, p. 148.

Chapter 21: Directed Donation and Other Options

P.266 Dr. Julian Schorr's comments on directed donation are taken from information he provided in March 1992.

P.266 The statement of Dr. Dennis Goldfinger is found in his paper, "The Case for Directed Donation," *Hastings Center Report.* April 1987;17:7.

P.268 In a study at Cedars Sinai Hospital in California, Dr. Dennis Goldfinger and Dr. Frederick Axelrod found just 2% of the patients transfused needed blood during the first four hours of hospitalization. Reported by Dr. Joseph Feldschuh, *Safe Blood*, The Fred Press, New York, NY. 1990, p. 156 and Notes p. 200.

P.271 The study concluding that women donors have less transmissible infections than men was by Corden et al., "Experience with 11,916 Designated Donors," *Transfusion.* 1986;26:484.

P.273 The AABB's recommendation of using homologous plasma only for documented clotting factor deficiencies was reported by Steven Gould, "Blood Components in Surgery," *News Briefs*, American Association of Blood Banks, Arlington, VA. May 1989.

P.274 Dr. Marcia Angell criticized unnecessary medical care, "Cost Containment and the Physician," in the *Journal of the American Medical Association.* 1985;254:1203.

P.275 The study concluding that coronary bypass surgery usually does not prolong life was by the Principle Investigators, "Coronary Artery Surgical Study," *Circulation.* 1983;68:939.

P.275 Dr. David Nash discusses the patients who benefit from bypass surgery in his book, *Medical Mayhem*, Walker and Company, New York, NY. 1985, pp. 101-104.

P.275 The study comparing heart patients who had bypass surgery with those who did not is by Graboys et al., "Results of a Second-Opinion Program for Coronary Artery Bypass Surgery," *Journal of the American Medical Association.* September 1987;258:12.

P.275-76 The increase in bypass surgery for those over 65 was reported by Terri Cotten, "Cost of Bypass Surgery Sparks Debate Over Its Use," *Gazette Telegraph*, August 19, 1990.

P.276 The finding that a second opinion could reduce bypass surgery by 50% was Graboys et al., "Results of a Second-Opinion Program for Coronary Artery Bypass Graft Surgery," Journal of the American Medical Association. September 1987;258:12.

P.276 The quote of Dr. David Nash is taken from his book, *Medical Mayhem*, Walker and Company, New York, NY. 1985, p. 88.

P.278 The statement that the elderly receive the bulk of the 23 million surgeries performed each year is from an article by Robin Marantz Henig, "The Unkindest Cut of All," AARP Bulletin. Washington, DC. September 1992.

P.278 The acknowledgement that the AIDS symptoms of older people are often misdiagnosed was from a brief report, "AIDS Knows No Age," in *Modern Maturity*, November 1991.

P.279 Dr. Walter Bortz's statement is from a letter he wrote to California State Senator John Doolittle in support of the Gann Blood Safety Act, July 12, 1989.

P.279 The statistic that 70% of the red cell transfusions are given to people older than 50 years of age is from Freidman et al. "Study of National Trends in Transfusion Practice." National Heart Institute, No. 1HB-92920, 1980.

P.279 The patient ages of the first 15 confirmed AIDS cases from HIV-tested blood were in a Letter to the Editor by Conley et al., "Transmission of AIDS from Blood Screened Negative for Antibody to HIV," *New England Journal of Medicine*. May 1992;326:1499.

P.280 Information on the French blood trial was taken from the following sources:

1. Rone Tempest, "Transfusions AIDS Tainted; Doctors on Trial," Los Angeles Times, July 21, 1992.

2. "French Official Knew of Tainted Blood," San Francisco Chronicle, July 22, 1992.

3. Marlise Simons, "Courtroom Anguish As France Tries 4 Over Tainted Blood," New York Times, July 30, 1992.

P.280 The Colorado Supreme Court ruling was reported by Wade Lambert and Milo Geyelin, "Ruling Opens Blood-Bank AIDS Liability," *Wall Street Journal*, April 27, 1992.

P.281 Information on the Quintana trial is from the following:

1. Howard Pankratz, "Doctor: AIDS Toll Avoidable," *Denver Post*, July 18, 1992.

2. Howard Pankratz, "Witness: Sex Query 'Unthinkable' in 83," *Denver Post*, July 27, 1992.

3. Dr. Harvey Klein was quoted by Howard Pankratz, "Screening Blood in 83 Had Danger, Court Told," *Denver Post*, July 30, 1992.

4. Howard Pankratz, "Doctor: Massive Research on AIDS Blood Testing Done," *Denver Post*, July 31, 1992.

5. Howard Pankratz, "$8 million Awarded at AIDS Trial," *Denver Post*, August 2, 1992.

P.281 The account of the Iowa lawsuit charging conspiracy by 1983 blood leaders was reported by Howard Pankratz, "Blood Banks Were Prudent, Doctor Testifies," *Denver Post*, July 29, 1992.

P.281-82 The inadequacy of the first Abbott HIV blood test was reported by John Crewdson, "Flaws in 1st AIDS Blood Test Probed," *Chicago Tribune*, January 26, 1992.

P.282   The deaths of the French blood victims were called "murder by bureaucracy" on the editorial page of the *Wall Street Journal*, August 5, 1992.

P.282   Dr. Jay Menitove presented his position on the responsibility of health agencies to warn of transfusion danger at the trial of Susie Quintana. Reported by Howard Pankratz, "Blood Banks Were Prudent, Doctor Testifies," *Denver Post*, July 29, 1992.

Useful Telephone Numbers

American Foundation for Safe Blood and Health Care   718-875-8991

Provides free information on safe transfusion therapies and is a clearing-house and network for persons who have contracted HIV/AIDS from a blood transfusion.

Medical Awareness Association   1-800-899-0005

Provides a hotline and free information on autologous blood transfusion to the public and to libraries, organizations, hospitals and doctor's offices.

American Association of Blood Banks   301-907-6977

You may call the association to determine the accreditation of autologous blood banks in your local area.

Idant Laboratories   212-223-4444

Provides frozen, long-term storage of autologous blood with pickup and delivery service to any part of the nation.

Institute of Bloodless Surgery   1-800-662-5663

A hotline for those whose religious beliefs do not allow blood transfusions. Increasingly used by patients seeking surgeons experienced in minimizing blood loss and dedicated to the use of autologous blood.

PSICOR   1-800-521-9757

Supplies hospitals lacking IAT capability with trained operators and machines that salvage the blood lost during surgery. Patients may call to determine if service is available in their locality but doctors or hospitals must make the arrangements. Or, you can call your local Red Cross which may also provide this service.

Glossary

A

AABB—American Association of Blood Banks. One of the two major blood banking trade organizations. The AABB takes a lead role in accreditation and in setting blood bank standards.

adverse immune transfusion reactions—Immune reactions that occur from the transfusion of homologous blood. If incompatible blood is administered, intravascular clumping and breakdown of red cells may cause a life-threatening illness. In addition to immediate hemolytic reactions, other reactions caused by homologous transfusion are: delayed hemolytic reactions, chill-fever reactions, allergic reactions, post-transfusion purpura, noncardiac pulmonary edema and graft-versus-host disease.

AIDS—Acquired immune deficiency syndrome. Caused by a retrovirus known as HIV which destroys the immune system.

albumin—A derivative of blood plasma used to treat burn victims and patients who are in shock. Albumin helps to keep fluid in the bloodstream.

American Red Cross—A nonprofit organization which engages in disaster relief and is the nation's largest collector of the blood used for transfusions. Although not technically a trade organization, it functions as one for over 50 Red Cross blood centers. The American Red Cross joins with the American Association of Blood Banks and the Council of Community Blood Centers to issue statements on blood policy.

anaphylactic shock—An allergic reaction which involves a collapse of the circulation and can result in death.

anemia—A reduction in the blood's red cells and/or hemoglobin. In cases of severe anemia, blood transfusion is administered.

anorexia—A loss of appetite which can result from depression and other illnesses.

antibody—A molecule that interacts with an antigen in an immune response against foreign invaders.

anticoagulant—A drug that prevents blood from clotting.

antigen—A foreign protein or substance that invokes the production of antibodies when it enters the body. For example, the immune system produces antibodies as a protective measure against viruses and bacteria which act as antigens.

apheresis—The process of removing a component such as plasma or platelets from a donor's blood and returning the remainder to the donor.

ARC—AIDS-related complex. The condition of being HIV-positive and suffering from AIDS-related illnesses that do not meet the criteria for full-blown AIDS classification. Some patients die from ARC and cannot be reported as AIDS cases.

artery—One of the vessels that carries blood from the heart to tissues throughout the body.

Ativan—A tranquilizer in the benzodiazepine drug group which treats nervousness and tension.

autologous (aw tŏl′ ō gŭs)—Related to self. An autologous transfusion is one that patients give themselves from blood they have predonated or from blood that has been salvaged during or after surgery.

autologous donation—A blood donation designated for the donor's own use.

autotransfusion—The process of self transfusion by use of the patient's own blood. The term autotransfusion is sometimes used interchangeably with IAT.

AZT—Azidothymidine. A drug that inhibits replication of the AIDS virus but does not cure the disease.

B

Bactrim—Trimethoprim-sulfamethorazole. A combination drug used to treat urinary tract infections and pneumocystis carinii pneumonia. Septra is another brand of the same drug combination.

benzodiazepines—A chemically similar group of drugs with a sedative action that works on the part of the brain that controls emotions. Addiction may become a major problem for those taking benzodiazepines.

biopsy—The removal of a small piece of living tissue which is examined under a microscope for diagnosis.

blood components—The elements into which blood may be broken—red cells, white cells, plasma and platelets. Plasma can then be divided down into derivatives and made into albumin, clotting factors or immune products.

blood group (also called blood type)—The classifying of a person's blood according to the presence or absence of specific antigens in it. The four major blood groups are A, B, AB and O. There are approximately 600 blood subtypes.

blood product—A medical product made from blood.

blood volume—The total amount of blood in a person's body.

C

candida albicans—A yeast infection that preys on those who have impaired immunity.

CAT scans—Computerized tomography (CT). Studies that focus X-rays on an area of the body to detect abnormalities. For example, brain scans are frequently performed on patients who have symptoms of mental dysfunction.

CCBC—Council of Community Blood Centers. One of the nation's major blood banking trade organizations.

CDC—Centers for Disease Control. The government agency that has the responsibility for tracking disease in the United States. The CDC compiles information and investigates the manner in which infectious diseases are spread.

cell saver—A machine that salvages blood lost during or after surgery and cleanses it for reinfusion to the patient.

central nervous system (CNS)—Includes the brain and spinal cord that control skeletal muscles and mental activities. Deterioration of the central nervous system is an early sign of AIDS.

cirrhosis—A potentially fatal condition in which liver cells are destroyed and replaced by nonfunctioning scar tissue. One of the causes of cirrhosis is hepatitis, a disease often transmitted by blood transfusion.

CMV—See **cytomegalovirus**.

crossmatching—Tests which determine blood compatibility between donor and recipient before a transfusion.

culture—The growing, in a lab, of organisms or cells taken from a patient so that identification can be made for diagnostic purposes.

cytomegalovirus (CMV)—A contagious disease that half the population has now been exposed to without developing serious disease.

However, CMV can cause serious illness in newborns or people with weakened immunity.

D

DDI—Dideoxyinosine. A drug cousin of AZT that inhibits the AIDS virus but is better tolerated by some patients than AZT.

dementia—A deterioration in mental function.

diagnosis—The established cause of an illness which enables proper treatment to be initiated.

directed donation (also called designated donation)—Blood donated by a donor that was chosen by an intended recipient and is reserved for the use of that recipient.

E

echocardiogram—A diagnostic test that uses ultrasound to visualize the heart.

ELISA—Enzyme-linked immunosorbent assay. A test that detects antibodies to infectious agents such as the AIDS virus.

endoscopy—An inspection of body organs for diagnostic purposes by looking through a tube having an optical system.

Epstein-Barr (EBV)—A virus associated with causing mononucleosis and other infections which can linger for years. EBV is rarely transmitted by transfusion and blood donations are not tested for it.

erythrocytes—See **red blood cells**.

erythropoietin—A hormone that stimulates bone marrow to reproduce red blood cells. Erythropoietin is now produced by genetic engineering and used as a drug to treat anemia.

F

Factor VIII—The clotting factor missing from the blood of most hemophiliacs. These hemophiliacs are either treated with Factor VIII from the pooled donations of thousands of plasma donors or from Factor VIII which is genetically engineered.

FDA—Food and Drug Administration. One of the agency's charges is the oversight of blood and blood product safety.

fibrillation—Abnormal rhythm of the heartbeat which, if prolonged can result in cardiac arrest.

fibrin—A protein which forms a mesh into which blood cells are entangled to form a clot.

fractionation—Separation of plasma into the derivatives used to make medicines.

free hemoglobin—A substance released from ruptured red blood cells which may cause kidney damage.

fresh-frozen plasma—Plasma frozen within a few hours after collection and stored without preservatives for up to one year.

G

gamma globulin—A blood protein consisting of many antibodies and used to boost immunity against viruses and bacteria.

geriatrics—The study of aging and the treatment of health problems associated with it.

germ—A microorganism, especially one that causes disease.

H

hallucination—A false perception having no relation to reality. A person who is hallucinating may hear, smell or see something that is not there.

hematocrit—A test that measures the percentage of red cells in blood. One of the yardsticks used to determine if a patient needs a blood transfusion. Normal hematocrit readings range from 40 to 50% for men and are slightly lower in women.

hemodilution—The process of drawing off a pint or two of a patient's blood before surgery and replacing it with saline solution so that fewer red cells will be lost as bleeding occurs. The drawn-off blood is reinfused when needed.

hemoglobin test—A measurement of the iron-containing protein in red blood cells which will be low if the patient is anemic. Normal hemoglobin levels for men range from 14 to 18 while normal levels for women are from 12 to 15.

hemolytic reaction—Destruction or rupture of blood cells which releases the contents of the red cells into the bloodstream. Hemolytic reactions range from mild to fatal.

hemophilia—A hereditary bleeding disorder caused by the absence of clotting factors in the blood. The disease occurs almost exclusively in males and is transmitted through normal mothers who carry the recessive gene.

hemorrhage—A loss of blood.

Heparin—An anticoagulant drug often used to prevent blood from clotting.

hepatitis—An inflammation of the liver caused by bacteria, chemicals or viruses. Illness may vary from mild to fatal. In the United States, blood transfusions have transmitted millions of viral hepatitis infections.

hepatitis B core antibody test—A test that indicates prior hepatitis B infection by detecting antibodies to the core of the hepatitis B virus.

hepatitis C—One of the viruses that causes non-A, non-B hepatitis. There is now a test for hepatitis C which blood banks are using on donations.

HIV—Human immunodeficiency virus. The retrovirus considered to be the infectious agent that causes AIDS. In the United States the virus was earlier known as HTLV-3 and in France as LAV.

homologous blood (hō mŏl′ ō gŭs)—Blood given to a transfusion recipient that was donated by another person and is compatible with the major blood types of the recipient. It is nearly impossible to get an identical match between donor and recipient blood because there are over 600 blood subtypes.

I

IAT—Intraoperative autologous transfusion. The process of collecting, cleansing and reinfusing the blood that a patient loses during surgery. In lay parlance, frequently referred to as blood recycling.

immune system—The body's defense mechanism against disease or other foreign substances.

incontinence—The involuntary, uncontrollable passage of urine or feces.

incubation period for AIDS—The time between the day of infection and when symptoms develop. May take 10 years or longer.

infectious agent—Any organism capable of producing disease. In lay parlance, a germ.

K

Kenalog—A steroid with anti-inflammatory action. May be prescribed as an ointment for skin rashes.

L

latent infection—One that is hidden and kept in check by a healthy immune system.

leukemia—A cancer of the blood characterized by unrestrained growth of white blood cells.

leukocytes—See **white blood cells.**

LIP—Lymphocytic interstitial pneumonitis. A chronic inflammation of the lungs common in children who have AIDS.

look-back program—An attempt to identify recipients of transfusions who received blood from donors who later tested positive for AIDS or hepatitis B.

long-term autologous blood storage—The freezing and storage of component blood units which are donated by individuals for their own possible future need. Red cells can be stored for at least 10 years and plasma for one to five years.

Lyme disease—A disease, usually spread by ticks, that may cause arthritis and other severe impairment. Lyme disease can be transmitted by transfusion but there is no effective screening test for blood bank use.

lymph nodes—Small nodes of lymphatic tissue which keep infectious agents and other particulate matter out of the bloodstream. Lymphadenopathy, an enlargement of lymph nodes, is an early sign of AIDS.

M

monodonor—A single donor who provides several blood components to a transfusion recipient, thus reducing the risk of viral infection and immune reactions. For example, one monodonor may provide all the platelets needed after heavy blood loss and eliminate single donations of platelets from as many as 10 donors.

myoclonic jerking—The condition of intermittent spasm and jerking of muscles.

N

NIH—National Institutes of Health.

nonprofit organizations—Companies that are exempt from paying taxes because they are intended to provide charitable service for the public good. In the United States the blood used for transfusions is supplied by nonprofit blood banks.

O

opportunistic infection—An infection that is kept under control by a healthy immune system but overwhelms AIDS patients and others with impaired immunity.

P

PCP—See **pneumecystis carinii pneumonia**.

Pentamidine—A drug used for the treatment of pneumocystis carinii pneumonia, especially for those patients who have adverse reactions to Bactrim and Septra. Pentamidine is also used as an aerosol mist and sprayed into the lungs as a preventive measure against PCP.

phenobarbital—A long-acting barbiturate used as a sedative and anti-convulsant.

plasma—The fluid part of the blood which contains proteins and blood cells.

plasma donors—Those who donate plasma. Most plasma is sold at commercial centers and made into medical products but it may also be given by volunteers at nonprofit blood banks.

plasmapheresis—The process of separating plasma from red cells and returning the red cells to the donor.

platelets—Small cells in blood which are essential for clot formation and controlling bleeding.

pleurisy—An inflammation of the membrane that enfolds the lungs.

pneumocystis carinii pneumonia (PCP)—A pneumonia caused by a protozoan which attacks immune suppressed individuals. Until the AIDS epidemic, there were very few cases of PCP in the nation. But during the past decade a high percentage of AIDS deaths have been due to pneumocystis.

postoperative autologous transfusion—Collection of the blood lost after surgery using the same techniques as intraoperative autologous transfusion (IAT). But the blood collected after surgery is usually filtered and returned to the patient without washing.

preoperative apheresis—The process of withdrawing platelet-rich plasma from a patient immediately before surgery for reinfusion as it is needed.

preoperative donation (also known as **autologous donation**)—Blood donations made by patients in the weeks before surgery and stored for their own use at the time of surgery.

prognosis—A prediction of the course of a disease and the chance for recovery.

R

reagent—A substance used in a test to detect the presence of another substance. The various reagents used in blood banking to test and type blood must be of the highest quality to ensure accurate results.

red blood cells (also called **erythrocytes**)—The cells in blood which carry oxygen and remove carbon dioxide.

Rh factor—A blood group factor in red blood cells capable of causing an intense immune reaction in people born Rh-negative.

S

saline solution—A sterile water and salt solution frequently used as a blood substitute until it can be determined if a transfusion is necessary.

sepsis—The presence in the blood stream of infectious organisms or their toxins.

Septra—Trimethoprim-sulfomethoxazole. A combination drug used to treat urinary tract infections and pneumocystis carinii pneumonia. Bactrim is another brand of the same drug combination.

standby collection canister—A simple device that suctions lost blood into a sterile canister and saves it. The device can be used during low blood loss surgeries so that blood can be washed and transfused back to the patient if it should be needed.

STD—Sexually transmitted disease.

surrogate test—A test that does not detect a specific disease but detects markers which may be associated with the disease.

T

T-cells—One of the groups of white blood cells necessary for a healthy immune system. Loss of T-cells results in a loss of immunity. The AIDS virus is a destroyer of T-cells.

transfusion—An infusion of blood or blood components into the bloodstream.

Tranxene—A tranquilizer in the benzodiazepine drug group that relieves anxiety and tension.

U

undertransfusion—Inadequate replacement of a patient's blood loss usually because of doctor concern over contamination in the blood supply.

unit—An inexact measurement of the blood and components used for transfusion. A unit of whole blood is just under a pint while a unit of red cells is the amount of red cells in one unit of whole blood. A unit of whole blood contains one component unit each of red cells, plasma and platelets.

V

vital signs—The signs of life—body temperature, heartbeat, respiration and blood pressure.

W

Western Blot—A very sensitive test that detects small amounts of antibodies. A positive HIV test result by the ELISA method must be confirmed by Western Blot to rule out a false positive.

white blood cells (also called **leukocytes**)—Cells that fight disease by ingesting foreign agents or producing antibodies.

window period for AIDS—The time between infection with the AIDS virus and seroconversion when antibodies begin to be produced by the body. During the window period a blood donor would be infectious and the test used by blood banks would not detect evidence of the virus. Until recently it was thought that the window period could be as long as three years, but it is now believed that the window period lasts from three weeks to six months. However, a few HIV-infected individuals may never produce detectable antibodies.

X

Xanax—A tranquilizer in the benzodiazepine drug group which acts on the brain to relieve anxiety and relax muscles. Xanax addiction is not uncommon and withdrawal symptoms include nausea, vomiting, trembling and seizures.

Index

Give the Gift of Consumer Awareness to Your Loved Ones, Friends and Colleagues!

ORDER FORM

YES, I want ____ copies of *The Blood Conspiracy* at $24.95 each, plus $3 shipping per book. (Colorado residents please include $1.00 state sales tax.) Canadian orders must be accompanied by a postal money order in U.S. funds.

____ Check/money order enclosed • Charge my ____ VISA ____ MC

Name _____ Phone_____

Organization _____

Address _____

City/State/Zip _____

Card # _____ Expires _____

Signature _____

Check your leading bookstore or call your credit card order to:
1-800-735-3256
Please make your check payable and return to:

Aspen Leaf Press
743 Gold Hill Place, Suite 297
P.O. Box 220
Woodland Park, CO 80866-0220